P9-DME-393

UNDERSTANDING HEALTH POLICY
A Clinical Approach

SIXTH EDITION

Thomas Bodenheimer, MD
Adjunct Professor
Department of Family & Community Medicine
University of California, San Francisco

Kevin Grumbach, MD
Professor and Chair
Department of Family & Community Medicine
University of California, San Francisco

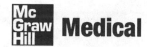
Medical

New York   Chicago   San Francisco   Lisbon   London   Madrid   Mexico City
Milan   New Delhi   San Juan   Seoul   Singapore   Sydney   Toronto

Understanding Health Policy: A Clinical Approach, Sixth Edition

2 3 4 5 6 7 8 9 0 DOC/DOC 17 16 15 14 13 12

ISBN 978-0-07-177052-1
MHID 0-07-177052-6
ISSN 1080-9465

Notice

Medicine is an ever-changing science. As new research and clinical experience broaden our knowledge, changes in treatment and drug therapy are required. The authors and the publisher of this work have checked with sources believed to be reliable in their efforts to provide information that is complete and generally in accord with the standards accepted at the time of publication. However, in view of the possibility of human error or changes in medical sciences, neither the authors nor the publisher nor any other party who has been involved in the preparation or publication of this work warrants that the information contained herein is in every respect accurate or complete, and they disclaim all responsibility for any errors or omissions or for the results obtained from use of the information contained in this work. Readers are encouraged to confirm the information contained herein with other sources. For example, and in particular, readers are advised to check the product information sheet included in the package of each drug they plan to administer to be certain that the information contained in this work is accurate and that changes have not been made in the recommended dose or in the contraindications for administration. This recommendation is of particular importance in connection with new or infrequently used drugs.

This book was set in Minion by Aptara®, Inc.
The editors were James Shanahan and Christina Thomas.
The production supervisor was Sherri Souffrance.
Project management was provided by Indu Jawwad, Aptara®, Inc.
The text designer was Alan Barnett.
RR Donnelley was printer and binder.

This book is printed on acid-free paper.

Contents

Preface

Understanding Health Policy: A Clinical Approach is a book about health policy as well as about individual patients and caregivers and how they interact with each other and with the overall health system. We, the authors, are practicing primary care physicians—one in a public hospital and clinic and the other, for many years, in a private practice. We are also analysts of our nation's health care system. In one sense, these two sides of our lives seem quite separate. When treating a patient's illness, it seems that health expenditures as a percentage of gross domestic product or variations in surgical rates between one city and another seem remote if not irrelevant—but they are neither remote nor irrelevant. Health policy affects the patients we see on a daily basis. Managed care referral patterns determine to which specialist we can send a patient, the coverage gaps for outpatient medications in the Medicare benefit package affects how we prescribe medications for our elderly patients, and differences in access to care between families on Medicaid and those with private coverage influences which patients ended up seeing one of us (in the private sector) and which the other (in a public setting). In *Understanding Health Policy*, we hope to bridge the gap separating the microworld of individual patient visits and the macrouniverse of health policy.

THE AUDIENCE

The book is primarily written for health science students—medical, nursing, nurse practitioner, physician assistant, pharmacy, social work, public health, and others—who will benefit from understanding the complex environment in which they will work. Physicians feature prominently in the text, but in the actual world of clinical medicine, patients' encounters with other health care givers are an essential part of their health care experience. Physicians would be unable to function without the many other members of the health care team. Patients seldom appreciate the contributions made to their well-being by public health personnel, research scientists, educators, and many other health-related professionals. We hope that the many nonphysician members of the clinical care, public health, and health science education teams as well as students aspiring to join these teams will find the book useful. Nothing can be accomplished without the combined efforts of everyone working in the health care field.

THE GOAL OF THE BOOK

Understanding Health Policy attempts to explain how the health care system works. We focus on basic principles of health policy in hopes that the reader will come away with a clearer, more systematic way of thinking about health care in the United States, its problems, and the alternatives for managing these problems. Most of the principles also apply to understanding health care systems in other nations.

Given the public's concerns about health care in the United States, the book concentrates on the failures of the system. We spend less time on the successful features because they need less attention. Only by recognizing the difficulties of the system can we begin to fix its problems. The goal of this book, then, is to help all of us understand the health care system so that we can better work in the system and change what needs to be changed.

CLINICAL VIGNETTES

In our attempt to unify the overlapping spheres of health policy and health care encounters by individuals, we use clinical vignettes as a central feature of the book. These short descriptions of patients, physicians, and other caregivers interacting with the health care system are based on our own experiences as physicians, the experiences of colleagues, or cases reported in the medical literature or popular press. Most of the people and institutions presented in the vignettes have been given fictitious names to protect privacy. Some names used are emblematic of the occupations, health problems, or attitudes portrayed in the vignettes; most do not have special significance.

OUR OPINIONS

In exploring the many controversial issues of health policy, our own opinions as authors inevitably color and shade the words we use and the conclusions we reach. We present several of our most fundamental values and perspectives here.

THE RIGHT TO HEALTH CARE

We believe that health care should be a right enjoyed equally by everyone. Certain things in life are considered essential. No one gets excited if someone is turned away from a movie or concert because he or she cannot afford a ticket. But sick people who are turned away from a medical practice can make headlines, and rightly so. A simple statement of the right to health care reads something like this: All people should have equal access to a reasonable level of appropriate health services, regardless of ability to pay.

In 2009, the United States entered into a fierce debate over whether health care should be a right. The debate focused on President Barack Obama's campaign to enact universal health insurance. Following a year of public ferment, Congress passed the Affordable Care Act, which goes a long way toward guaranteeing health care as a right. Yet, at the time of writing this edition of *Understanding Health Policy,* the controversy continues with challenges to implementation of the Affordable Care Act.

THE IMPERATIVE TO CONTAIN COSTS

We believe that limits must be placed on the costs of health care. Cost controls can be imposed in a manner that does relatively little harm to the health of the public. The rapidly rising costs of health care are in part created by scientific advances that spawn new, expensive technologies. Some of these technologies truly improve health care, some are of little value or harmful, and others are of benefit to some patients but are inappropriately used for patients whom they do not benefit. Eliminating medical services that produce no benefit is one path to "painless" cost control (see Chapter 8).

Reduction in the rapidly rising cost of administering the health care system is another route to painless cost containment. Administrative excess wastes money that could be spent for useful purposes, either within or outside the health care sector. While large bureaucracies do have the advantage of creating jobs, the nation and the health care system have a great need for more socially rewarding and productive jobs (eg, home health aides, drug rehabilitation counselors, childcare workers, and many more) that could be financed from funds currently used for needless administrative tasks.

There is a growing consensus that health care cost increases are bad for the economy. Employers complain that the high cost of health insurance for employees reduces international competitiveness. If government health expenditures continue their rapid rise, other publicly financed programs essential to the nation's economy (eg, education and transportation) will be curtailed and the unsustainable government budget deficits will strain the future of the nation's well-being.

Rising costs are harmful to everyone because they make health services and health insurance unaffordable. Many companies are shifting more health care costs onto their employees. As government health budgets balloon, cutbacks are inevitable, generally hurting the elderly and the poor. Individuals with no health insurance or inadequate coverage have a far harder time paying for care as costs go up. As a general rule, when costs go up, access goes down.

For these reasons, we believe that health care costs should be contained, using strategies that do the least harm to the health of the population.

THE NEED FOR POPULATION-BASED MEDICINE

Most physicians, nurses, and other health professionals are trained to provide clinical care to individuals. Yet clinical care is not the only determinant of health status; standard of living and public health measures have an even greater influence on the health of a population (see Chapter 3). Health care, then, should have another dimension:

concern for the population as a whole. Individual physicians may be first-rate in caring for their patients' heart attacks, but may not worry enough about the prevalence of hypertension, smoking, elevated cholesterol levels, uncontrolled diabetes, and lack of exercise in their city, in their neighborhood, or among the group of patients enrolled in their practices. For years, clinical medicine has divorced itself from the public health community, which does concern itself with the health of the population. We believe that health caregivers should be trained to add a population orientation to their current role of caring for individuals.

ACKNOWLEDGMENTS

We could not have written this book by ourselves. The circumstances encountered by hundreds of our patients and dozens of our colleagues provided the insights we needed to understand and describe the health care system. Any inaccuracies in the book are entirely our responsibility. Our warmest thanks go to our families, who have provided both encouragement and patience.

Earlier versions of Chapters 2, 4, 5, 8, 9, and 16 were published serially as articles in the *Journal of the American Medical Association* (1994;272:634–639, 1994;272:971–977, 1994;272:1458–1464, 1995;273:160–167, 1995;274:85–90, and 1996;276:1025–1031) and are published here with permission (copyright, 1994, 1995, and 1996, American Medical Association).

CONCLUSION

This is a book about health policy. As such, we will cite technical studies and will make cross-national generalizations. We will take matters of profound personal meaning—sickness, health, providing of care to individuals in need—and discuss them using the detached language of "inputs and outcomes," "providers and consumers," and "cost-effectiveness analysis." As practicing physicians, however, we are daily reminded of the human realities of health policy. *Understanding Health Policy: A Clinical Approach* is fundamentally about the people we care for: the uninsured janitor enduring the pain of a gallbladder attack because surgery might leave him in financial ruin, or the retired university professor who sustains a stroke and whose life savings are disappearing in nursing home bills uncovered by her Medicare or private insurance plans.

Almost every person, whether a mother on public assistance, a working father, a well-to-do physician, or a millionaire insurance executive, will someday become ill, and all of us will die. Everyone stands to benefit from a system in which health care for all people is accessible, affordable, appropriate in its use of resources, and of high quality.

Thomas Bodenheimer
Kevin Grumbach
San Francisco, California
February, 2012

Introduction: The Paradox of Excess and Deprivation

Louise Brown was an accountant with a 25-year history of diabetes. Her physician taught her to monitor her glucose at home, and her dietician helped her follow a diabetic diet. Her diabetes was brought under good control. Diabetic retinopathy was discovered at yearly eye examinations, and periodic laser treatments of her retina prevented loss of vision. Ms. Brown lived to the age of 88, a success story of the US health care system.

Angela Martini grew up in an inner-city housing project, never had a chance for a good education, became pregnant as a teenager, and has been on public assistance while caring for her four children. Her Medicaid coverage allows her to see her family physician for yearly physical examinations. A breast examination located a suspicious lesion, which was found to be cancer on biopsy. She was referred to a surgical breast specialist, underwent a mastectomy, was treated with a hormonal medication, and has been healthy for the past 15 years.

For people with private or public insurance who have access to health care services, the melding of high-quality primary and preventive care with appropriate specialty treatment can produce the best medical care in the world. The United States is blessed with thousands of well-trained physicians, nurses, pharmacists, and other health caregivers who compassionately provide up-to-date medical attention to patients who seek their assistance. This is the face of the health care system in which we can take pride. Success stories, however, are only part of the reality of health care in the United States.

EXCESS AND DEPRIVATION

The health care system in the United States has been called "a paradox of excess and deprivation" (Enthoven and Kronick, 1989). Some persons receive too little care because they are uninsured, inadequately insured, or have Medicaid coverage that many physicians will not accept.

James Jackson's Medicaid benefits were terminated because of state cutbacks. At age 34, he developed abdominal pain but did not seek care for 10 days because he had no insurance and feared the cost of treatment. He began to vomit, became weak, and was finally taken to an emergency room by his cousin. The physician diagnosed a perforated ulcer with peritonitis and septic shock. The illness had gone on too long; Mr. Jackson died on the operating table. Had he received prompt medical attention, his illness would likely have been cured.

Betty Yee was a 68-year-old woman with angina, high blood pressure, and diabetes. Her total bill for medications, which were only partly covered under her Medicare plan, came to $200 per month. She was unable to afford the medications, her blood pressure went out of control, and she suffered a stroke. Ms. Yee's final lonely years were spent in a nursing home; she was paralyzed on her right side and unable to speak.

Mary McCarthy became pregnant but could not find an obstetrician who would accept her Medicaid card. After 7 months, she began to experience severe headaches, went to the emergency room, and was found to have hypertension and pre-eclampsia. She delivered a stillborn baby.

While some people cannot access the care they need, others receive too much care that is costly and may be harmful.

At age 66, Daniel Taylor noticed that he was getting up to urinate twice each night. It did not bother him much. His family physician sent him to a urologist, who found that his prostate was enlarged (though with no signs of cancer) and recommended surgery. Mr. Taylor did not want surgery. He had a friend with the same symptoms whose urologist had said that surgery was not needed. Since Mr. Taylor never questioned doctors, he went ahead with the procedure anyway. After the surgery he became incontinent of urine.

Consuelo Gonzalez had a minor pain in her back, which was completely relieved by over-the-counter acetaminophen. She went to the doctor just to make sure the pain was nothing serious, and it was not. The physician gave Ms. Gonzalez a stronger medicine, indomethacin, to take three times a day. The indomethacin caused a bleeding ulcer requiring a 9-day hospital stay at a cost of $27,000 to her health insurer.

▶ Too Little Care

In 2009, over 50 million people in the United States had no health insurance. Many are victims of the changing economy, which has shifted from a manufacturing economy based on highly paid full-time jobs with good fringe benefits, toward a service economy with lower-paying jobs that are often part-time and have poor or no benefits (Renner and Navarro, 1989). Three-fourths of uninsured adults are employed. Lack of insurance is not simply a problem of the poor but has also become a middle-class phenomenon, particularly for families of people who are self-employed or work in small establishments. Many people with health insurance have inadequate coverage. In 2007, 45% of adults could not get needed care because they could not afford to pay the bills (Collins et al, 2008).

▶ Too Much Care

According to health services expert Robert Brook (1989):

> *...almost every study that has seriously looked for overuse has discovered it, and virtually every time at least double-digit overuse has been found. If one could extrapolate from the available literature, then perhaps one-fourth of hospital days, one-fourth of procedures, and two-fifths of medications could be done without. (Brook, 1989)*

A 1998 report estimated that 20%–30% of patients continue to receive care that is not appropriate (Schuster et al, 1998). A 2003 study found that elderly patients in some areas of the country receive 60% more services—hospital days, specialty consultations, and medical procedures—than similar patients in other areas; the patients receiving fewer services had the same mortality rates, quality of care, access to care, and patient satisfaction as those receiving more services (Fisher et al, 2003a and 2003b). In 2009, health care quality expert Brent James estimated that half of all health care dollars are wasted (James, 2009).

THE PUBLIC'S VIEW OF THE HEALTH CARE SYSTEM

Health care in the United States encompasses a wide spectrum, ranging from the highest-quality, most compassionate treatment of those with complex illnesses, to the turning away of the very ill because of lack of an ability to pay; from well-designed protocols for prevention of illness to inappropriate high-risk surgical procedures performed on uninformed patients. While the past three decades have been witness to major upheavals in health care, one fundamental truth remains: the United States has the least universal, most costly health care system in the industrialized world (Davis et al, 2010).

Many people view the high costs of care and the lack of universal access as indicators of serious failings in the health care system. In 2009, only 15% of people in the United States believed that the system was working well (Blendon et al, 2009). In 2010, 33% of Americans reported not seeing a doctor or not filling a prescription due to costs, a prevalence of access problems considerably higher than that in other developed nations (Schoen et al, 2010).

UNDERSTANDING THE CRISIS

In order to correct the weaknesses of the health care system while maintaining its strengths, it is necessary to understand how the system works. How is health care financed? What are the causes and consequences of incomplete access to care? How are physicians paid, and what is the effect of their mode of reimbursement on health care costs? How are health care services organized and quality of care enhanced? Is sufficient attention paid to the prevention of illness, and what are different strategies for preventing illness?

How can the problems of health care be solved? Does the health reform law enacted by Congress in 2010 provide the answer? Can costs be controlled in a manner that does not reduce access? Can access be expanded in a manner that does not increase costs? How have other nations done it—or attempted to do it? How might the health care system in the United States change in the future?

REFERENCES

Blendon RJ et al. The American public and the next phase of the health care debate. *N Engl J Med.* 2009;361:e48.

Brook RH. Practice guidelines and practicing medicine. *JAMA.* 1989;262:3027.

Collins SR et al. *Losing Ground: How the Loss of Adequate Health Insurance Is Burdening Working Families.* New York: Commonwealth Fund; 2008.

Davis K et al. *Mirror, Mirror on the Wall.* New York: Commonwealth Fund; 2010.

Enthoven A, Kronick R. A consumer-choice health plan for the 1990s. *N Engl J Med.* 1989;320:29.

James BC. A conversation with Brent C James, MD. Health reform debate overlooks physician–patient dynamic. *Managed Care.* December 2009:18(12):31.

Fisher ES et al. The implications of regional variations in Medicare spending. Part 1: The content, quality, and accessibility of care. *Ann Intern Med.* 2003a;138:273.

Fisher ES et al. The implications of regional variations in Medicare spending. Part 2: Health outcomes and satisfaction with care. *Ann Intern Med.* 2003b;138:288.

Renner C, Navarro V. Why is our population of uninsured and underinsured persons growing? The consequences of the "deindustrialization" of the United States. *Int J Health Serv.* 1989;19:433.

Schoen C et al. How health insurance design affects access to care and costs, by income, in eleven countries. *Health Aff (Millwood).* 2010;29:2323.

Schuster M et al. How good is the quality of health care in the United States? *Milbank Q.* 1998;76:517.

Paying for Health Care

Health care is not free. Someone must pay. But how? Does each person pay when receiving care? Do people contribute regular amounts in advance so that their care will be paid for when they need it? When a person contributes in advance, might the contribution be used for care given to someone else? If so, who should pay how much?

Health care financing in the United States evolved to its current state through a series of social interventions. Each intervention solved a problem but in turn created its own problems requiring further intervention. This chapter will discuss the historical process of the evolution of health care financing.

MODES OF PAYING FOR HEALTH CARE

The four basic modes of paying for health care are out-of-pocket payment, individual private insurance, employment-based group private insurance, and government financing (Table 2–1). These four modes can be viewed both as a historical progression and as a categorization of current health care financing.

▶ Out-of-Pocket Payments

Fred Farmer broke his leg in 1911. His son ran 4 miles to get the doctor, who came to the farm to splint the leg. Fred gave the doctor a couple of chickens to pay for the visit. His great-grandson, Ted, who is uninsured, broke his leg in 2011. He was driven to the emergency room, where the physician ordered an x-ray and called in an orthopedist who placed a cast on the leg. The cost was $1800.

One hundred years ago, people like Fred Farmer paid physicians and other health care practitioners in cash or through barter. In the first half of the twentieth century, out-of-pocket cash payment was the most common method of reimbursement. This is the simplest mode of financing—direct purchase by the consumer of goods and services (Figure 2–1).

People in the United States purchase most consumer items, from DVD players to haircuts, through direct out-of-pocket payments. This is not the case with health care (Arrow, 1991; Evans, 1984), and one may ask why health care is not considered a typical consumer item.

Need versus Luxury

Whereas a DVD player is considered a luxury, health care is regarded as a basic human need by most people.

For 2 weeks, Marina Perez has had vaginal bleeding and has felt dizzy. She has no insurance and is terrified that medical care might eat up her $500 in savings. She scrapes together $100 to see her doctor, who finds that her blood pressure falls to 90/50 mm Hg upon standing and that her hematocrit is 26%. The doctor calls Marina's sister Juanita to drive her to the hospital. Marina gets into the car and tells Juanita to take her home.

If health care is a basic human right, then people who are unable to afford health care must have a payment mechanism available that is not reliant on out-of-pocket payments.

Table 2–1. Health care financing in 2009[a]

Type of Payment	Percentage of National Health Expenditures, 2009
Out-of-pocket payment	12%
Individual private insurance	3%
Employment-based private insurance	31%[b]
Government financing	47%
Other	7%
Total	100%

Principal Source of Coverage	Percentage of Population, 2009
Uninsured	17%
Individual private insurance	5%
Employment-based private insurance	48%
Government financing	30%
Total	100%

Source: Data extracted from Martin A et al. Recession contributes to slowest annual rate of increase in health spending in five decades. *Health Affairs.* 2011;30:11–22; US Census Bureau: *Income, Poverty, and Health Insurance Coverage in the United States, 2009.* p. 60–238, September, 2010.
[a]Because private insurance tends to cover healthier people, the percentage of expenditures is far less than the percentage of population covered. Public expenditures are far higher per population because the elderly and disabled are concentrated in the public Medicare and Medicaid programs.
[b]This includes private insurance obtained by federal, state, and local employees, which is in part purchased by tax funds.

Unpredictability of Need and Cost

Whereas the purchase of a DVD player is a matter of choice and the price is known to the buyer, the need for and cost of health care services are unpredictable. Most people do not know if or when they may become severely ill or injured or what the cost of care will be.

> Jake has a headache and visits the doctor, but he does not know whether the headache will cost $100 for a physician visit plus the price of a bottle of ibuprofen, $1000 for an MRI, or $100,000 for surgery and irradiation for brain cancer.

The unpredictability of many health care needs makes it difficult to plan for these expenses. The medical costs associated with serious illness or injury usually exceed a middle-class family's savings.

Patients Need to Rely on Physician Recommendations

Unlike the purchaser of a DVD player, a person in need of health care may have little knowledge of what he or she is buying at the time when care is needed.

> Jenny develops acute abdominal pain and goes to the hospital to purchase a remedy for her pain. The physician tells her that she has acute cholecystitis or a perforated ulcer and recommends hospitalization, an abdominal CT scan, and upper endoscopic studies. Will Jenny, lying on a gurney in the emergency room and clutching her abdomen with one hand, use her other hand to leaf through a textbook of internal medicine to determine whether she really needs these services, and should she have brought along a copy of Consumer Reports to learn where to purchase them at the cheapest price?

Health care is the foremost example of asymmetry of information between providers and consumers (Evans, 1984). A patient with abdominal pain is in a poor position to question a physician who is ordering laboratory tests, x-rays, or surgery. When health care is

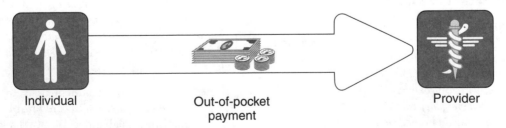

▲ **Figure 2–1.** Out-of-pocket payment is made directly from patient to provider.

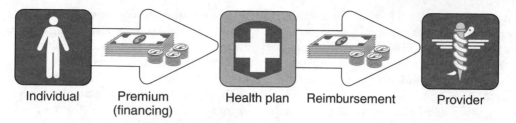

▲ **Figure 2–2.** Individual private insurance. A third party, the insurance plan (health plan), is added, dividing payment into a financing component and a reimbursement component.

elective, patients can weigh the pros and cons of different treatment options, but even so, recommendations may be filtered through the biases of the physician providing the information. Compared with the voluntary demand for DVD players (the influence of advertising notwithstanding) the demand for health services is partially involuntary and is often physician- rather than consumer-driven.

For these reasons among others, out-of-pocket payments are flawed as a dominant method of paying for health care services. Because the direct purchase of health services became increasingly difficult for consumers and was not meeting the needs of hospitals and physicians to be reliably paid, health insurance came into being.

▶ Individual Private Insurance

Bud Carpenter is self-employed. He recently purchased a health insurance policy from his insurance broker for his family. To pay the $500 monthly premium, he had to work some extra jobs on weekends, and the $2500 deductible meant he would still have to pay quite a bit of his family's medical costs out of pocket. Mr. Carpenter preferred to pay these costs rather than take the risk of spending the money saved for his children's college education on a major illness. When his son became ill with leukemia and the hospital bill reached $80,000, Mr. Carpenter appreciated the value of health insurance. Nonetheless he had to feel disgruntled when he read a newspaper story listing his insurance company among those that paid out on average less than 60 cents for health services for every dollar collected in premiums.

With private health insurance, a third party, the insurer, is added to the patient and the health care

provider, who are the two basic parties of the health care transaction. While the out-of-pocket mode of payment is limited to a single financial transaction, private insurance requires two transactions—a premium payment from the individual to an insurance plan (also called a health plan), and a reimbursement payment from the insurance plan to the provider (Figure 2–2). In nineteenth-century Europe, voluntary benefit funds were set up by guilds, industries, and mutual societies. In return for paying a monthly sum, people received assistance in case of illness. This early form of private health insurance was slow to develop in the United States. In the early twentieth century, European immigrants set up some small benevolent societies in US cities to provide sickness benefits for their members. During the same period, two commercial insurance companies, Metropolitan Life and Prudential, collected 10–25 cents per week from workers for life insurance policies that also paid for funerals and the expenses of a final illness. The policies were paid for by individuals on a weekly basis, so large numbers of insurance agents had to visit their clients to collect the premiums as soon after payday as possible. Because of the huge administrative costs, individual health insurance never became a dominant method of paying for health care (Starr, 1982). In 2009, individual policies provided health insurance for only 5% of the US population (see Table 2–1).

▶ Employment-Based Private Insurance

Betty Lerner and her schoolteacher colleagues each paid $6 per year to Prepaid Hospital in 1929. Ms. Lerner suffered a heart attack and was hospitalized at no cost. The following year Prepaid Hospital built a new wing and raised the teachers' prepayment to $12.

Rose Riveter retired in 1961. Her health insurance premium for hospital and physician care, formerly paid by her employer, had been $25 per month. When she called the insurance company to obtain individual coverage, she was told that premiums at age 65 cost $70 per month. She could not afford the insurance and wondered what would happen if she became ill.

The development of private health insurance in the United States was impelled by the increasing effectiveness and rising costs of hospital care. Hospitals became places not only in which to die, but also in which to get well. However, many patients were unable to pay for hospital care, and this meant that hospitals were unable to attract "customers."

In 1929, Baylor University Hospital agreed to provide up to 21 days of hospital care to 1500 Dallas schoolteachers such as Betty Lerner if they paid the hospital $6 per person per year. As the Great Depression deepened and private hospital occupancy in 1931 fell to 62%, similar hospital-centered private insurance plans spread. These plans (anticipating health maintenance organizations [HMOs]) restricted care to a particular hospital. The American Hospital Association built on this prepayment movement and established statewide Blue Cross hospital insurance plans allowing free choice of hospital. By 1940, 39 Blue Cross plans controlled by the private hospital industry had enrolled over 6 million people. The Great Depression reduced the amount patients could pay physicians out of pocket, and in 1939, the California Medical Association set up the first Blue Shield plan to cover physician services. These plans, controlled by state medical societies, followed Blue Cross in spreading across the nation (Starr, 1982; Fein, 1986).

In contrast to the consumer-driven development of health insurance in European nations, coverage in the United States was initiated by health care providers seeking a steady source of income. Hospital and physician control over the "Blues," a major sector of the health insurance industry, guaranteed that reimbursement would be generous and that cost control would remain on the back burner (Law, 1974; Starr, 1982).

The rapid growth of employment-based private insurance was spurred by an accident of history. During World War II, wage and price controls prevented companies from granting wage increases, but allowed the growth of fringe benefits. With a labor shortage, companies competing for workers began to offer health insurance to employees such as Rose Riveter as a fringe benefit. After the war, unions picked up on this trend and negotiated for health benefits. The results were dramatic: Enrollment in group hospital insurance plans grew from 12 million in 1940 to 142 million in 1988.

With employment-based health insurance, employers usually pay most of the premium that purchases health insurance for their employees (Figure 2–3). However, this flow of money is not as simple as it looks. The federal government views employer premium payments as a tax-deductible business expense. The government does not treat the health insurance fringe benefit as taxable income to the employee, even though the payment of premiums could be interpreted as a form of employee income. Because each premium dollar of employer-sponsored health insurance results in a reduction in taxes collected, the government is in essence subsidizing employer-sponsored health insurance. This subsidy is enormous, estimated at $260 billion per year (Gruber, 2010).

The growth of employment-based health insurance attracted commercial insurance companies to the

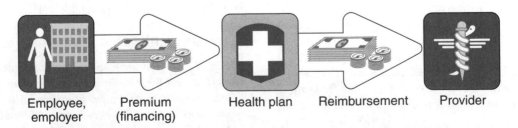

▲ **Figure 2–3.** Employment-based private insurance. In addition to the direct employer subsidy, indirect government subsidies occur through the tax-free status of employer contributions for health insurance benefits.

health care field to compete with the Blues for customers. The commercial insurers changed the entire dynamic of health insurance. The new dynamic was called **experience rating.** (The following discussion of experience rating can be applied to individual as well as employment-based private insurance.)

Healthy Insurance Company insures three groups of people—a young healthy group of bank managers, an older healthy group of truck drivers, and an older group of coal miners with a high rate of chronic illness. Under experience rating, Healthy sets its premiums according to the experience of each group in using health services. Because the bank managers rarely use health care, each pays a premium of $200 per month. Because the truck drivers are older, their risk of illness is higher, and their premium is $400 per month. The miners, who have high rates of black lung disease, are charged a premium of $600 per month. The average premium income to Healthy is $400 per member per month.

Blue Cross insures the same three groups and needs the same $400 per member per month to cover health care plus administrative costs for these groups. Blue Cross sets its premiums by the principle of community rating. For a given health insurance policy, all subscribers in a community pay the same premium. The bank managers, truck drivers, and mine workers all pay $400 per month.

Health insurance provides a mechanism to distribute health care more in accordance with human need rather than exclusively on the basis of ability to pay. To achieve this goal, funds are redistributed from the healthy to the sick, a subsidy that helps pay the costs of those unable to purchase services on their own.

Community rating achieves this redistribution in two ways:

1. Within each group (bank managers, truck drivers, and mine workers), people who become ill receive benefits in excess of the premiums they pay, while people who remain healthy pay premiums while receiving few or no health benefits.

2. Among the three groups, the bank managers, who use less health care than their premiums are worth, help pay for the miners, who use more health care than their premiums could buy.

Experience rating is far less redistributive than community rating. Within each group, those who become ill are subsidized by those who remain well, but among the different groups, healthier groups (bank managers) do not subsidize high-risk groups (mine workers). Thus the principle of health insurance, which is to distribute health care more in accordance with human need rather than exclusively on the ability to pay, is weakened by experience rating (Light, 1992).

In the early years, Blue Cross plans set insurance premiums by the principle of community rating, whereas commercial insurers used experience rating as a "weapon" to compete with the Blues (Fein, 1986). Commercial insurers such as Healthy Insurance Company could offer cheaper premiums to low-risk groups such as bank managers, who would naturally choose a Healthy commercial plan at $200 over a Blue Cross plan at $400. Experience rating helped commercial insurers overtake the Blues in the private health insurance market. While in 1945 commercial insurers had only 10 million enrollees, compared with 19 million for the Blues, by 1955 the score was commercials 54 million and the Blues 51 million.

Many commercial insurers would not market policies to such high-risk groups as mine workers, leaving Blue Cross with high-risk patients who were paying relatively low premiums. To survive the competition from the commercial insurers, Blue Cross had no choice but to seek younger, healthier groups by abandoning community rating and reducing the premiums for those groups. In this way, many Blue Cross and Blue Shield plans switched to experience rating. Without community rating, older and sicker groups became less and less able to afford health insurance.

From the perspective of the elderly and those with chronic illness, experience rating is discriminatory. Healthy persons, however, might have another viewpoint on the situation and might ask why they should voluntarily transfer their wealth to sicker people through the insurance subsidy. The answer lies in the unpredictability of health care needs. When purchasing health insurance, an individual does not know if he or she will suddenly change from a state of good health to one of illness. Thus, *within a group,* people are willing to risk paying for health insurance, even though they may not use it. *Among different groups,* however, healthy people have no economic incentive to voluntarily pay for community rating and subsidize another group of sicker people. This is why community rating cannot survive in a market-driven competitive private insurance system (Aaron, 1991).

The most positive aspect of health insurance—that it assists people with serious illness to pay for their care—has also become one of its main drawbacks—the difficulty in controlling costs in an insurance environment. With direct purchase, the "invisible hand" of each individual's ability to pay holds down the price and quantity of health care. However, if a patient is well insured and the cost of care causes no immediate fiscal pain, the patient will use more services than someone who must pay for care out of pocket. In addition, particularly before the advent of fee schedules, health care providers could increase fees more easily if a third party was available to foot the bill.

Thus health insurance was originally an attempt by society to solve the problem of unaffordable health care under an out-of-pocket payment system, but its very capacity to make health care more affordable created a new problem. If people no longer had to pay out of their own pockets for health care, they would use more health care; and if health care providers could charge insurers rather than patients, they could more easily raise prices, especially during the era when the major insurers (the Blues) were controlled by hospitals and physicians. The solution of insurance fueled the problem of rising costs. As private insurance became largely experience rated and employment based, persons who had low incomes, who were chronically ill, or who were elderly found it increasingly difficult to afford private insurance.

▶ Government Financing

In 1984 at age 74 Rose Riveter developed colon cancer. She was now covered by Medicare, which had been enacted in 1965. Even so, her Medicare premium, hospital deductible expenses, physician copayments, short nursing home stay, and uncovered prescriptions cost her $2700 the year she became ill with cancer.

Employment-based private health insurance grew rapidly in the 1950s, helping working people and their families to afford health care. But two groups in the population received little or no benefit: the poor and the elderly. The poor were usually unemployed or employed in jobs without the fringe benefit of health insurance; they could not afford insurance premiums. The elderly, who needed health care the most and whose premiums had been partially subsidized by community rating, were hard hit by the trend toward experience rating. In the late 1950s, less than 15% of the elderly had any health insurance (Harris, 1966). Only one program could provide affordable care for the poor and the elderly: tax-financed government health insurance.

Government entered the health care financing arena long before the 1960s through such public programs as municipal hospitals and dispensaries to care for the poor and through state-operated mental hospitals. But only with the 1965 enactment of Medicare (for the elderly) and Medicaid (for the poor) did public insurance payments for privately operated health services become a major feature of health care in the United States. Medicare Part A (Table 2–2) is a hospital insurance plan for the elderly financed largely through social security taxes from employers and employees. Medicare Part B (Table 2–3) insures the elderly for physician services and is paid for by federal taxes and monthly premiums from the beneficiaries. Medicare Part D, enacted in 2003, offers prescription drug coverage and is paid for by federal taxes and monthly premiums from beneficiaries. Medicaid (Table 2–4) is a program run by the states that is funded by federal and state taxes, which pays for the care of certain low-income groups. In 2009, Medicare and Medicaid expenditures totaled $502 and $374 billion, respectively (Martin et al, 2011).

With its large deductibles, copayments, and gaps in coverage, Medicare paid for only 48% of the average beneficiary's health care expenses in 2006 (Kaiser Family Foundation, 2010a). Most of the 47 million Medicare beneficiaries (2010) have supplemental coverage. In 2010, nearly 30% of beneficiaries had additional coverage from their previous employment, about 20% purchased supplemental private insurance (called "Medigap" plans), 24% were enrolled in the Medicare Advantage program, and 19% were enrolled in both Medicare and Medicaid (Kaiser Family Foundation, 2010b).

The Medicare Modernization Act (MMA) of 2003 made two major changes in the Medicare program: the expansion of the role of private health plans (the Medicare Advantage program, Part C) and the establishment

Table 2–2. Summary of Medicare Part A, 2011

Who is eligible?

Upon reaching the age of 65 years, people who are eligible for Social Security are automatically enrolled in Medicare Part A whether or not they are retired. A person who has paid into the Social Security system for 10 years and that person's spouse are eligible for Social Security. People who are not eligible for Social Security can enroll in Medicare Part A by paying a monthly premium.

People under the age of 65 who are totally and permanently disabled may enroll in Medicare Part A after they have been receiving Social Security disability benefits for 24 months. People with chronic renal disease requiring dialysis or a transplant may also be eligible for Medicare Part A without a 2-year waiting period.

How is it financed?

Financing is through the Social Security system. Employers and employees each pay to Medicare 1.45% of wages and salaries. Self-employed people pay 2.9%. The 2010 Accountable Care Act increases the rate for higher-income taxpayers (incomes greater than $200,000 for individuals or $250,000 for couples) from 1.45% to 2.35% starting in 2013.

What services are covered?[a]

Services	Benefit	Medicare Pays
Hospitalization	First 60 days[b] 61st to 90th day[b] 91st to 150th day[c] Beyond 90 days if lifetime reserve days are used up	All but a $1132 deductible per spell of illness All but $283/day All but $566/day Nothing
Skilled nursing facility	First 20 days 21st to 100th day Beyond 100 days	All All but $141.50/day Nothing
Home health care	100 visits per spell of illness	100% for skilled care as defined by Medicare regulations
Hospice care	As long as a doctor certifies person suffers from a terminal illness	100% for most services, copays for outpatient drugs and coinsurance for inpatient respite care
Unskilled nursing home care	Care that is mainly custodial is not covered	Nothing

[a]For patients in Medicare Advantage plans, covered services and patient responsibility for payment changes based on the specifics of each Medicare Advantage plan.

[b]Part A benefits are provided by each "spell of illness" rather than for each year. A "spell of illness" begins when a beneficiary enters a hospital and ends 60 days after discharge from the hospital or from a skilled nursing facility.

[c]Beyond 90 days, Medicare pays for 60 additional days only once in a lifetime ("lifetime reserve days").

of a prescription drug benefit (Part D). Under the Medicare Advantage program, a beneficiary can elect to enroll in a private health plan contracting with Medicare, with Medicare subsidizing the premium for that private health plan rather than paying hospitals, physicians, and other providers directly as under Medicare Parts A and B. Beneficiaries joining a Medicare Advantage plan sacrifice some degree of freedom of choice of physician and hospital in return for lower out-of-pocket payments and are only allowed to receive care from health care providers who are connected with that plan. Two-thirds of Medicare Advantage plans are health maintenance organizations (HMOs) (see Chapter 6). In order to channel more patients into

Medicare Advantage plans, the MMA provided generous payments to those plans, with the result that they cost the federal government 14% more than the government paid for health care services for similar Medicare beneficiaries in the traditional Part A and Part B programs. The 2010 health care reform law passed by the Obama Administration (the Accountable Care Act) reduced payments to Medicare Advantage plans with the goal of saving the Medicare program $136 billion over the following 10 years (Kaiser Family Foundation, 2010c).

Medicare Part D provides partial coverage for prescription drugs. In 2010, 82% of Part D was financed through tax revenues, with 10% coming from

Table 2–3. Summary of Medicare Part B, 2011

Who is eligible?
People who are eligible for Medicare Part A who elect to pay the Medicare Part B premium of $115.40 per month. Some low-income persons are not required to pay the premium. Higher-income beneficiaries (over $85,000 for individual, $170,000 for couple) have higher premiums related to income.

How is it financed?
Financing is in part by general federal revenues (personal income and other federal taxes) and in part by Part B monthly premiums.

What services are covered?[a]

Services	Benefit	Medicare Pays
Medical expenses Physician services Physical, occupational, and speech therapy Medical equipment Diagnostic tests (no coinsurance for laboratory services)	All medically necessary services	80% of approved amount after a $162 annual deductible
Preventive care	Pap smears; mammograms; colorectal/prostate cancer, cardiovascular and diabetes screening; pneumococcal and influenza vaccinations; yearly physical examinations	Included in medical expenses, with deductible, and for some services the copayment, waived
Outpatient medications	Partially covered under Medicare Part D	All except for premium, deductible, coinsurance, and "donut hole," which vary by drug plan
Eye refractions, hearing aids, dental services	Not covered	Nothing

[a]For patients in Medicare Advantage plans, covered services and patient responsibility for payment changes based on the specifics of each Medicare Advantage plan.

beneficiary premiums (Kaiser Family Foundation, 2010a). As of 2010, 59% of Medicare beneficiaries had enrolled in the voluntary Medicare Part D program. Part D has been criticized because (1) there are major gaps in coverage, (2) coverage has been farmed out to private insurance companies rather than administered by the federal Medicare program, and (3) the government is not allowed to negotiate with pharmaceutical companies for lower drug prices. These 3 features of the program have caused confusion for beneficiaries, physicians, and pharmacists and a high cost for the program. Beneficiaries desiring Medicare Part D can

Table 2–4. Summary of Medicaid, 2011

Medicaid is a federal program administered by the states, with the federal government paying between 50% and 76% of total Medicaid costs; the federal contribution is greater for states with lower per capita incomes. The federal government requires that certain categories of low-income people be enrolled in state Medicaid programs (Kaiser Family Foundation, 2010d):

1. Low-income families with children who meet certain eligibility requirements;
2. Most elderly, disabled, and blind individuals who receive cash assistance under the federal Supplemental Security Income (SSI) program;
3. Children under age 6 and pregnant women whose family income is at or below 133% of the federal poverty level; and
4. Schoolaged children (6-18) whose family income is at or below the federal poverty level. In 2011, the federal poverty level was $22,350 for a family of 4. States may offer Medicaid eligibility to other categories of low-income people.

The federal government requires that a broad set of services be covered under Medicaid, including hospital, physician, laboratory, x-ray, prenatal, preventive, nursing home, and home health services, although these services can be restricted through federal waivers.

enroll in one of 1500 stand-alone private prescription drug plans or receive their Part D coverage through a Medicare Advantage plan. Different plans cover different medications and require different premiums, deductibles, and coinsurance payments. The standard plan in 2010 had a $310 yearly deductible and 25% coinsurance up to an initial coverage limit of $2830 in total drug costs, after which coverage stops until the beneficiary has spent $4550 out of pocket (excluding premiums) for prescription drugs. Above $4550, coverage resumes with 5% coinsurance. The coverage gap, called the "donut hole," becomes a major problem for patients with chronic illness needing several medications. The Accountable Care Act of 2010 gradually reduces the amounts beneficiaries must pay in the donut hole.

In 2009, the trustees of the Medicare program estimated that the Part A trust fund would be depleted by 2017. The Accountable Care Act, by raising social security payments and reducing expenditures, has extended Medicare's solvency through 2029.

The Medicaid program (Table 2–4) is jointly administered by the federal and state governments. Although designed for low-income Americans, not all poor people are eligible for Medicaid. In addition to being poor, Medicaid has required that people also meet "categorical" eligibility criteria such as being a young child, pregnant, elderly, or disabled. Medicaid enrollment is growing dramatically, increasing from 32 million to 58 million people between 2000 and 2010 (9 million of whom are "dual eligibles" receiving both Medicare and Medicaid). The Accountable Care Act includes a huge expansion of Medicaid starting in 2014, eliminating the categorical eligibility criteria and offering the program to all citizens and legal residents with family income below 133% of the federal poverty line. The additional 16 million people on Medicaid will be financed largely by the federal government at a cost of over $40 billion per year in new dollars (see Chapter 15).

From 2000 to 2010, Medicaid expenditures rose from $200 billion to $374 billion. To slow down this expenditure growth, the federal government ceded to states enhanced control over Medicaid programs through Medicaid waivers, which allow states to reduce the number of people eligible for Medicaid, make alterations in the scope of covered services, require Medicaid recipients to pay part of their costs, and obligate Medicaid recipients to enroll in managed care plans (see Chapter 4). In 2010, over half of Medicaid recipients were enrolled in managed care plans. Because Medicaid pays physicians an average of 72% of Medicare fees, the majority of adult primary care physicians limit the number of Medicaid patients they will see; these patients are increasingly concentrated in academic health centers and community health centers.

In 1997, the federal government created the State Children's Health Insurance Program (SCHIP), a companion program to Medicaid. SCHIP covers children in families with incomes at or below 200% of the federal poverty level, but above the Medicaid income eligibility level. States legislating a SCHIP program receive generous federal matching funds and can administer SCHIP through Medicaid or by creating a separate program. In 2009, almost 8 million children were enrolled in the program.

Government health insurance for the poor and the elderly added a new factor to the health care financing equation: the taxpayer (Figure 2–4). With government-financed health plans, the taxpayer can interact with the health care consumer in two distinct ways:

1. The social insurance model, exemplified by Medicare, allows only those who have paid a certain amount of social security taxes to be eligible for Part A and only those who pay a monthly premium to receive benefits from Part B. As with private insurance, social insurance requires people to make a contribution in order to receive benefits.

2. The contrasting model is the Medicaid public assistance model, in which those who contribute (taxpayers) may not be eligible for benefits (Bodenheimer and Grumbach, 1992).

It must be remembered that private insurance contains a subsidy: redistribution of funds from the healthy to the sick. Tax-funded insurance has the same subsidy and usually adds another: redistribution of funds from upper- to lower-income groups. Under this double subsidy, exemplified by Medicare and Medicaid, healthy middle-income employees generally pay more in social security payments and other taxes than they receive in health services, whereas unemployed, disabled, and lower-income elderly persons tend to receive more in health services than they contribute in taxes.

The advent of government financing improved financial access to care for some people, but, in turn,

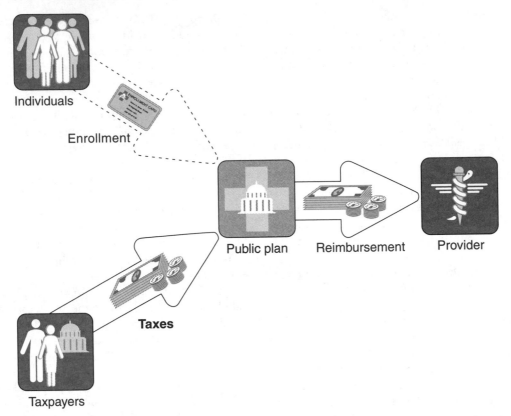

▲ **Figure 2–4.** Government-financed insurance. Under the social insurance model (eg, Medicare Part A), only individuals paying taxes into the public plan are eligible for benefits. In other models (eg, Medicaid), an individual's eligibility for benefits may not be directly linked to payment of taxes into the plan.

aggravated the problem of rising costs. The federal government and state governments have responded by attempting to limit Medicare and Medicaid payments to physicians and hospitals. At the same time, the rising costs of private insurance continue to place employment-based coverage out of the fiscal reach of many employers and employees.

THE BURDEN OF FINANCING HEALTH CARE

Different methods of financing health care place different burdens on the various income levels of society. Payments are classified as **progressive** if they take a rising percentage of income as income increases, **regressive** if they take a falling percentage of income as income increases, and **proportional** if the ratio of payment to income is the same for all income classes (Pechman, 1985).

What principle should underlie the choice of revenue source for health care? A central purpose of the health care system is to maintain and improve the health of the nation's population. As discussed in Chapter 3, rates of mortality and disability are far higher for low-income people than for the wealthy. Burdening low-income families with high levels of payments for health care (ie, regressive payments) reduces their disposable income, amplifies the ill effects of poverty, and thereby worsens their health. It makes little sense to finance a health care system—whose purpose is to improve health—with payments that worsen health. Thus, regressive payments could be considered "unhealthy."

Rita Blue earns $10,000 per year for her family of 4. She develops pneumonia, and her out-of-pocket health costs come to $1000, 10% of her family income.

Cathy White earns $100,000 per year for her family of 4. She develops pneumonia, and her out-of-pocket health costs come to $1000, 1% of her family income.

Out-of-pocket payments are a regressive mode of financing. According to the 1987 National Medical Care Expenditure Survey, out-of-pocket payments took 12% of the income of families in the nation's lowest-income quintile, compared with 1.2% for families in the wealthiest 5% of the population (Bodenheimer and Sullivan, 1997). This pattern is confirmed by the 2000 Medical Expenditure Panel Survey (MEPS, 2003). Many economists and health policy experts would consider this regressive burden of payment as unfair. Aggravating the regressivity of out-of-pocket payments is the fact that lower-income people tend to be sicker and thus have more out-of-pocket payments than the wealthier and healthier.

Jim Hale is a young, healthy, self-employed accountant whose monthly income is $6000, with a health insurance premium of $200, or 3% of his income.

Jack Hurt is a disabled mine worker with black lung disease. His income is $1800 per month, of which $400 (22%) goes for his health insurance.

Experience-rated private health insurance is a regressive method of financing health care because increased risk of illness tends to correlate with reduced income. If Jim Hale and Jack Hurt were enrolled in a community-rated plan, each with a premium of $300, they would respectively pay 5% and 17% of their incomes for health insurance. With community rating, the burden of payment is regressive, but less so than with experience rating.

Most private insurance is not individually purchased but rather obtained through employment. How is the burden of employment-linked health insurance premiums distributed?

Jill is an assistant hospital administrator. To attract her to the job, the hospital offered her a package of salary plus health insurance of $6500 per month. She chose to take $6200 in salary, leaving the hospital to pay $300 for her health insurance.

Bill is a nurse's aide, whose union negotiated with the hospital for a total package of $2800 per month; of this amount $2500 is salary and $300 pays his health insurance premium.

Do Jill and Bill pay nothing for their health insurance? Not exactly. Employers generally agree on a total package of wages and fringe benefits; if Jill and Bill did not receive health insurance, their pay would probably go up by nearly $300 per month. That is why employer-paid health insurance premiums are generally considered deductions from wages or salary, and thus paid by the employee (Blumberg et al, 2007). For Jill, health insurance amounts to only 5% of her income, but for Bill it is 12%. The MEPS corroborates the regressivity of employment-based health insurance; in 2001–2003, premiums took an average of 10.9% of the income of families in between 100% and 200% of the federal poverty line compared with 2.3% for those above 500% of poverty (Blumberg et al, 2007).

Larry Lowe earns $10,000 and pays $410 in federal and state income taxes, or 4.1% of his income.

Harold High earns $100,000 and pays $12,900 in income taxes, or 12.9% of his income.

The progressive income tax is the largest tax providing money for government-financed health care. Most other taxes are regressive (eg, sales and property taxes), and the combined burden of all taxes that finance health care is roughly proportional (Pechman, 1985).

In 2009, 46% of health care expenditures were financed through out-of-pocket payments and premiums, which are regressive, while 47% was funded through government revenues (Martin et al, 2011), which are proportional. The sum total of health care financing is regressive. In 1999, the poorest quintile of households spent 18% of income on health care, while the highest-income quintile spent only 3% (Cowan et al, 2002). Overall, the US health care system is financed in a manner that is unhealthy.

CONCLUSION

Neither Fred Farmer nor his great-grandson Ted had health insurance, but the modern-day Mr. Farmer's predicament differs drastically from that of his ancestor. Third-party financing of health care has fueled an expansive health care system that offers treatments unimaginable a century ago, but at tremendous expense.

Each of the four modes of financing health care developed historically as a solution to the inadequacy of the previous modes. Private insurance provided protection to patients against the unpredictable costs of medical care, as well as protection to providers of care against the unpredictable ability of patients to pay. But the private insurance solution created three new, interrelated problems:

1. The opportunity for health care providers to increase fees to insurers caused health services to become increasingly unaffordable for those with inadequate insurance or no insurance.

2. The employment-based nature of group insurance placed people who were unemployed, retired, or working part-time at a disadvantage for the purchase of insurance, and partially masked the true costs of insurance for employees who did receive health benefits at the workplace.

3. Competition inherent in a deregulated private insurance market gave rise to the practice of experience rating, which made insurance premiums unaffordable for many elderly people and other medically needy groups.

To solve these problems, government financing was required, but government financing fueled an even greater inflation in health care costs.

As each "solution" was introduced, health care financing improved for a time. But rising costs have jeopardized private and public coverage for many people and made services unaffordable for those without a source of third-party payment. The problems of each financing mode, and the problems created by each successive solution, have accumulated into a complex crisis characterized by inadequate access for some and high costs for everyone.

REFERENCES

Aaron HJ. *Serious and Unstable Condition: Financing America's Health Care*. Washington, DC: Brookings Institution; 1991.

Arrow KJ. Uncertainty and the welfare economics of medical care. *Am Econ Rev*. 1963;53:941.

Blumberg LJ et al. Setting a standard of affordability for health insurance coverage. *Health Affairs*. 2007;26:w463-w473.

Bodenheimer T, Grumbach K. Financing universal health insurance: Taxes, premiums, and the lessons of social insurance. *J Health Polit Policy Law*. 1992;17:439.

Bodenheimer T, Sullivan K. The logic of tax-based financing for health care. *Int J Health Services*. 1997;27:409.

Cowan CA et al. Burden of health care costs: Businesses, households, and governments, 1987–2000. *Health Care Financ Rev*. 2002;23:131.

Evans RG. *Strained Mercy*. Toronto, Ontario, Canada: Butterworths; 1984.

Fein R. *Medical Care, Medical Costs*. Cambridge, MA: Harvard University Press; 1986.

Gruber J. The tax exclusion for employer-sponsored health insurance. *National Bureau of Economic Research*; February 2010. www.nber.org/papers/w15766. Accessed November 11, 2011.

Harris R. *A Sacred Trust*. New York, NY: New American Library; 1966.

Kaiser Family Foundation. Medicare Spending and Financing. 2010a. www.kff.org. Accessed August 3, 2011.

Kaiser Family Foundation. Medicare at a Glance. 2010b. www.kff.org. Accessed August 3, 2011.

Kaiser Family Foundation. Medicare Advantage 2010 Data Spotlight. 2010c. www.kff.org. Accessed August 3, 2011.

Kaiser Family Foundation. The Medicaid Program at a Glance. 2010d. www.kff.org. Accessed August 3, 2011.

Law SA. *Blue Cross: What Went Wrong?* New Haven, CT: Yale University Press; 1974.

Light DW. The practice and ethics of risk-rated health insurance. *JAMA*. 1992;267:2503.

Martin A et al. Recession contributes to slowest annual rate of increase in health spending in five decades. *Health Affairs*. 2011;30:11.

Medical Expenditure Panel Survey. Health insurance coverage of the civilian non-institutionalized population, first half of 2002. Agency for Healthcare Research and Quality, June 2003. www.meps.ahrq.gov. Accessed November 11, 2011.

Pechman JA. *Who Paid the Taxes, 1966–1985*. Washington, DC: Brookings Institution; 1985.

Starr P. *The Social Transformation of American Medicine*. New York, NY: Basic Books; 1982.

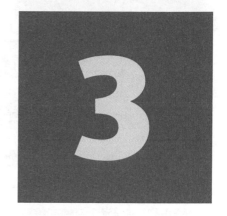

Access to Health Care

Access to health care is the ability to obtain health services when needed. Lack of adequate access for millions of people is a crisis in the United States.

Access to health care has two major components. First and most frequently discussed is ability to pay. Second is the availability of health care personnel and facilities that are close to where people live, accessible by transportation, culturally acceptable, and capable of providing appropriate care in a timely manner and in a language spoken by those who need assistance. The first and longest portion of this chapter dwells on financial barriers to care. The second portion touches on nonfinancial barriers. The final segment explores the influences other than health care (in particular, socioeconomic status and race) that are important determinants of the health status of a population.

FINANCIAL BARRIERS TO HEALTH CARE

▶ Lack of Insurance

Ernestine Newsome was born into a low-income working family living in South Central Los Angeles. As a young child, she rarely saw a physician and was behind on her childhood immunizations. When Ernestine was 7 years old, her mother began working for the telephone company, and this provided the family with health insurance. Ernestine went to a neighborhood physician for regular checkups. When she reached 19, she left home and began work as a part-time secretary. She was no longer eligible for her family's health insurance coverage, and her new job did not provide insurance. She has not seen a physician since starting her job.

Health insurance coverage, whether public or private, is a key factor in making health care accessible. In 1980, 25 million people were uninsured, but by 2009 the number had increased to 51 million (Table 3–1 and Figure 3–1) (US Census Bureau, 2010). The particular pattern of uninsurance is related to the employment-based nature of health care financing. Most people, like Ernestine Newsome, obtain health insurance when employers voluntarily decide to offer group coverage to employees and their families and their employers help pay for the costs of health insurance. People whose employers choose not to provide health insurance, are self-employed, or are unemployed are left to fend for themselves outside of the employer-sponsored group health insurance market, with the result that many are uninsured. Often people without employment-based insurance are not eligible for public programs such as Medicare and Medicaid, and are unable to purchase individual private coverage because they cannot afford the premiums.

Between the 1930s and mid-1970s, because of the growth of private health insurance and the 1965 passage of Medicare and Medicaid, the number of uninsured persons declined steadily, but since 1976, the number has been growing. The single most important factor explaining the growing number of uninsured is a 25-year trend of decreasing private insurance coverage in the United States. Virtually all people aged 65 and older are covered by Medicare, and the number of people enrolled in Medicaid has increased. However, a dwindling proportion of children and working age adults are covered by private insurance, exposing the limitations of the employment-linked system of private insurance in the

Table 3–1. Estimated principal source of health insurance, 2009

	Number of People (millions)	Population (%)
Medicare[a]	43	14
Medicaid/SCHIP	49	16
Employment-based private insurance	146	48
Individual private insurance	15	5
Uninsured	51	17
Total United States population	304	

Source: US Census Bureau. Income, Poverty, and Health Insurance Coverage in the United States, 2009; pp. 60–238, September 2010.
[a]For people with Medicare plus private insurance or Medicaid, Medicare is considered the principal source of insurance. The Medicaid and private insurance figures do not count Medicare beneficiaries who also have Medicaid or private insurance.

United States. If the 2010 health care reform law, the Accountable Care Act, is fully implemented, the number of uninsured people is expected to drop from 51 million to 22 million (Buettgens et al, 2010).

Why People Lack Insurance?

Joe Fortuno dropped out of high school and went to work for Car Doctor auto body shop in 2003. His employer paid the full cost of health insurance for

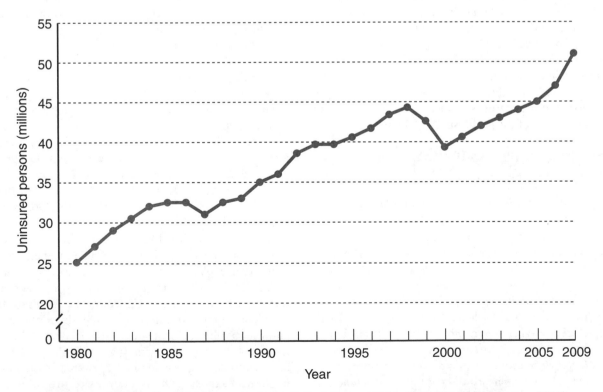

Figure 3–1. Number of uninsured persons in the United States, 1980 to 2009 (US Census Bureau, 2010).

Joe and his family. Joe's younger cousin Pete Luckless got a job working at an auto mechanic shop in 2005. The company did not offer health insurance benefits. In 2008, Car Doctor, after experiencing a doubling of health insurance premium rates over the prior few years, began requiring that its employees pay $150 per month for the employer-sponsored health plan. Joe could not afford the monthly payments and lost his health insurance.

Why has private health insurance coverage decreased over the past decades, creating the uninsurance crisis? There are several explanations:

1. The skyrocketing cost of health insurance has made coverage unaffordable for many businesses and individuals. From 2000 to 2010, employer-sponsored health insurance premiums rose by 114%. In 2010, the average annual cost of health insurance, including employer and employee contributions, was $5049 for individuals and $13,770 for families (Claxton et al, 2010). Some employers responded to rising health insurance costs by dropping insurance policies for their workers. Many employers have shifted more of the cost of health insurance premiums and health services onto their employees, resulting in employees dropping health coverage because of unaffordability. On average, employee contributions represent 19% of the premium for individual employee coverage and 30% for family coverage, though some employees have to pay more than half of the premium for family coverage (Claxton et al, 2010). Low-income workers are hit especially hard by the combination of rising insurance costs and declining employer subsidies.

Jean Irons worked for Bethlehem Steel as a clerk and her fringe benefits included health insurance. Bethlehem Steel was bought by a global corporation and her plant moved to another country. She found a job as a food service worker in a small restaurant. Her pay decreased by 35%, and the restaurant did not provide health insurance.

2. During the past few decades, the economy in the United States has undergone a major transition. The number of highly paid, largely unionized, full-time manufacturing workers with employer-sponsored health insurance has declined, and the workforce has shifted toward more low-wage, increasingly part-time, nonunionized service, and clerical workers whose employers are less likely to provide insurance (Renner and Navarro, 1989). Between 1980 and 2006, the number of workers in the manufacturing sector decreased by 30% while the number working in the service sector increased by 75%. From 1957 to 2000, the percentage of workers with part-time jobs—generally without health benefits—increased from 12% to 21%.

These two factors—increasing health care costs and a changing labor force—eroded private insurance coverage. One countervailing trend has been a major expansion of public insurance coverage through the Medicaid and State Children's Health Insurance Program (SCHIP) programs. Without these changes, many more millions of Americans would currently be uninsured.

Sally Lewis worked as a receptionist in a physician's office. She received health insurance through her husband, who was a construction worker. They got divorced, she lost her health insurance, and her physician employer told her he could not provide her with health insurance because of the cost.

3. The link of private insurance with employment inevitably produces interruptions in coverage because of the unstable nature of employment. People who are laid off from their jobs or who leave jobs because of illness may also lose their insurance. Family members insured through the workplace of a spouse may lose their insurance in cases of divorce, job loss, or death of the working family member. People who leave their employment may be eligible to pay for continued coverage under their group plan for 18 months, as stipulated in the Consolidated Omnibus Budget Reconciliation Act of 1985 (COBRA), with the requirement that they pay the full cost of the premium; however, many people cannot afford the premiums, which may exceed $1000 per month for a family.

The often transient nature of employment-linked insurance is compounded by difficulties in maintaining eligibility for Medicaid. Small increases in family income can mean that families no longer qualify for Medicaid. The net result is that millions of people cycle in and out of the ranks of the uninsured every month. A total of 87 million people, 29% of the entire US population,

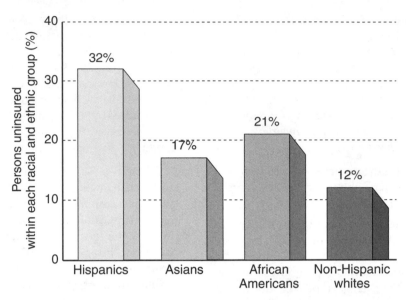

▲ **Figure 3–2.** Percentage of population lacking health insurance by race and ethnicity in 2009 (US Census Bureau, 2010).

went without health insurance for all or part of the 2-year period 2007–2008 (Families USA, 2009). Health insurance may be a fleeting benefit.

Who Are the Uninsured?

In 2009, 12% of non-Hispanic whites were uninsured, compared with 21% of African Americans, 17% of Asians, and 32% of Latinos (Figure 3–2). Twenty-seven percent of individuals with annual household incomes less than $25,000 were uninsured, compared with 9% of individuals with household incomes of $75,000 or more (Figure 3–3) (US Census Bureau, 2010).

Morris works for a corner grocery store that employs five people. Morris once asked the owner whether the employees could receive health insurance through their work, but the owner said it was too expensive. Morris, his wife, and their three kids are uninsured.

Norris, a shipyard worker, was laid off 3 years ago, and at age 60 is unable to get another job. He lives on county general assistance of $400 per month, but is ineligible for Medicaid because he is not a parent, not older than 65, and not disabled. He is uninsured.

The uninsured can be divided into two major categories: the employed uninsured (Morris) and the unemployed uninsured (Norris). Seventy-five percent of the uninsured are employed or the spouses and children of those who work. Most of the jobs held by the employed uninsured are low paying, in small firms, and may be part time (Figures 3–4 and 3–5). Twenty-five percent of the uninsured are unemployed, often with incomes below the poverty line, but like Norris are ineligible for Medicaid.

Does Health Insurance Make a Difference?

Two US senators are debating the issue of access to health care. One decries the stigma of uninsurance and claims that people without insurance receive less care and suffer worse health than those with insurance. The other disagrees, claiming that hospitals and physicians deliver large amounts of charity care, which allows uninsured people to receive the services they need.

To resolve this debate, the US Congress Office of Technology Assessment (1992) conducted a comprehensive review to determine whether health insurance makes a difference in the use of health care and in

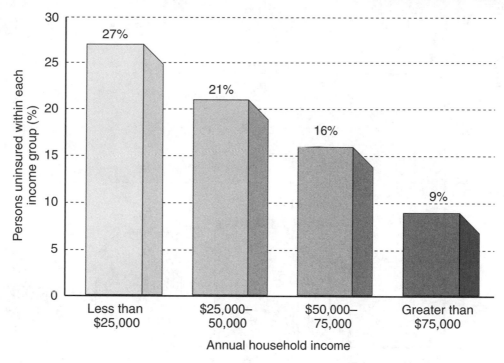

▲ **Figure 3–3.** Lack of insurance by income in 2009 (US Census Bureau, 2010).

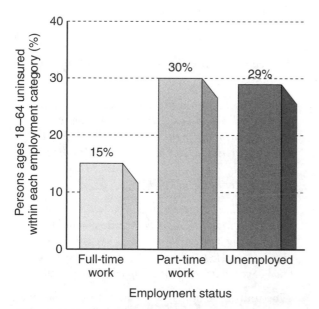

▲ **Figure 3–4.** Lack of insurance by employment status in 2009 (US Census Bureau, 2010).

health outcomes. The findings, corroborated by the Institute of Medicine (2002), proved that people lacking health insurance receive less care and have worse health outcomes.

Health Insurance and Use of Health Services

> *Percy, a child whose parents were both employed but not insured, was refused admission by a private hospital for treatment of an abscess. Outpatient treatment failed, and his mother attempted to admit Percy to other area hospitals, which also refused care. Finally an attorney arranged for the original hospital to admit the child; the parents then owed the hospital $6000.*

Access to health care is most simply measured by the number of times a person uses health care services. Commonly used data are numbers of physician visits, hospital days, and preventive services received.

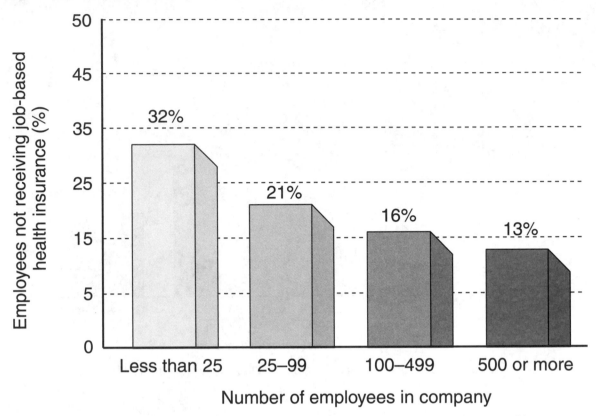

▲ **Figure 3–5.** Lack of job-based insurance by size of employer in 2007 (Kaiser Family Foundation, Health Insurance Coverage in America, 2008, www.kff.org).

In addition, access can be quantified by surveys in which respondents report whether or not they failed to seek care or delayed care when they felt they needed it. In 2009, 56% of uninsured adults, compared with 10% of those with insurance, had no usual source of care, 32%, compared with 8% of those with insurance, postponed seeking care due to cost, and 26%, compared with 4% for those with insurance, went without needed care due to cost (Kaiser Family Foundation, 2010a).

Health Insurance and Health Outcomes

Dan Sugarman noticed that he was urinating a lot and feeling weak. His friend told him that he had diabetes and needed medical care, but lacking health insurance, Mr. Sugarman was afraid of the cost. Eight days later, his friend found him

in a coma. He was hospitalized for diabetic keto-acidosis.

Penny Evans worked in a Nevada casino. She was uninsured and ignored a growing mole on her chest. After many months of delay, she saw a dermatologist and was diagnosed with malignant melanoma, which had metastasized. She died 2 years later at the age of 44.

Leo Morelli, a hypertensive patient, was doing well until his company relocated to Mexico and he lost his job. Lacking both paycheck and health insurance, he became unable to afford his blood pressure medications. Six months later, he collapsed with a stroke.

The uninsured suffer worse health outcomes than those with insurance. Compared with insured persons, the uninsured like Mr. Sugarman have more avoidable hospitalizations; like both Mr. Sugarman and Ms. Evans, they tend to be diagnosed at later stages of life-threatening illnesses, and they are on average more seriously ill when hospitalized (American College of Physicians, 2000). Higher rates of hypertension and cervical cancer and lower survival rates for breast cancer among the uninsured, compared with those with insurance, are associated with less frequent blood pressure screenings, Pap smears, and clinical breast examinations (Ayanian et al, 2000). People without insurance have greater rates of uncontrolled hypertension, diabetes, and elevated cholesterol than those with insurance (Wilper et al, 2009). Most significantly, people who lack health insurance suffer a higher overall mortality rate than those with insurance. After adjusting for age, sex, education, poorer initial health status, and smoking, it was found that lack of insurance alone increased the risk of dying by 25% (Franks et al, 1993). The Institute of Medicine estimated that lack of health insurance accounts for 18,000 deaths annually in the United States (Institute of Medicine, 2004).

Does Medicaid Make a Difference?

Medicaid, the federal and state public insurance plan, has made great strides in improving access to care for two-thirds of people with incomes below the federal poverty level, but Medicaid has its limitations.

Medicaid and Use of Health Services

Concepcion Ortiz lived in a town of 25,000 persons. When she became pregnant, her sister told her that she was eligible for Medicaid, which she obtained. She called each obstetrician in town and none would take Medicaid patients. When she reached her sixth month, she became desperate.

For those people with Medicaid coverage, access to care is by no means guaranteed. Medicaid pays physicians far less than does Medicare or private insurance with the result that many physicians do not accept Medicaid patients.

As a rule, people with Medicaid have a level of access to medical care that is intermediate between those without insurance and those with private insurance. Compared with uninsured people, those with Medicaid are more likely to have a regular source of medical care and are less likely to report delays in receiving care.

But these access measures for Medicaid recipients are not as good as for people with private insurance (Kaiser Family Foundation, 2010a).

Medicaid and Health Outcomes

Health outcomes for Medicaid recipients lag behind those for privately insured people. Compared with privately insured people, Medicaid recipients have lower rates of immunizations, screening for breast and cervical cancer, hypertension and diabetes control, and timeliness of prenatal care. (Landon et al, 2007). Medicaid patients with cancer have their disease detected at significantly later stages than privately insured patients, with the delays in diagnosis comparable for uninsured and Medicaid patients (Halpern et al, 2007). Persons with Medicaid are sometimes relegated, with the uninsured, to the lowest tier of the health care system.

▶ Underinsurance

Health insurance does not guarantee financial access to care. Many people are underinsured; that is, their health insurance coverage has limitations that restrict access to needed services (Table 3–2). An estimated 20% of insured Americans between the ages of 19 and 64 were underinsured in 2007, up from 12% in 2003 (Gabel et al, 2009).

Limits to Insurance Coverage

In 2007, 71% of privately insured people with low incomes and substantial medical expenditures were underinsured. This number is rising as health care costs rise and insurance coverage becomes less comprehensive (Gabel et al, 2009). In 2007, 62% of bankruptcies in the United States were caused by inability to pay medical bills; 75% of these individuals had health insurance at the onset of their illness (Himmelstein et al, 2009).

Table 3–2. Categories of underinsurance

Limits to insurance coverage
Insurance deductibles and copayments
Gaps in Medicare coverage
Lack of coverage for long-term care

Insurance Deductibles and Copayments

Eva Stefanski works as a legal secretary and has a Blue Cross high-deductible health plan policy with a $2500 deductible. Last year, she failed to show up for her mammogram appointment because she did not have $150 to pay for the test. This year, she also decides to forego making an appointment for her periodic pap test.

For people with low or moderate incomes, insurance deductibles and copayments may represent a substantial financial problem. From 2006 to 2010, the percent of people with employer-sponsored insurance having a deductible of $1000 or more for single (not family) coverage grew from 10% to 27%. In 2010, 13% of insured employees (up from 4% in 2006) had high-deductible insurance plans, with families paying an average deductible of $3500 plus the employee premium contribution and copayments (Claxton et al, 2010).

Gaps in Medicare Coverage

Corazon Estacio suffers from angina, congestive heart failure, and high blood pressure, in addition to diabetes. She takes 17 pills per day: four each of glyburide and metformin, three isosorbide, two carvedilol and two furosemide, and one each of benazepril and aspirin. Because of the deductibles and the "doughnut hole" in her Medicare Part D plan, her yearly medication bill comes to $3840.

Ferdinand Foote was covered by Medicare and had no Medigap, Medicare Advantage, or Medicaid coverage. He was hospitalized for peripheral vascular disease caused by diabetes and a non-healing infected foot ulcer. He spent 4 days in the acute hospital and 1 month in the skilled nursing facility and made weekly physician visits following his discharge. The costs of illness not covered by Medicare included a $1132 deductible for acute hospital care, a $141.50 per day copayment for days 21 to 30 of the skilled nursing facility stay, a $162 physician deductible, and a 20% ($12) physician copayment per visit for 12 visits. The total came to $2853 not including the cost of uncovered outpatient medications.

Medicare paid for only 48% of the average beneficiary's health care expenses in 2006 (Kaiser Family Foundation, 2010b). For the 5% of beneficiaries in poorest health, uncovered costs in 2004 averaged $7646, up 48% from 1992 (Riley, 2008). As discussed in Chapter 2, Medicare Part D requires beneficiaries to continue shouldering large out-of-pocket expenses for their medications, a situation that is expected to improve with the Accountable Care Act of 2010.

Lack of Coverage for Long-Term Care

Victoria and Gus Pappas had $80,000 in the bank when Gus had a stroke. After his hospitalization, he was still paralyzed on the right side and unable to speak or swallow. After 18 months in the nursing home, most of the $80,000 was gone. At that point, Medicaid picked up the nursing home costs.

Medicare paid only 20% of the elderly's nursing home bills in 2009, and private insurance policies picked up only an additional 8% (see Chapter 12). Many elderly families spend their life savings on long-term care, qualifying for Medicaid only after becoming impoverished.

The Effects of Underinsurance

Does underinsurance represent a serious barrier to the receipt of medical care? The famous Rand Health Insurance Experiment compared nonelderly individuals who had health insurance plans with no out-of-pocket costs and those who had plans with varying amounts of patient cost sharing (deductibles or copayments). The study found that cost sharing reduces the rate of ambulatory care use, especially among the poor, and that patients with cost-sharing plans demonstrate a reduction in both appropriate and inappropriate medical visits. For low-income adults, the cost-sharing groups received Pap smears 65% as often as the free-care group. Hypertensive adults in the cost-sharing groups had higher diastolic pressures, and children had higher rates of anemia and lower rates of immunization (Brook et al, 1983; Lohr et al, 1986; Lurie et al, 1987).

In 2003, underinsured adults aged 19 to 64 with health problems were much more likely than well-insured adults to skip recommended tests or follow-up, forego seeing a physician when they felt sick, and fail to fill a prescription on account of cost (Schoen et al, 2005). In 2006, 20% of Medicare beneficiaries with

Part D coverage did not fill, or delayed filling, a prescription due to inability to pay the uncovered costs (Neuman et al, 2007). In summary, lack of comprehensive insurance reduces access to health care services and may contribute to poorer health outcomes.

NONFINANCIAL BARRIERS TO HEALTH CARE

Nonfinancial barriers to health care include inability to access care when needed, language, literacy, and cultural differences between patients and health caregivers, and factors of gender and race. Excellent discussions of these issues can be found in the book "Medical Management of Vulnerable and Underserved Patients" (King and Wheeler, 2007).

▶ Lack of Prompt Access

Medical practices often fail to provide their patients with access at the time when the patient needs care. This problem has worsened with the growing shortage of primary care practitioners. In 2008, 28% of Medicare beneficiaries without a primary care physician reported difficulty finding such a physician, a 17% increase from 2006. Thirty-one percent of privately insured patients had an unwanted delay in obtaining an appointment for routine care in 2008. In 2006, only 27% of adults with a usual source of care could easily contact their physician by phone, obtain care or advice after hours, and experience timely office visits. After Massachusetts passed its health insurance expansion in 2006, demand for primary care increased without an increase in supply, resulting in the average wait time to see a primary care internist increasing from 17 days in 2005 to 31 days in 2008. Fewer primary care physicians are accepting Medicaid patients, and inappropriate emergency department visits are growing, especially for Medicaid patients, due to inability to access timely primary care (Bodenheimer and Pham, 2010).

▶ Gender and Access to Health Care

Olga Madden is angry. Her male physician had not listened. He told her that her incontinence was from too many childbirths and that she would have to live with it. She had questions about the hormones he was prescribing, but he always seemed too busy, so she never asked. Ms. Madden calls her HMO and gets the names of two female physicians, a female physician assistant, and a nurse practitioner. She calls them. Their receptionists tell her that none of them is accepting new patients; they are all too busy.

Access problems for women often begin with finding a physician who communicates effectively. Women are 50% more likely than men to report leaving a physician because of dissatisfaction with their care, and they are more than twice as likely to report that their physician "talked down" to them or told them their problems were "all in their head" (Leiman et al, 1997). Female physicians have a more patient-centered style of communicating and spend more time with their patients than do male physicians (Roter and Hall, 2004). In a study of patients with insurance coverage for Pap smears and mammograms, the patients of female physicians were almost twice as likely to receive a Pap smear and 1.4 times as likely to have a mammogram than the patients of male physicians (Lurie et al, 1993).

Physicians are less likely to counsel women than men about cardiac prevention—diet, exercise, and weight reduction. After having a heart attack, women are less likely than men to receive recommended diagnostic tests and are less likely to be prescribed recommended aspirin and beta-blockers (Agency for Healthcare Research and Quality, 2005).

Because women are more likely than men to have a chronic condition, women use more chronic medications and are more likely than men not to fill a prescription because of cost. Because more women than men are Medicaid recipients, they are more likely to be turned away from physicians who do not accept Medicaid. Fewer than one-third of women of reproductive age have received counseling about emergency contraception, sexually transmitted diseases, or domestic violence (Kaiser Family Foundation, 2005b).

For those women who wish to terminate a pregnancy, access to abortions is limited in many areas of the country. In 2009, 87% of US counties had no identifiable abortion provider. While women have reduced access to certain kinds of care, an equally serious problem may be instances of inappropriate care. A study conducted in a managed-care medical group in California found that 70% of hysterectomies were inappropriate (Broder et al, 2000).

Race and Access to Health Care

Jose is suffering. The pain from his fractured femur is excruciating, and the emergency department physician has given him no pain medication. In the next room, Joe is asleep. He has received 10 mg of morphine for his femur fracture.

At a California emergency department, 55% of Latino patients with extremity fractures received no pain medication compared with 26% of non-Latino whites. This marked difference in treatment was attributable not to insurance status but to ethnicity (Todd et al, 1993). African American patients similarly receive poorer pain control than whites (Todd et al, 2000).

Because a far higher proportion of minorities than whites is uninsured, has Medicaid coverage, or is poor, access problems are amplified for these groups. African Americans and Latinos in the United States are less likely to have a regular source of care or to have had a physician visit in the past year (King and Wheeler, 2007). Racial and ethnic differences in access to care are not always a matter of differences in financial resources and insurance coverage. Studies have shown that African Americans and Latinos receive fewer services even when compared with non-Hispanic whites who have the same level of health insurance and income (Agency for Healthcare Research and Quality, 2009).

Studies have also detected such disparities in quality of care. Looking at 38 measures of quality for such conditions as diabetes, asthma, HIV/AIDS, cardiac care, and cancer, African Americans receive poorer quality of care than whites for 66% of these quality measures; American Indians and Alaska Natives and Latinos also have lower quality indicators (King and Wheeler, 2007).

Neighborhoods that have high proportions of African American or Latino residents have far fewer physicians practicing in these communities. African American and Latino primary care physicians are more likely than white physicians to locate their practices in underserved communities (Komaromy et al, 1996).

What explains these disparities in access to care across racial and ethnic groups that are not fully accounted for by differences in insurance coverage and socioeconomic status? Several hypotheses have been proposed. Cultural differences may exist in patients' beliefs about the value of medical care and attitudes toward seeking treatment for their symptoms. However, differences in patient preferences do not account for substantial amounts of the racial variations seen in cardiac surgery rates (Mayberry et al, 2000). A related factor may be ineffective communication between patients and caregivers of differing races, cultures, and languages. African Americans are more likely than whites to report that their physicians did not properly explain their illness and its treatment (LaVeist et al, 2000). Access barriers related to communication problems may be particularly acute for the subset of Latino patients for whom Spanish is the primary language. However, language issues do not fully account for access barriers faced by Latinos. In the study of emergency department pain medication cited previously, even Latinos who spoke English as their primary language were much less likely than non-Latino whites to receive pain medication.

Because many of these hypotheses do not satisfactorily explain the observed racial disparities in access to care, an important consideration is whether racism may also contribute to these patterns (King and Wheeler, 2007). Medicine in the United States has not escaped the nation's legacy of institutionalized racism toward many minority groups. Many hospitals, including institutions in the North, were for much of the twentieth century either completely segregated or had segregated wards, with inferior facilities and services available to nonwhites. Explicit segregation policies persisted in many hospitals until a few decades ago. Racial barriers to entry into the medical profession gave rise to the establishment of black medical schools such as the Howard, Morehouse, and Meharry schools of medicine. Although such overt racism is a diminishing feature of medicine in the United States, more insidious and often unconscious forms of discrimination may continue to color the interactions between patients and their caregivers and influence access to care for minorities (Van Ryn, 2002).

THE RELATION BETWEEN HEALTH CARE AND HEALTH STATUS

Access to health care does not by itself guarantee good health. A complex array of factors, only one of which is health care, determines whether a person is healthy or not.

Ace Banks is 48, an executive vice president, with four grandparents who lived past 90 years of age and parents alive and well in their late 70s. Mr. Banks went to an Ivy League college where he was a star athlete. He has never seen a physician except for a sprained ankle.

Keith Cole is a coal miner who at age 48 developed pneumonia. He had excellent health insurance through his union and went to see the leading pulmonologist in the state. He was hospitalized but became less and less able to breathe because the pneumonia was severely complicated by black lung disease, which he contracted through his job. He received high-quality care in the intensive care unit at a fully insured cost of $65,000, but he died.

Bill Downes, an African American man, knew that his father was killed by high blood pressure and his mother died of diabetes. Mr. Downes spent his childhood in poverty living with eight children at his grandmother's house. He had little to eat except what was provided at the school lunch program, a diet heavily laden with cheese and butter. To support the family, he left school at age 15 and got a job. At age 24, he was diagnosed with high blood pressure and diabetes. He did not smoke and was meticulous in following the diet prescribed by his physician. He had private health insurance through his job as a security guard and was cared for by a professor of medicine at the medical school. In spite of excellent medical care, his glucose and cholesterol levels and blood pressure were difficult to control, and he developed retinopathy, kidney failure, and coronary heart disease. At age 48, he collapsed at work and died of a heart attack.

▶ Health Status and Income

The gap between the rich and the poor has widened markedly in the United States. Between 1952 and 2005, the proportion of pretax income reported by the wealthiest decile of the population increased from 31% to 44%; the share of income for the richest 1% doubled from 8% in 1980 to 17% in 2005. At the same time, income is decreasing for the great majority of households (Woolf, 2007). As the stories of Ace Banks, Keith Cole, and Bill Downes suggest, the health of an individual or a population is influenced less by medical care than by broad socioeconomic factors such as income and education (Braveman et al, 2010). People in the United States with incomes above four times the poverty level live on average 7 years longer than those with incomes below the poverty level (Table 3–3). The mortality rate for heart disease among laborers is more than twice the rate for managers and professionals. The incidence of cancer increases as family income decreases, and survival rates are lower for low-income cancer patients. Higher infant mortality rates are linked to low income and low educational level. Not only does the income level of individuals affect their health and life expectancy, the way in which income is distributed within communities also appears to influence the overall health of the population. In the United States, overall mortality rates are higher in states that have a more unequal distribution of income, with greater concentration of wealth in upper income groups (Lochner et al, 2001). Some social scientists have concluded that the toxic health effects of social inequality in developed nations result from the psychosocial stresses of social hierarchies and social oppression, not simply from material deprivation (Kawachi and Kennedy, 1999).

Table 3–3. Income, race, and life expectancy in years (at age 25)[a]

Race	Income as Percent of Federal Poverty Level (FPL)			
	≤100% FPL	101%–200% FPL	201%–400% FPL	≥401% FPL
Black	45.5	48.0	50.7	52.6
White	49.0	51.4	53.8	55.8

[a]Life expectancy in years indicates the average additional years of life expected for individuals in each group at age 25 and is calculated from data in the National Mortality Longitudinal Survey, 1988–1998 as reported in Braveman PA et al. Socioeconomic disparities in health in the United States: What the patterns tell us. Am J Public Health. 2010;100:S186–S196.

Table 3–4. Life expectancy in years

In 1950	Women	Men
White	72.2	66.5
African American	62.9	59.1
In 2006		
White	80.6	75.7
African American	76.5	69.7

Source: US Department of Health and Human Services. *Health United States* 2009. www.cdc.gov.

Health Status and Race

African Americans experience dramatically worse health than white Americans. Life expectancy is lower for African Americans than for other racial and ethnic groups in the United States (Table 3–4). Infant mortality rates among African Americans are more than double those for whites (Table 3–5), and the relative disparity in infant mortality has widened during the past decade. Mortality rates for African Americans exceed those for whites for 7 of the 10 leading causes of death in the United States, including the most common killers in the US population—heart disease, strokes, and cancer (Table 3–6) (US Department of Health and Human Services, 2009). African American men younger than 45 years have 10 times the likelihood of dying of hypertension than white men in the same age group. Although the incidence of breast cancer is lower in African American women than in white women, in African American women this disease is diagnosed at a more advanced stage of illness, and thus they are more

Table 3–5. Infant mortality, 2006 (per 1000 live births)

White, non-Latino	5.6
African American	13.3
Latino	5.6
Asian or Pacific Islander	4.8
American Indian or Alaska Native	8.4

Source: US Department of Health and Human Services. *Health United States* 2009. www.cdc.gov.

Table 3–6. Age-adjusted death rates per 100,000 population, 2006

	White	African American
Malignant neoplasms (cancer)	179.9	217.4
Coronary heart disease	134.2	161.6
Stroke	41.7	61.6

Source: US Department of Health and Human Services. *Health United States* 2009. www.cdc.gov.

likely to die of breast cancer (Institute of Medicine, 2003; Halpern et al, 2007).

Native Americans are another ethnic group with far poorer health than that of whites. Native Americans younger than 45 years have far higher death rates than whites of comparable age, and the Native American infant mortality rate is 50% higher than the rate of whites (US Department of Health and Human Services, 2009).

Latinos and Asians and Pacific Islanders are minority groups characterized by great diversity. Health status varies widely between Cuban Americans, who tend to be more affluent, and poor Mexican American migrant farm workers, as well as between Japanese families, who are more likely to be middle class, and Laotians, who are often indigent. Compared with whites, Latinos have markedly higher death rates for diabetes and the acquired immune deficiency syndrome. Overall, Latinos have lower age-adjusted mortality rates than whites because of less cardiovascular disease and cancer. Asians in the United States have lower death rates than whites for all age groups (US Department of Health and Human Services, 2009).

Some of the differences in mortality rates of African Americans and Native Americans compared with whites are related to the higher rates of poverty among these minority groups. In 2009, the white poverty rate was 12% compared with 26% for African Americans, and 25% for Latinos (US Census Bureau, 2010). However, even compared with whites in the same income class, African Americans as a group have inferior health status. Although mortality rates decline with rising income among both African Americans and whites, at any given income level, the mortality rate for African Americans is consistently higher than the rate for whites (Table 3–3). Thus, social factors and stresses related to race itself seem to contribute to the relatively poorer health of African Americans. The inferior health outcomes among African Americans, such as higher mortality rates for heart disease, cancer, and stroke, are in part explained by the lower rate of access to health services among this group.

If lower income is associated with poorer health, and if Latinos tend to be poorer than non-Latino whites in the United States, then why do Latinos have overall lower mortality rates than non-Latino whites? This is possibly related to the fact that many Latinos are immigrants, and foreign-born people often have lower mortality rates than people born in the United States at the same level of income (Abraido-Lanza et al, 1999; Goel et al, 2004). This phenomenon is often referred to as the "healthy immigrant" effect. If this is the case, mortality rates for Latinos may rise as a higher proportion of their population is born in the United States.

CONCLUSION

Health outcomes are determined by multiple factors. Socioeconomic status appears to be the dominant influence on health status; yet medical care and public health interventions are also extremely important (King and Wheeler, 2007). The advent of the polio vaccine markedly reduced the number of paralytic polio cases. From 1970 to 2004, age-adjusted death rates from stroke decreased by more than 100%—a successful result of hypertension diagnosis and treatment. Early prenatal care can prevent low-birth-weight and infant deaths. Irradiation and chemotherapy have transformed the prognosis of some cancers (eg, Hodgkin disease) from a certain fatal outcome toward complete cure. A 1980 study of mortality rates in 400 counties in the United States found that after controlling for income, education, cigarette consumption, and prevalence of disability, a 10% increase in per capita medical care expenditures was associated with a reduced average mortality rate of 1.57% (Roemer, 1991). Moreover, the health care system provides patients with chronic disease welcome relief from pain and suffering and helps them to cope with their illnesses. Access to health care does not guarantee good health, but without such access health is certain to suffer.

REFERENCES

Abraido-Lanza AF et al. The Latino mortality paradox: A test of the "salmon bias" and healthy migrant hypothesis. *Am J Public Health.* 1999;89:1543.

Agency for Healthcare Research and Quality. *Women's Health Care in the United States.* May 2005. www.ahrq.gov.

Agency for Healthcare Research and Quality. National Healthcare Disparities Report, 2009. www.ahrq.gov.

Ayanian JZ et al. Unmet needs of uninsured adults in the United States. *JAMA.* 2000;284:2061.

Bodenheimer T, Pham HH. Primary care: Current problems and proposed solutions. *Health Aff (Millwood).* 2010:29:799.

Braveman PA et al. Socioeconomic disparities in health in the United States: What the patterns tell us. *Am J Public Health.* 2010;100:S186–S196.

Broder MS et al. The appropriateness of recommendations for hysterectomy. *Obstet Gynecol.* 2000;95:199.

Brook RH et al. Does free care improve adults' health? *N Engl J Med.* 1983;309:1426.

Buettgens M et al. *Why the Individual Mandate Matters.* Urban Institute Web Site. December 2010. www.urban.org.

Claxton G et al. Health benefits in 2010: Premiums rise modestly, workers pay more toward coverage. *Health Aff (Millwood).* 2010;29:1942.

Families USA. *Americans at Risk. One in Three Uninsured.* March 2009. www.familiesusa.org.

Franks P et al. Health insurance and mortality. *JAMA.* 1993;270:737.

Gabel JR et al. Trends in underinsurance and the affordability of employer coverage, 2004–2007. *Health Aff (Millwood).* 2009; 28:w595.

Goel MS et al. Obesity among US immigrant subgroups by duration of residence. *JAMA.* 2004;292:2860.

Halpern MT et al. Insurance status and stage of cancer at diagnosis among women with breast cancer. *Cancer.* 2007;110:231.

Himmelstein DU et al. Medical bankruptcy in the United States, 2007. *Am J Med.* 2009;122:741.

Institute of Medicine. *Care Without Coverage: Too Little, Too Late.* Washington, DC: National Academies Press; 2002.

Institute of Medicine. *Unequal Treatment.* Washington, DC: National Academies Press; 2003.

Institute of Medicine. *Insuring America's Health.* Washington, DC: National Academies Press; 2004.

Kaiser Family Foundation. The Uninsured and the Difference Health Insurance Makes. September 2010a. www.kff.org.

Kaiser Family Foundation. Medicare Spending and Financing. 2010b. www.kff.org.

Kaiser Family Foundation: *Women and Health Care.* Menlo Park, CA: Kaiser Family Foundation; July 2005. www.kff.org.

Kawachi I, Kennedy BP. Income inequality and health: Pathways and mechanisms. *Health Serv Res.* 1999;34:215.

King TE, Wheeler MB. *Medical Management of Vulnerable and Underserved Patients.* New York, NY: McGraw-Hill; 2007.

Komaromy M et al. The role of Black and Hispanic physicians in providing health care for underserved populations. *N Engl J Med.* 1996;334:1305.

Landon BE et al. Quality of care in Medicaid managed care and commercial health plans. *JAMA.* 2007;298:1674.

LaVeist TA et al. Attitudes about racism, medical mistrust, and satisfaction with care among African American and white cardiac patients. *Med Care Res Rev.* 2000;57(Suppl 1):146.

Leiman JM et al. *Selected Facts on U.S. Women's Health: A Chart Book.* New York: The Commonwealth Fund; 1997.

Lochner K et al. State-level income inequality and individual mortality risk: A prospective, multilevel study. *Am J Public Health.* 2001;91:385.

Lohr KN et al. Use of medical care in the Rand Health Insurance Experiment. *Med Care.* 1986;24(Suppl):S1.

Lurie N et al. Preventive care: Do we practice what we preach? *Am J Public Health.* 1987;77:801.

Lurie N et al. Preventive care for women: Does the sex of the physician matter? *N Engl J Med.* 1993;329:478.

Mayberry RM et al. Racial and ethnic differences in access to medical care. *Med Care Res Rev.* 2000;57(Suppl 1):108.

Neuman P et al. Medicare prescription drug benefit progress report. *Health Aff (Millwood).* 2007;26:w630.

Renner C, Navarro V. Why is our population of uninsured and underinsured persons growing? The consequences of the "deindustrialization" of the United States. *Int J Health Serv.* 1989;19:433.

Riley GF. Trends in out-of-pocket healthcare costs among older community-dwelling Medicare beneficiaries. *Am J Manag Care.* 2008;14:692.

Roemer MI. *National Health Systems of the World.* New York: Oxford University Press; 1991.

Roter DL, Hall JA. Physician gender and patient-centered communication. *Annu Rev Public Health.* 2004;25:497.

Schoen et al. Insured but not protected: How many adults are underinsured? *Health Affairs Web Exclusive.* June 14, 2005: w5–289. http://content.healthaffairs.org. Accessed November 11, 2011.

Todd KH et al. Ethnicity and analgesic practice. *Ann Emerg Med.* 2000;35:11.

Todd KH et al. Ethnicity as a risk factor for inadequate emergency department analgesia. *JAMA.* 1993;269: 1537.

US Census Bureau. Income, Poverty, and Health Insurance Coverage in the United States, 2009; pp. 60–238, September, 2010.

US Congress, Office of Technology Assessment. *Does Health Insurance Make a Difference?* OTA-BP-H-99. US Government Printing Office; 1992.

US Department of Health and Human Services. *Health United States 2009.* www.cdc.gov.

Van Ryn M. Research on the provider contribution to race/ethnicity disparities in medical care. *Med Care.* 2002;40(Suppl):I-140.

Wilper et al. Hypertension, diabetes, and elevated cholesterol among insured and uninsured U.S. adults. *Health Aff (Millwood).* 2009;28:1151.

Woolf SH. Future health consequences of the current decline in US household income. *JAMA.* 2007;298:1931.

Reimbursing Health Care Providers

Chapter 2 described the different modes of financing health care: out-of-pocket payments, individual health insurance, employment-based health insurance, and government financing. Each of these mechanisms attempted to solve the problem of unaffordable care for certain groups, but each "solution" in turn created new problems by stimulating rapid rises in health care costs. One of the factors contributing to this inflation was reimbursement of physicians and hospitals by insurance companies and government programs. Therefore, new methods of reimbursement have been tried as one way of lowering the growth rate in health care costs.

Dr. Mary Young has recently finished her family medicine residency and joined a small group practice, PrimaryCare. On her first day, she has the following experiences with health care financing: her first patient is insured by Blue Shield; Primary Care is paid a fee for the physical examination and for the electrocardiogram (ECG) performed. Dr. Young's second patient requires the same services, for which PrimaryCare receives no payment but is forwarded $10 for each month that the patient is enrolled in the practice. In the afternoon, a hospital utilization review physician calls Dr. Young, explains the diagnosis-related group (DRG) payment system, and suggests that she send home a patient hospitalized with pneumonia. In the evening, she goes to the emergency department, where she has agreed to work two shifts per week for $85 per hour.

During the course of a typical day, some physicians will be involved with four or five distinct types of reim-

bursement. This chapter will describe the different ways in which physicians and hospitals are paid. Although reimbursement has many facets, from the setting of prices to the processing of claims, this discussion will focus on one of its most basic elements: establishing the unit of payment. This basic principle must be grasped before one can understand the key concept of physician-borne risk.

UNITS OF PAYMENT

Methods of payment can be placed along a continuum that extends from the least to the most aggregated unit. The methods range from the simplest (one fee for one service rendered) to the most complex (one payment for many types of services rendered), with many variations in between (Table 4–1).

▶ Definitions of Methods of Payment

Fee-for-Service Payment

The unit of payment is the visit or procedure. The physician or hospital is paid a fee for each office visit, ECG, intravenous fluid, or other service or supply provided. This is the only form of payment that is based on individual components of health care. All other reimbursement modes aggregate or group together several services into one unit of payment.

Payment by Episode of Illness

The physician or hospital is paid one sum for all services delivered during one illness, as is the case with global surgical fees for physicians and DRGs for hospitals.

Table 4–1. Units of payment

	Least Aggregated				Most Aggregated
	Procedure	Day	Episode of Illness	Patient	Time
Physician	Fee-for-service	—	Surgical or obstetric fee Physician DRG	Capitation	Salary
Hospital	Fee-for-service	Per diem	Hospital DRG	Capitation	Global budget

DRG, diagnosis-related group.

Per Diem Payments to Hospitals

The hospital is paid for all services delivered to a patient during 1 day.

Capitation Payment

One payment is made for each patient's care during a month or year.

Payment for All Services Delivered to All Patients within a Certain Time Period

This includes global budget payment of hospitals and salaried payment of physicians.

▶ Managed Care Plans

Traditionally physicians and hospitals have been paid on a fee-for-service basis. The development of managed care plans introduced changes in the methods by which hospitals and physicians are paid, for the purpose of controlling costs. Managed care is discussed in more detail in Chapter 6; in this chapter, only those aspects needed to understand physician and hospital reimbursement will be considered.

There are three major forms of managed care: fee-for-service practice with utilization review, preferred provider organizations (PPOs), and health maintenance organizations (HMOs).

Fee-for-Service Reimbursement with Utilization Review

This is the traditional type of payment, with the addition that the third-party payer (whether private insurance company or government agency) assumes the power to authorize or deny payment for expensive medical interventions such as hospital admissions, extra hospital days, and surgeries.

Preferred Provider Organizations

PPOs are loose-knit organizations in which insurers contract with a limited number of physicians and hospitals who agree to care for patients, usually on a discounted fee-for-service basis with utilization review.

Health Maintenance Organizations

HMOs are organizations whose patients are required (except in emergencies) to receive their care from providers within that HMO. There are several types of HMOs which are discussed in Chapter 6. Some HMOs pay physicians and hospitals by more highly bundled units of payment (eg, per diem, capitation, or salary).

METHODS OF PHYSICIAN PAYMENT

▶ Payment per Procedure: Fee-for-Service

Roy Sweet, a patient of Dr. Weisman, is seen for recent onset of diabetes. Dr. Weisman spends 20 minutes performing an examination, fingerstick blood glucose test, urinalysis, and ECG. Each service has a fee set by Dr. Weisman: $92 for a complex visit, $8 for a fingerstick glucose test, $15 for a urinalysis, and $70 for an ECG. Because Mr. Sweet is uninsured, Dr. Weisman reduces the total bill from $185 to $90.

In 1988, Dr. Lenz, an ophthalmologist, requested that Dr. Weisman do a medical consultation for Gertrude Rales, who developed congestive heart failure and arrhythmias following cataract surgery. Dr. Weisman took 90 minutes to perform the consultation and was paid $100 by Medicare. Dr. Lenz had spent 90 minutes on the surgery plus pre- and *postoperative care and received $1600 from Medicare. In 1998, Dr. Weisman did a similar consultation for Dr. Lenz and received $130; Dr. Lenz was sent $900 for the operation.*

Melissa High, a Medicaid recipient, makes three visits to Dr. Weisman for hypertension. He bills Medicaid $92 for one complex visit and $52 each for two shorter visits. He is paid $26 per visit, 40% of his total charges. Under Medicaid, Dr. Weisman may not bill Ms. High for the balance of his fees.

Dr. Weisman contracted with Blue Cross to care for its PPO patients at 70% of his normal fee. Rick Payne, a PPO patient, comes in with a severe headache and is found to have left arm weakness and hyperreflexia. Dr. Weisman is paid $84.40 for a complex visit. Before a magnetic resonance imaging (MRI) scan can be ordered, the PPO must be asked for authorization.

Traditionally, private physicians have been reimbursed by patients and insurers through the fee-for-service mechanism. Before the passage of Medicare and Medicaid, physicians often discounted fees for elderly or poor patients, and even afterward many physicians have continued to assist uninsured people in this way.

Private insurers, as well as Medicare and Medicaid in the early years, usually reimbursed physicians according to the usual, customary, and reasonable (UCR) system, which allowed physicians a great deal of latitude in setting fees. As cost containment became more of a priority, the UCR approach to fees was largely supplanted by payer-determined fee schedules. An example of this is Melissa High's three visits, which incurred charges of $196 of which Medicaid paid only $78 ($26 per visit).

In the early 1990s, Medicare moved to a fee schedule determined by a resource-based relative-value scale (RBRVS). With this system, fees (which vary by geographic area) are set for each service by estimating the time, mental effort and judgment, technical skill, physical effort, and stress typically related to that service (Bodenheimer et al, 2007). The RBRVS system made a somewhat feeble attempt to correct the bias of physician payment that has historically paid for surgical and other procedures at a far higher rate than primary care and cognitive services. In 1998, Dr. Weisman was paid nearly 15% of Dr. Lenz's surgery fee, compared with 6% of that fee in 1988, before the advent of RBRVS.

PPO managed care plans often pay contracted physicians on a discounted fee-for-service basis and require prior authorization for expensive procedures.

With fee-for-service payments, physicians have an economic incentive to perform more services because more services bring in more payments (see Chapter 10). The fee-for-service incentive to provide more services contributed to the rapid rise in health care costs in the United States (Relman, 2007).

▶ Payment per Episode of Illness

Dr. Nick Belli removes Tom Stone's gallbladder and is paid $1300 by Blue Cross. Besides performing the cholecystectomy, Dr. Belli sees Mr. Stone three times in the hospital and twice in his office for postoperative visits. Because surgery is paid by means of a global fee, Dr. Belli may not bill separately for the visits, which are included in his $1300 cholecystectomy fee.

Joan Flemming complains of having had coughing, fever, and green sputum for 1 week. Dr. Violet Gramm analyzes a sputum smear and orders a chest x-ray and makes the diagnosis of pneumonia. She treats Ms. Flemming as an outpatient with azithromycin, checking her once a week for 3 weeks. With the experimental episode-based system, Dr. Gramm is paid one fee for all services and procedures involved in treating Ms. Flemming's pneumonia.

Surgeons usually receive a single payment for several services (the surgery itself and postoperative care) that have been grouped together, and obstetricians are paid in a similar manner for a delivery plus pre- and postnatal care. This bundling together of payments is often referred to as reimbursement at the unit of the case or episode.

With payment by episode, surgeons have an economic incentive to limit the number of postoperative visits because they do not receive extra payment for extra visits. On the other hand, they continue to have an incentive to perform more surgeries, as with the traditional fee-for-service system. Some health care experts recommend paying physicians through an episode-based system similar to that used by Medicare for hospital reimbursement (Pham et al, 2010). Under such a system one fee would be paid for one episode of illness, no matter how many times the patient visited the physician.

At this point, it is helpful to introduce the important concept of risk. Risk refers to the potential to lose money, earn less money, or spend more time without additional payment on a reimbursement transaction. With the traditional fee-for-service system, the party paying the bill (insurance company, government agency, or patient) absorbs all the risk; if Dr. Weisman sees Rick Payne ten times rather than five times for his headaches, Blue Cross pays more money and Mr. Payne spends more in copayments. Bundling of services transfers a *portion* of the risk from the payer to the physician; if Dr. Belli sees Tom Stone ten times rather than five times for follow-up after cholecystectomy, he does not receive any additional money. However, Blue Cross is also partially at risk; if more Blue Cross enrollees require gallbladder surgery, Blue Cross is responsible for more $1300 payments. As a general rule, the more services bundled into one payment, the larger the share of financial risk that is shifted from payer to provider. (*Payer* is a general term referring to whomever pays the bill; in Chapter 16, a distinction is made between purchasers of health insurance such as employers, and insurers, who can both be payers.)

▶ Payment per Patient: Capitation

Capitation payments (per capita payments or payments "by the head") are monthly payments made to a physician for each patient signed up to receive care from that physician—generally a primary care physician. The essence of capitation is a shift in financial risk from insurers to providers. Under fee-for-service, patients who require expensive health services cost their health plan more than they pay the plan in insurance premiums; the insurer is at risk and loses money. Physicians and hospitals who provide the care earn more money for treating ill people. In a 180-degree role reversal, capitation frees insurers of risk by transferring risk to providers. An HMO that pays physicians via capitation has little to fear in the short run from patients who become ill. The HMO pays a fixed sum no matter how many services are provided. The providers, in contrast, earn no additional money yet spend a great deal of time and incur large office and hospital expenditures to care for people who are sick. (In the long term, HMOs do want to limit services in order to reduce provider pressure for higher capitation payments.)

Certain methods have been developed to mitigate the financial risk associated with capitation payment. One method involves reintroducing fee-for-service payments for specified services. Such types of services provided but not covered within the capitation payment are called *carve-outs;* their reimbursement is "carved out" of the capitation payment and paid separately. Pap smears, immunizations, office ECGs, and minor surgical procedures may be carved out and paid on a fee-for-service basis.

A common method of managing risk is called "risk-adjusted capitation." For physicians paid by capitation, patients with serious illnesses require a great deal more time without any additional payment, creating an incentive to sign up healthy patients and avoid those who are sick. Risk-adjusted capitation provides higher monthly payments for elderly patients and for those with chronic illnesses. However, risk adjustment poses a major challenge. Researchers have investigated measures for risk-adjusting capitation payments by appraising an individual's state of health or risk of needing health care services (Brown et al, 2010).

Capitation has potential merits as a way to control costs by providing an alternative to the inflationary tendencies of fee-for-service payment. In addition, capitation has been advocated for its potential beneficial influence on the organization of care. Capitation payments require patients to register with a physician or group of physicians. The clear enumeration of the population of patients in a primary care practice offers advantages for monitoring appropriate use of services and planning for these patients' needs. Capitation also potentially allows for more flexibility at the practice level in how to most effectively and efficiently organize and deliver services. For example, fee-for-service typically only pays for an in-person visit with a physician; under capitation payment, a physician could substitute "virtual visits" such as e-mail and telephone contacts for in-person visits for following up on blood pressure or diabetes control, or delegate routine preventive care tasks to nurses or medical assistants in the practice, without experiencing a financial disincentive for these alternative ways of delivering care. Capitation also explicitly defines—in advance—the amount of money available to care for an enrolled population of patients, providing a better framework for rational allocation of resources and innovation in developing better modes of delivering services. For a large group of primary care physicians, the sheer size of the aggregated capitation payments provides clout and flexibility over how to best arrange ancillary and specialty services.

Capitation with Two-Tiered Structures

Jennifer is a young woman in England who develops an ear infection; her general practitioner, Dr. Walter Liston, sees her and prescribes antibiotics. Jennifer pays no money at the time of the visit and receives no bill. Dr. Liston is paid the British equivalent of $12 per month to care for Jennifer, no matter how many times she requires care. When Jennifer develops appendicitis and requires an x-ray and surgical consultation, Dr. Liston sends her to the local hospital for these services; payment for these referral services is incorporated into the hospital's operating budget paid for separately by the National Health Service.

British System—Capitation payments to physicians in the United States are complicated, as will shortly be seen. But in the United Kingdom, they have traditionally been simple (see Chapter 14). Under the traditional British National Health Service, each person enrolls with a general practitioner, who becomes the primary care physician (PCP). For each person on the general practitioner's list, the physician receives a monthly capitation payment. The more patients on the list, the more money the physician earns. Patients are required to route all nonemergency medical needs through the general practitioner "gatekeeper," who when necessary makes referrals for specialist services or hospital care. Patients can freely change from one general practitioner to another. This simple arrangement, illustrated in Figure 4–1, is referred to as a two-tiered capitation structure. One tier is the health plan (the government in the case of the UK) and the other tier the individual PCP or a small number of physicians in group practice.

United States System—In the United States, capitation payment is associated with HMO plans and not with traditional or PPO insurance. Some HMO plans have two-tiered structures, with HMOs paying capitation fees directly to PCPs (Figure 4–1). However, capitation payment in US managed care organizations more often involves a three-tiered structure.

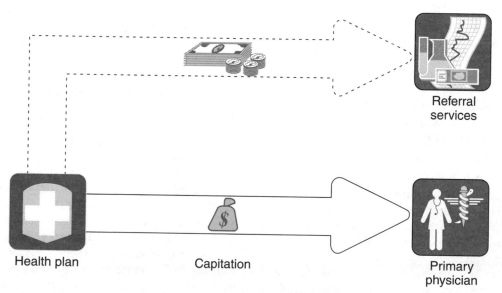

Referral services

Health plan

Capitation

Primary physician

▲ **Figure 4–1.** Two-tiered capitated payment structures. The health plan pays the primary care physician by capitation and pays for referral services (eg, x-rays and specialist consultations) through a different reimbursement stream.

CHAPTER 4

Capitation with Three-Tiered Structures

In three-tiered structures, HMOs do not pay capitation fees directly to individual physicians or small group practices, but instead rely on an intermediary administrative structure for processing these payments (Robinson and Casalino, 1995). In one variety of such three-tiered structures (Figure 4–2A), physicians remain in their own private offices but join together into physician groups called independent practice associations (IPAs).

> *George is enrolled through his employer in Smart-Care, an HMO run by Smart Insurance Company. SmartCare has contracted with two IPAs to provide physician services for its enrollees in the area where George lives. George has chosen to receive his care from Dr. Bunch, a PCP affiliated with one of these IPA groups, CapCap Associates IPA. Smart-Care pays CapCap Associates a $60 monthly capitation fee on George's behalf for all physician and related outpatient services. CapCap Associates in turn pays Dr. Bunch a $15 monthly capitation fee to serve as George's primary care physician.*

> *George develops symptoms of urinary obstruction consistent with benign prostatic hyperplasia. Dr. Bunch orders some laboratory tests and refers George to a urologist for cystoscopy. The laboratory and the urologist bill CapCap Associates on a fee-for-service basis and are paid by the IPA from a pool of money (called a risk pool) that the IPA has set aside for this purpose from the capitation payments CapCap Associates receives from Smart-Care. At the end of the year, CapCap Associates has money left over in this diagnostic and specialist services risk pool. CapCap Associates distributes this surplus revenue to its PCPs as a bonus.*

Sorting out the flow of payments and nature of risk sharing becomes difficult in this type of three-tiered capitation structure. In most three-tiered HMOs, the financial risk for diagnostic and specialist services is borne by the overall IPA organization and spread among all the participating PCPs in the IPA. In the 1980s and 1990s, the CapCap Associates type of IPA often provided financial incentives to PCPs to limit the use of diagnostic and specialist services by returning to these physicians any surplus funds that remain at the end of the year. This method of reimbursement is known as capitation-plus-bonus payment. The less frequent the use of diagnostic and specialist services, the higher the year-end bonus for IPA physician gatekeepers. This arrangement came under criticism as representing a conflict of interest for PCPs because their personal income was increased by denying diagnostic and specialty services to their patients (Rodwin, 1993). More recently some managed care organizations have begun to tie bonus payments to quality measures—"pay for performance"—rather than to cost control (see Chapter 10). A considerable price must be paid for setting up a three-tiered structure because administrative costs are substantial for both the health plan and the IPA.

> *George's brother Steve works for the same company as George and also has SmartCare insurance. Steve, however, obtains his primary care from a physician in the other SmartCare IPA plan, Cap-Fee Associates. Like CapCap Associates, CapFee Associates is an IPA that receives $60 per month in capitation fees for every patient enrolled. Unlike CapCap Associates, CapFee Associates pays its PCPs on a fee-for-service basis.*

Three-tiered IPA structures become even more confusing when the unit of reimbursement differs across tiers. In the CapCap Associates model, capitation is the basic payment method for both the IPA as a whole and its constituent primary care physicians. However, in the CapFee Associates model the IPA receives capitation payments from the health insurance plan but then reimburses its participating PCPs on a fee-for-service basis (Figure 4–2B). Under this arrangement, the fees billed by the IPA physicians may well exceed the amount of money the IPA has received from the insurance plan on a capitated basis to pay for physician and related outpatient services. To reduce this risk, many IPAs of the CapFee Associates type pay their physicians only a portion, perhaps 60%, of a predetermined fee schedule and withhold the other 40%. If money is left over at the end of the year, the physicians receive a portion of the withheld money.

With the CapFee system, the IPA is the main entity at risk because provision of more services can cause the IPA to lose money. But individual physicians are also partially at risk because if expenditures by the IPA are high, they will not receive the withheld funds. The economic incentive for individual primary care physicians is a mixed one. It is to the physician's financial advantage to schedule as many patient visits as possible because

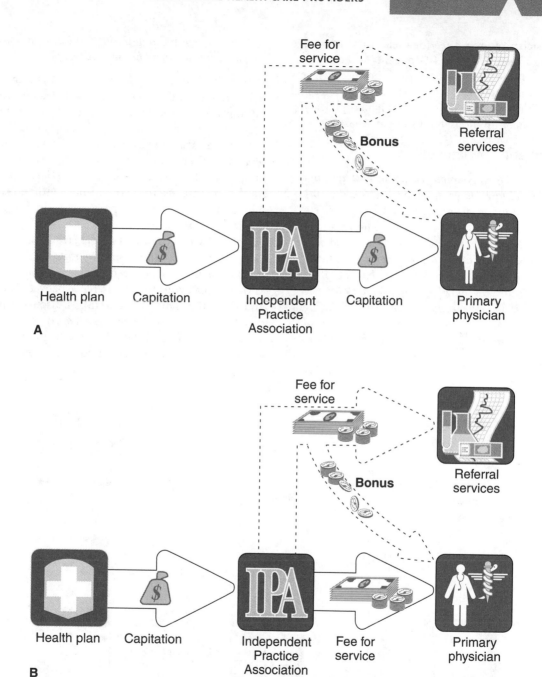

▲ **Figure 4–2.** Three-tiered capitated payment structures. **(A)** The CapCap Associates type of arrangement, in which primary physicians receive a capitation payment plus a bonus from the IPA if there is an end-of-the-year surplus in the pool for paying for referral services. **(B)** The CapFee Associates type of arrangement, in which the IPA receives capitation payments from the health plans, but pays its primary care physicians on a fee-for-service basis.

the physician receives a fee for each visit. But a large number of visits overall by IPA patients, as well as high use of laboratory and x-ray studies and specialist services, will deplete the IPA budget, thereby increasing the possibility that the IPA could go bankrupt, leaving its physicians with thousands of unpaid charges.

▶ Payment per Time: Salary

Dr. Joyce Parto is employed as an obstetrician-gynecologist by a large staff model HMO. She considers the financial security and lack of business worries in her current work setting an improvement over the stresses she faced as a solo fee-for-service practitioner before joining the HMO. However, she has some concerns that the other obstetricians are allowing the hospital's obstetric house staff to manage most of the deliveries during the night, and wonders if the lack of financial incentives to attend deliveries may be partly to blame. She is also annoyed by the bureaucratic hoops she has to jump through to cancel an afternoon clinic to attend her son's school play.

In contrast with traditional private physicians, physicians in the public sector (municipal, Veterans Health Administration and military hospitals, state mental hospitals), and in community clinics are usually paid by salary. Salaried practice aggregates payment for all services delivered during a month or year into one lump sum. Managed care has brought salaried practice to the private sector, sometimes with a salary-plus-bonus arrangement, particularly in integrated medical groups and group and staff model HMOs (see Chapter 6). Group and staff model HMOs bring physicians and hospitals under one organizational roof.

The distinction between staff and group model HMOs is analogous to the difference between the two- and three-tiered IPA model HMOs discussed previously. The staff model HMO is a two-tiered payment structure, with an HMO insurance plan directly employing physicians on a salaried basis (Figure 4–3A).

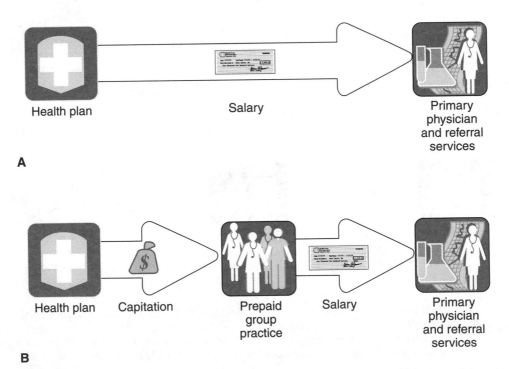

A

B

▲ **Figure 4–3.** Salaried payment. **(A)** In the staff model HMO, the plan directly employs physicians. **(B)** In the group model HMO, a "prepaid group practice" receives capitation payments from the plan and then reimburses its physicians by salary.

In the group model HMO, the HMO insurance plan contracts on a capitated basis with an intermediary physician group, which in turn pays its individual physicians a salary (Figure 4–3B).

HMO physicians paid purely by salary bear little if any individual financial risk; the HMO or physician group is at risk if expenses are too great. To manage risk, administrators at group and staff model HMOs may place constraints on their physician employees, such as scheduling them for a high volume of patient visits or limiting the number of available specialists. Salaried physicians are at risk of not getting extra pay for extra work hours. For a physician paid an annual salary without allowances for overtime pay, a high volume of complex patient visits may turn an 8-hour day into a 12-hour day with no increase in income. HMOs and medical groups may offer bonuses to salaried physicians if overall expenses are less than the amounts budgeted for these expenses or if the physician performs high quality care (pay for performance).

METHODS OF HOSPITAL PAYMENT

▶ Payment per Procedure: Fee-for-Service

Kwin Mock Wong is hospitalized for a bleeding ulcer. At the end of his 4-day stay, the hospital sends a $14,000 seven-page itemized hospital bill to Blue Cross, Mr. Wong's insurer.

In the past, insurance companies made fee-for-service payments to private hospitals based on the principle of "reasonable cost," a system under which hospitals had a great deal of influence in determining the level of payment. Because the American Hospital Association and Blue Cross played a large role in writing reimbursement regulations for Medicare, that program initially paid hospitals according to a similar reasonable cost formula (Law, 1974). More recently, private and public payers concerned with cost containment have begun to question hospital charges and negotiate lower payments, or to shift financial risk toward the hospitals by using per diem, DRG, or capitation payments.

▶ Payment per Day: Per Diem

John Johnson, an HMO patient, with a severe headache is admitted to the hospital. During his 3-day stay, he undergoes MRI scanning, lumbar puncture, and cerebral arteriography, procedures that are all costly to the hospital in terms of personnel and supplies. The hospital receives $4800, or $1600 per day from the HMO; Mr. Johnson's stay costs the hospital $7200.

Tom Thompson, in the same HMO, is admitted for congestive heart failure. He receives intravenous furosemide for 3 days and his condition improves. Diagnostic testing is limited to a chest x-ray, ECG, and basic blood work. The hospital receives $4800; the cost to the hospital is $4200.

Many insurance companies and Medicaid plans contract with hospitals for per diem payments rather than paying a fee for each itemized service (room charge, MRI, arteriogram, chest x-ray, and ECG). The hospital receives a lump sum for each day the HMO patient is in the hospital. The insurer may send a utilization review nurse to the hospital to review the charts of its patients, and if the nurse decides that a patient is not acutely ill, the HMO may stop paying for additional days.

Per diem payments represent a bundling of all services provided for one patient on a particular day into one payment. With traditional fee-for-service payment, if the hospital performs several expensive diagnostic studies, it makes more money because it charges for each study, whereas with per diem payment the hospital receives no additional money for expensive procedures. Per diem bundling of services into one fee removes the hospital's financial incentive because it loses, rather than profits, by performing expensive studies.

With per diem payment, the insurer continues to be at risk for the number of days a patient stays in the hospital because it must pay for each additional day. However, the hospital is at risk for the number of services performed on any given day because it incurs more costs without additional payment when it provides more services. It is in the insurer's interest to conduct utilization reviews to reduce the number of hospital days, but the insurer is less concerned about how many services are performed within each day; that fiscal concern has been transferred to the hospital.

▶ Payment per Episode of Hospitalization: Diagnosis-Related Groups

Bill is a 67-year-old man who enters the hospital for acute pulmonary edema. He is treated with *furosemide and oxygen in the emergency room, spends 36 hours in the hospital, and is discharged. The cost to the hospital is $5200. The hospital receives a $7000 DRG payment from Medicare.*

Will is an 82-year-old man who enters the hospital for acute pulmonary edema. In spite of repeated treatments with furosemide, captopril, digoxin, and nitrates, he remains in heart failure. He requires telemetry, daily blood tests, several chest x-rays, electrocardiograms, and an echocardiogram, and is finally discharged on the ninth hospital day. His hospital stay costs $23,000 and the hospital receives $7000 from Medicare.

The DRG method of payment for Medicare patients started in 1983. Rather than pay hospitals on a fee-for-service basis, Medicare pays a lump sum for each hospital admission, with the size of the payment dependent on the patient's diagnoses. The DRG system has gone one step further than per diem payments in bundling services into one payment. While per diem payment lumps together all services performed during one day, DRG reimbursement lumps together all services performed during one hospital episode. (Although an episode of illness may extend beyond the boundaries of the acute hospitalization [eg, there may be an outpatient evaluation preceding the hospitalization and transfer to a nursing facility for rehabilitation afterward], the term *episode* under the DRG system refers only to the portion of the illness actually spent in the acute care hospital.)

With the DRG system, the Medicare program is at risk for the number of admissions, but the hospital is at risk for the length of hospital stay and the resources used during the hospital stay. Medicare has no financial interest in the length of stay, which (except in unusually long "outlier" stays) does not affect Medicare's payment. In contrast, the hospital has an acute interest in the length of stay and in the number of expensive procedures performed; a long, costly hospitalization such as Will's produces a financial loss for the hospital, whereas a short stay yields a profit. Hospitals therefore conduct internal utilization review to reduce the costs incurred by Medicare patients.

▶ Payment per Patient: Capitation

Jane is enrolled in Blue Cross HMO, which contracts with Upscale Hospital to care for Jane if she requires hospitalization. Upscale receives $60 per month as a capitation fee for each patient enrolled in the HMO. Jane is healthy, and during the 36 months that she is an HMO member, the hospital receives $2160, even though Jane never sets foot in the hospital.

Wayne is also enrolled in Blue Cross HMO. Twenty-four months following his enrollment, he contracts Pneumocystis carinii pneumonia, and in the following 12 months he spends 6 weeks in Upscale Hospital at a cost of $35,000. Upscale receives a total of $2160 (the $60 capitation fee per month for 36 months) for Wayne's care.

With capitation payment, hospitals are at risk for admissions, length of stay, and resources used; in other words, hospitals bear all the risk and the insurer, usually an HMO, bears no risk. Capitation payment to hospitals has almost disappeared as a method of payment.

▶ Payment per Institution: Global Budget

Don Samuels, a member of the Kaiser Health Plan, suffers a sudden overwhelming headache and is hospitalized for 1 week at Kaiser Hospital in Oakland, California, for an acute cerebral hemorrhage. He goes into a coma and dies. No hospital bill is generated as a result of Mr. Samuels' admission, and no capitation payments are made from any insurance plan to the hospital.

Kaiser Health Plan is a large integrated delivery system that in some regions of the United States operates its own hospitals. Kaiser hospitals are paid by the Kaiser Health Plan through a global budget: a fixed payment is made for all hospital services for 1 year. Global budgets are also used in Veterans Health Administration, Department of Defense, and local municipal or county hospitals in the United States, as well as being a standard payment method in Canada and many European nations. In managed care parlance, one might say that the hospital is entirely at risk because no matter how many patients are admitted and how many expensive services are performed, the hospital must figure out how to stay within its fixed budget. Global budgets represent the most extensive bundling of services: Every service performed on every patient during 1 year is aggregated into one payment.

CONCLUSION

During the 1990s, the push for cost containment created a movement to change—in two ways—how physicians and hospitals are paid:

1. Private insurers, Medicare, and Medicaid often replaced fee-for-service payment, which encourages use of more services, with reimbursement mechanisms that place economic pressure on physicians and hospitals to limit the number and cost of services offered. The bundling of services into one payment tends to shift financial risk away from payers toward physicians and hospitals.

2. Whereas levels of payment were formerly set largely by providers themselves (reasonable cost reimbursement for hospitals and usual, customary, and reasonable fees for physicians), payment levels are increasingly determined by negotiation between payers and providers or by fee schedules set by payers.

The second of these trends appears to be a permanent feature of provider payment. But the first change, the substitution of capitation and other bundled mechanisms in place of fee-for-service, was largely reversed for physician payment, although more bundled forms of payment are still common for hospital reimbursement. Fee-for-service made a comeback. However, with the accelerating health cost crisis, a great deal of discussion has been taking place since 2010 about reintroducing alternatives to fee for service.

One of the challenges in designing an optimal payment system is striking the right balance between economic incentives for overtreatment and undertreatment (Casalino, 1992). The British National Health Service has traditionally mixed units of payment for general practitioners, paying a global budget for overhead costs (eg, office rent and staff), a capitation payment for each patient enrolled in the practice, and fee-for-service payments selectively for preventive services (eg, vaccinations and Pap tests) and some home visits in order to encourage provision of these items. In the United States, some managed care organizations are following the British example, creating blended payments for physicians that include elements of both capitation and fee for service (Robinson, 1999). This innovation has the potential to balance overtreatment and undertreatment incentives.

REFERENCES

Bodenheimer T et al. The primary care-specialty income gap: Why it matters. *Ann Intern Med.* 2007;146:301.

Brown J et al. Does Risk Adjustment Reduce Selection in the Private Health Insurance Market?, 2010. www.wcas.northwestern.edu/csio/Conferences/DugganPaper.pdf. Accessed November 23, 2011.

Casalino LP. Balancing incentives: How should physicians be reimbursed? *JAMA.* 1992;267:403.

Law SA. *Blue Cross: What Went Wrong?* New Haven, CT: Yale University Press; 1974.

Pham HH et al. Episode-Based Payments: Charting a Course for Health Care Payment Reform. Center for Studying Health System Change Policy Analysis, January 2010. www.hschange.com.

Relman A. *Second Opinion: Rescuing America's Health Care.* New York: Public Affairs; 2007.

Robinson JC. Blended payment methods in physician organizations under managed care. *JAMA.* 1999;282:1258.

Robinson JC, Casalino LP. The growth of medical groups paid through capitation in California. *N Engl J Med.* 1995;333:1684.

Rodwin MA. *Medicine, Money, and Morals: Physicians' Conflicts of Interest.* New York, NY: Oxford University Press; 1993.

How Health Care Is Organized—I: Primary, Secondary, and Tertiary Care

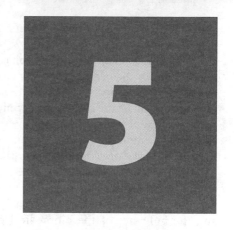

Frank Hope has walked with a limp since contracting polio in the 1940s. When he watches his daughter run after her young toddler, he feels a sense of gratitude that the era of vaccination has protected his child and grandchild from such a disabling infection. He recalls the excitement that gripped the nation as the Salk polio vaccine was first tested and then adopted into widespread use. In Frank's mind, these types of scientific breakthroughs attest to the wonders of the US health care system.

Frank's grandson attends a day-care program. Ruby, a 3-year-old girl in the program, was recently hospitalized for a severe asthma attack complicated by pneumococcal pneumonia. She spent 2 weeks in a pediatric intensive care unit, including several days on a respirator. Ruby's mother works full-time as a bus driver while raising three children. She has comprehensive private health insurance through her job but finds it difficult to keep track of all her children's immunization schedules and to find a physician's office that offers convenient appointment times. She takes Ruby to an evening-hours urgent care center when Ruby has some wheezing but never sees the same physician twice. Ruby never received all her pneumococcal vaccinations or consistent prescription of a steroid inhaler to prevent a severe asthma attack. Ruby's mother blames herself for her child's hospitalization.

People in the United States rightfully take pride in the technologic accomplishments of their health care system. Innovations in biomedical science have almost eradicated scourges such as polio and measles and have allowed such marvels as organ transplantation, "knifeless" gamma-ray surgery for brain tumors, and intensive care technology that saves the lives of children with asthma complicated by pneumonia. Yet for all its successes, the health care system also has its failures. For example, asthma is the most common cause of hospitalization in childhood (Akinbami et al, 2009). Proper medical care can markedly reduce the frequency of severe asthma symptoms and of asthma hospital admissions. In cases such as Ruby's, the failure to prevent severe asthma flare-up is not related to financial barriers, but rather reflects organizational problems, particularly in the delivery of primary care and preventive services.

The organizational task facing all health care systems is one of "assuring that the right patient receives the right service at the right time and in the right place" (Rodwin, 1984). An additional criterion could be ". . . and by the right caregiver." The fragmented care Ruby received for her asthma is an example of this challenge. Who is responsible for planning and ensuring that every child receives the right service at the right time? Can an urgent care center or an in-store clinic at Wal-Mart designed for episodic needs be held accountable for providing comprehensive care to all patients passing through its doors? Should parents be expected to make appointments for routine visits at medical offices and clinics, or should public health nurses travel to homes and day-care centers to provide preventive services out in the community? What is the proper balance between intensive care units that provide life-saving services to critically ill patients and primary care services geared toward less dramatic medical and preventive needs?

The previous chapters have emphasized financial transactions in the health care system. In this chapter and the following one, the organization of the health care system will be the main focus. While considerable debate has dwelled on how to improve financial access to care, less emphasis has been given to the question "access to what?" In this chapter, organizational systems will be viewed through a wide-angle lens, with emphasis on such broad concepts as the relationship between primary, secondary, and tertiary levels of care, and the influence of the biomedical paradigm and medical professionalism in shaping US health care delivery. In Chapter 6, a zoom lens will be used to focus on specific organizational models that have appeared (often only to disappear) in this country over the past century.

MODELS OF ORGANIZING CARE

▶ Primary, Secondary, and Tertiary Care

One concept is essential in understanding the topography of any health care system: the organization of care into primary, secondary, and tertiary levels. In the Lord Dawson Report, an influential British study written in 1920, the author (1975) proposed that each of the three levels of care should correspond with certain unique patient needs.

1. Primary care involves common health problems (eg, sore throats, diabetes, arthritis, depression, or hypertension) and preventive measures (eg, vaccinations or mammograms) that account for 80% to 90% of visits to a physician or other caregiver.

2. Secondary care involves problems that require more specialized clinical expertise such as hospital care for a patient with acute renal failure.

3. Tertiary care, which lies at the apex of the organizational pyramid, involves the management of rare and complex disorders such as pituitary tumors and congenital malformations.

Two contrasting approaches can be used to organize a health care system around these levels of care: (1) the carefully structured Dawson model of regionalized health care and (2) a more free-flowing model.

1. One approach uses the Dawson model as a scaffold for a highly structured system. This model is based on the concept of regionalization: the organization and coordination of all health resources and services within a defined area (Bodenheimer, 1969). In a regionalized system, different types of personnel and facilities are assigned to distinct tiers in the primary, secondary, and tertiary levels, and the flow of patients across levels occurs in an orderly, regulated fashion. This model emphasizes the primary care base.

2. An alternative model allows for more fluid roles for caregivers, and more free-flowing movement of patients, across all levels of care. This model tends to place a higher value on services at the tertiary care apex than at the primary care base.

Although most health care systems embody elements of both models, some gravitate closer to one polarity or the other. The British National Health Service (NHS) and some large integrated delivery systems in the United States resemble the regionalized approach, while US health care as a whole traditionally followed the more dispersed format.

▶ The Regionalized Model: The Traditional British National Health Service

Basil, a 60-year-old man living in a London suburb, is registered with Dr. Prime, a general practitioner in his neighborhood. Basil goes to Dr. Prime for most of his health problems, including hay fever, back spasms, and hypertension. One day, he experiences numbness and weakness in his face and arm. By the time Dr. Prime examines him later that day, the symptoms have resolved. Suspecting that Basil has had a transient ischemic attack, Dr. Prime prescribes aspirin and refers him to the neurologist at the local hospital, where a carotid artery sonogram reveals high-grade carotid stenosis. Dr. Prime and the neurologist agree that Basil should make an appointment at a London teaching hospital with a vascular surgeon specializing in head and neck surgery. The surgeon recommends that Basil undergo carotid endarterectomy on an elective basis to prevent a major stroke. Basil returns to Dr. Prime to discuss this recommendation and inquires whether the operation could be performed at a local hospital closer to home. Dr. Prime informs him that only a handful of London hospitals are equipped to perform this type of specialized operation. Basil schedules his operation in London and several months later has an uncomplicated carotid endarterectomy. Following the operation, he returns to Dr. Prime for his ongoing care.

The British NHS has traditionally typified a relatively regimented primary—secondary—tertiary care structure (Figure 5–1).

1. For physician services, the primary care level is virtually the exclusive domain of general practitioners (commonly referred to as GPs), who practice in small- to medium-sized groups and whose main responsibility is ambulatory care. Two-thirds of all physicians in the United Kingdom are GPs.

2. The secondary tier of care is occupied by physicians in such specialties as internal medicine, pediatrics, neurology, psychiatry, obstetrics and gynecology, and general surgery. These physicians are located at hospital-based clinics and serve as consultants for outpatient referrals from GPs, in turn routing most patients back to GPs for ongoing care needs. Secondary-level physicians also provide care to hospitalized patients.

3. Tertiary care subspecialists such as cardiac surgeons, immunologists, and pediatric hematologists are located at a few tertiary care medical centers.

Hospital planning follows the same regionalized logic as physician services. District hospitals are local facilities equipped for basic inpatient services. Regional tertiary care medical centers handle highly specialized inpatient care needs.

Planning of physician and hospital resources within the NHS occurs with a population focus. GP groups provide care to a base population of 5000 to 50,000

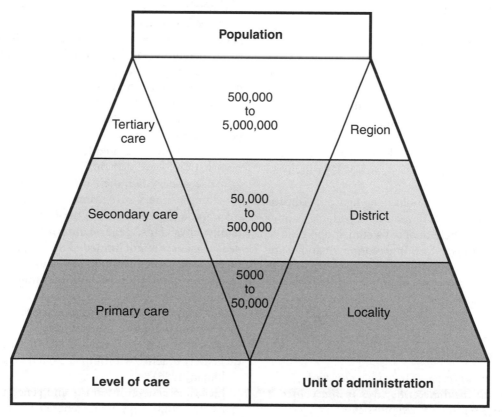

▲ **Figure 5–1.** Organization of services under the traditional National Health Service model in the United Kingdom. Care is organized into distinct levels corresponding to specific functions, roles, administrative units, and population bases.

persons, depending on the number of GPs in the practice. District hospitals have a catchment area population of 50,000 to 500,000, while tertiary care hospitals serve as referral centers for a population of 500,000 to 5 million (Fry, 1980).

Patient flow moves in a stepwise fashion across the different tiers. Except in emergency situations, all patients are first seen by a GP, who may then steer patients toward more specialized levels of care through a formal process of referral. Patients may not directly refer themselves to a specialist.

While nonphysician health professionals, such as nurses, play an integral role in staffing hospitals at the secondary and tertiary care levels, especially noteworthy is the NHS' multidisciplinary approach to primary care. GPs work in close collaboration with practice nurses (similar to nurse practitioners in the United States), home health visitors, public health nurses, and midwives (who attend most deliveries in the United Kingdom). Such teamwork, along with accountability for a defined population of enrolled patients and universal health care coverage, helps to avert such problems as missed childhood vaccinations. Public health nurses visit all homes in the first weeks after a birth to provide education and assist with scheduling of initial GP appointments. A national vaccination tracking system notifies parents about each scheduled vaccination and alerts GPs and public health nurses if a child has not appeared at the appointed time. As a result, more than 85% of British preschool children receive a full series of immunizations. (The British NHS is discussed at greater length in Chapter 14.)

A number of other nations, ranging from industrialized countries in Scandinavia to developing nations in Latin America, have adopted a similar approach to organizing health services. In developing nations, the primary care tier relies more on community health educators and other types of public health personnel than on physicians.

▶ The Dispersed Model: Traditional United States Health Care Organization

Polly Seymour, a 55-year-old woman with private health insurance who lives in the United States, sees several different physicians for a variety of problems: a dermatologist for eczema, a gastroenterologist for recurrent heartburn, and an orthopedist for tendinitis in her shoulder. She may ask her gastroenterologist to treat a few general medical problems, such as borderline diabetes. On occasion, she has gone to the nearby hospital emergency department for treatment of urinary tract infections. One day, Polly feels a lump in her breast and consults a gynecologist. She is referred to a surgeon for biopsy, which indicates cancer. After discussing treatment options with Polly, the surgeon performs a lumpectomy and refers her to an oncologist and radiation therapy specialist for further therapy. She receives all these treatments at a local hospital, a short distance from her home.

The US health care system has had a far less structured approach to levels of care than the British NHS. In contrast to the stepwise flow of patient referrals in the United Kingdom, insured patients in the United States, such as Polly Seymour, have traditionally been able to refer themselves and enter the system directly at any level. While many patients in the United Kingdom have a primary care physician (PCP) to initially evaluate all their problems, many people in the United States have become accustomed to taking their symptoms directly to the specialist of their choice.

One unique aspect of the US approach to primary care has been to broaden the role of internists and pediatricians. While general internists and general pediatricians in the United Kingdom and most European nations serve principally as referral physicians in the secondary tier, their US counterparts share in providing primary care. Moreover, the overlapping roles among "generalists" in the United States (GPs, family physicians, general internists, and general pediatricians) are not limited to the outpatient sector. PCPs in the United States have assumed a number of secondary care functions by providing substantial amounts of inpatient care. Only recently has the United States moved toward the European model that removes inpatient care from the domain of PCPs and assigns this work to "hospitalists"—physicians who exclusively practice within the hospital (Wachter and Goldman, 1996).

Including general internists and general pediatricians, the total supply of generalists amounts to approximately one-third of all physicians in the United States, a number well below the 50% or more found in

Canada and many European nations (Starfield, 1998). To fill in the primary care gap, some physicians at the tertiary care level in the United States have also acted as PCPs for some of their patients. In contrast to physicians, nurse practitioners and physician assistants are more likely to work in primary care settings and are a key component of the nation's clinical workforce.

US hospitals are not constrained by rigid secondary and tertiary care boundaries. Instead of a pyramidal system featuring a large number of general community hospitals at the base and a limited number of tertiary care referral centers at the apex, hospitals in the United States each aspire to offer the latest in specialized care. In most urban areas, for example, several hospitals compete with each other to perform open heart surgery, organ transplants, radiation therapy, and high-risk obstetric procedures. The resulting structure resembles a diamond more than a pyramid, with a small number of hospitals (mostly rural) that lack specialized units at the base, a small number of elite university medical centers providing highly superspecialized referral services at the apex, and the bulk of hospitals providing a wide range of secondary and tertiary services in the middle.

▶ Which Model Is Right?

Critics of the US health care system find fault with its "top-heavy" specialist and tertiary care orientation and lack of organizational coherence. Analyses of health care in the United States over the past half century abound with such descriptions as "a nonsystem with millions of independent, uncoordinated, separately motivated moving parts," "fragmentation, chaos, and disarray," and "uncontrolled growth and pluralism verging on anarchy" (Somers, 1972; Halvorson and Isham, 2003). The high cost of health care has been attributed in part to this organizational disarray. Quality of care may also suffer. For example, when many hospitals each perform small numbers of surgical procedures such as coronary artery bypass grafts, mortality rates are higher than when such procedures are regionalized in a few higher-volume centers (Grumbach et al, 1995).

Defenders of the dispersed model reply that pluralism is a virtue, promoting flexibility and convenience in the availability of facilities and personnel. In this view, the emphasis on specialization and technology is compatible with values and expectations in the United States, with patients placing a high premium on direct access to specialists and tertiary care services, and on autonomy in selecting caregivers of their choice for a particular health care need. Similarly, the desire for the latest in hospital technology available at a convenient distance from home competes with plans to regionalize tertiary care services at a limited number of hospitals.

▶ Balancing the Different Levels of Care

Dr. Billie Ruben completed her residency training in internal medicine at a major university medical center. Like most of her fellow residents, she went on to pursue subspecialty training, in her case gastroenterology. Dr. Ruben chose this career after caring for a young woman who developed irreversible liver failure following toxic shock syndrome. After a nerve-racking, touch-and-go effort to secure a donor liver, transplantation was performed and the patient made a complete recovery.

Upon completion of her training, Dr. Ruben joined a growing subspecialty practice at Atlantic Heights Hospital, a successful private hospital in the city. Even though the metropolitan area of 2 million people already has two liver transplant units, Atlantic Heights has just opened a third such unit, feeling that its reputation for excellence depends on delivering tertiary care services at the cutting edge of biomedical innovation. In her first 6 months at the hospital, Dr. Ruben participates in the care of only two patients requiring liver transplantation. Most of her patients seek care for chronic, often ill-defined abdominal pain and digestive problems. As Dr. Ruben begins seeing these patients on a regular basis, she starts to give preventive care and treat nongastrointestinal problems such as hypertension and diabetes. At times she wishes she had experienced more general medicine during her training.

Advocates of a stronger role for primary care in the United States believe that it is too important to be considered an afterthought in health planning. In this view, overemphasis on the tertiary care apex of the pyramid creates a system in which health care resources are not well matched to the prevalence and incidence of health problems in a community. In an article entitled "The Ecology of Medical Care" published more than four decades ago, Kerr White recorded the monthly prevalence of illness for a general population of 1000 adults (White et al, 1961). In this group, 750 experienced one or more illnesses or injuries during the month. Of these patients, 250 visited a physician at least once during the month, nine were admitted to a hospital, and only one was referred to a university medical center. Dr. White voiced concern that the training of health care professionals at tertiary care–oriented academic medical centers gave trainees like Dr. Billie Ruben an unrepresentative view of the health care needs of the community.

Serious questions can be raised about the nature of the average medical student's experience, and perhaps that of some of this student's clinical teachers, with the substantive problems of health and disease in the community. In general, this experience must be both limited and unusually biased if, in a month, only 0.0013 of the "sick" adults. . . . or 0.004 of the patients . . . . in a community are referred to university medical centers. . . . Medical, nursing, and other students of the health professions cannot fail to receive unrealistic impressions of medicine's task in contemporary Western society. . . . (White et al, 1961)

Updating Kerr White's findings, Larry Green found precisely the same patterns four decades later (Green et al, 2001).

An English GP, John Fry (1980) conducted a related study of the ecology of care, in which he systematically recorded the types of health problems that brought patients to his office in the 1970s. Because of the GP's function as a gatekeeper under the NHS, Dr. Fry's investigation provides a close approximation of the full incidence and prevalence of diseases requiring medical attention among his population of registered patients (Table 5–1). The dominant pathology in this unselected population consisted of minor ailments (many of which would have improved without treatment), chronic conditions such as hypertension and arthritis, and gradations of mental illness. The incidence of new cancers was relatively rare, and only a handful of patients manifested complex syndromes such as multiple sclerosis. Although the specific pattern of illnesses differs for a US family physician practicing in the 21st century compared with the pattern for a British GP in the 1970s (eg, human immunodeficiency virus infection and Alzheimer disease do not appear in Table 5–1), the general pattern remains true. Dr. Fry's

study confirms the adage that "common disorders commonly occur and rare ones rarely happen."

Although these analyses suggest that most health needs can be met at the primary care level, this observation should not imply that most health care resources should be devoted to primary care. The minority of patients with severe or complicated conditions requiring secondary or tertiary care will command a much larger share of health care resources per capita than the majority of people with less dramatic health care needs. Treating a patient with liver failure costs a great deal more than treating a patient for a sore throat. Even in the United Kingdom, where the 65% of physicians who are GPs provide 60% of all ambulatory care, expenditures on their services account for less than 10% of the overall NHS budget, whereas the cost of inpatient and outpatient hospital care at the secondary and tertiary levels consumes nearly two-thirds of the budget. Thus, the pyramidal shape shown in Figure 5–1 better represents the distribution of health care problems in a community than the apportionment of health care expenditures. While almost all industrialized nations devote a dominant share of health care resources to secondary and tertiary care, the ecologic view reminds us that most people have health care needs at the primary care level.

▶ The Functions and Value of Primary Care

Dr. O. Titus Wells has cared for all six of Bruce and Wendy Smith's children. As a family physician whose practice includes obstetrics, Dr. Wells attended the births of all but one of the children. The Smiths' 18-month-old daughter Ginny has had many ear infections. Even though this is a common problem, Dr. Wells finds that it presents a real medical challenge. Sometimes examination of Ginny's ears indicates a raging infection and at other times shows the presence of middle ear fluid, which may or may not represent a bona fide bacterial infection. He tries to reserve antibiotics for clear-cut cases of bacterial otitis. He feels it is important that he be the one to examine Ginny's ears because her eardrums never look entirely normal and he knows what degree of change is suspicious for a genuinely new infection.

When Ginny is 2 years old, Dr. Wells recommends to the Smiths that she see an otolaryngologist and

Table 5–1. Persons per year seeking care in a general practitioner practice with a registered population of 2500, according to problem

	Persons per Year Seeking Care		Persons per Year Seeking Care
Minor illness		*Major illness*	
General disorders		Pneumonia	20
Upper respiratory infections	600	Severe depression	10
Skin disorders	325	Suicide attempt	3
Emotional problems	300	Suicide	1 in 4 years
Gastrointestinal disorders	300	Acute myocardial infarction	8
Accidents	200	Acute appendicitis	5
Specific disorders		Acute strokes	5
Acute tonsillitis	100	New cancers	5
Acute otitis media	75	Lung	2 per year
Acute urinary infections	50	Breast	1 per year
"Acute back" syndrome	50	Large bowel	2 every 3 years
Migraine headache	25	Stomach	1 every 2 years
Hay fever	25	Prostate	1 every 2 years
Preventive care needs	300	Cervix	1 every 4 years
(eg, immunization, check-up,		Brain	1 every 10 years
prenatal care)		Lymphoma	1 every 15 years
		Thyroid	1 every 20 years
		Chronic illness	
		Chronic arthritis	100
		Chronic psychiatric problems	60
		High blood pressure	50
		Obesity	40
		Chronic bronchitis	35
		Chronic heart failure	30
		Cancers (new and old)	30
		Asthma	25
		Peptic ulcers	20
		Coronary artery disease	20
		Cerebrovascular disease	15
		Epilepsy	10
		Diabetes	10
		Thyroid disease	7
		Parkinsonism	3
		Multiple sclerosis	1
		Chronic renal disease	less than 1

Source: Reproduced with permission from Fry J. Primary care. In: Fry J, ed. *Primary Care.* London, England: William Heinemann; 1980.

audiologist to check for hearing loss and language impairment. The audiograms show modest diminution of hearing in one ear. The otolaryngologist informs the Smiths that ear tubes are an option. At Ginny's return visit with Dr. Wells, he discusses the pros and cons of tube placement with the Smiths. He also uses the visit as an opportunity to encourage Mrs. Smith to quit smoking, mentioning that research has shown that exposure to tobacco smoke may predispose children to ear infections.

Barbara Starfield, one of the world's foremost scholars in the field of primary care, conceptualized the key tasks of primary care as (1) first contact care, (2) longitudinality, (3) comprehensiveness, and (4) coordination. Dr. Wells' care of the Smith family illustrates these essential features of primary care. He is the first-contact physician performing the initial evaluation when Ginny or other family members develop symptoms of illness. *Longitudinality* (or *continuity*) refers to sustaining a patient–caregiver relationship over time. Dr. Wells' familiarity with Ginny's condition helps him to better discern an acute infection. Comprehensiveness consists of the ability to manage a wide range of health care needs, in contrast with specialty care, which focuses on a particular organ system or procedural service. Dr. Wells' comprehensive, family-oriented care makes him aware that Mrs. Smith's smoking cessation program is an important part of his treatment plan for Ginny. Coordination builds upon longitudinality. Through referral and follow-up, the primary care provider integrates services delivered by other caregivers. These tasks performed by Dr. Wells meet the definition of primary care as defined by the Institute of Medicine: "Primary care is the provision of integrated, accessible health care services by clinicians who are accountable for addressing a large majority of personal health care needs, developing sustained partnerships with patients, and practicing in the context of family and community" (Institute of Medicine, 1996).

A functional approach helps characterize which health care professionals truly fill the primary care niche. Among physicians in the United States, family physicians, general internists, and general pediatricians typically provide first contact, longitudinal, comprehensive, coordinated care. Emergency medicine physicians provide first contact care that may be relatively comprehensive for acute problems, but they do not provide continuity of care or coordinate care for patients on an ongoing basis. Some obstetrician-gynecologists provide first contact and longitudinal care, but usually only for reproductive health conditions; it is the rare obstetrician-gynecologist who is trained and inclined to comprehensively care for the majority of a woman's health needs throughout the lifespan (Rivo et al, 1994). Similarly, a patient with kidney failure or a patient with cancer may have a strong continuity of care relationship with a nephrologist or an oncologist, but these medical subspecialists rarely assume responsibility for comprehensive care of clinical problems outside of their specialty area or coordinate most ancillary and referral services (Rosenblatt et al, 1998).

In addition to physicians, many generalist nurse practitioners and physician assistants in the United States deliver the four key Starfield functions and serve as primary care providers for their patients. Research performed in a selected number of practices have demonstrated comparable quality of care for patients treated by primary care physicians and nurse practitioners (Horrocks et al, 2002).

Studies have found that the core elements of good primary care advance the "triple aims" of health system improvement: better patient experiences, better patient outcomes, and lower costs (Starfield, 1998). For example, continuity of care is associated with greater patient satisfaction, higher use of preventive services, reductions in hospitalizations, and lower costs (Saultz and Albedaiwi, 2004; Saultz and Lochner, 2005). There is evidence that having a regular source of care results in better control of hypertension and less reliance on emergency department services (Shea et al, 1992). A Canadian study found that children undergoing tonsillectomy were more likely to have the operation performed for appropriate indications when they were referred to the otolaryngologist by a pediatrician than when care was directly sought from the otolaryngologist (Roos, 1979). Persons whose care meets a primary care–oriented model have better perceived access to care are more likely to receive recommended preventive services, are more likely to adhere to treatment, and are more satisfied with their care (Bindman et al, 1996; Stewart et al, 1997; Safran et al, 1998). International comparisons have indicated that nations with a greater primary care orientation tend to have more satisfied patients and better performance on health indicators such as infant mortality, life expectancy, and total health expenditures (Starfield et al, 2005). Within the United States, states with more PCPs per capita have lower total mortality rates, lower heart disease and cancer mortality rates, and higher life expectancy at birth compared with states having fewer PCPs, adjusting for other factors such as age and per capita income. In contrast, increases in specialist supply are associated with greater costs but not improved quality (Starfield et al, 2005). In an analysis of quality and cost of care across states for Medicare beneficiaries, Baicker and Chandra (2004) found that states with more PCPs per capita had lower per capita Medicare costs and higher quality. States with more specialists per capita had lower quality and higher per capita Medicare expenditures.

▶ Care Coordination and "Gatekeeping"

Polly Seymour, described earlier in the chapter, feels terrible. Every time she eats, she feels nauseated and vomits frequently. She has lost 8 pounds, and her oncologist is worried that her breast cancer has spread. She undergoes blood tests, an abdominal

CT scan, and a bone scan, all of which are normal. She returns to her gastroenterologist, who tells her to stop the ibuprofen she has been taking for tendinitis. Her problem persists, and the gastroenterologist performs an endoscopy, which shows mild gastric irritation. A month has passed, $3000 has been spent, and Polly continues to vomit.

Polly's friend Martha recommends a nurse practitioner who has been caring for Martha for many years and who, in Martha's view, seems to spend more time talking with patients than do many physicians. Polly makes an appointment with the nurse practitioner, Sara Steward. Ms. Steward takes a complete history, which reveals that Polly is taking tamoxifen for her breast cancer and that she began to take aspirin after stopping the ibuprofen. Ms. Steward explains that either of these medications can cause vomiting and suggests that they be stopped for a week. Polly returns in a week, her nausea and vomiting resolved. Ms. Steward then consults with Polly's oncologist, and together they decide to restart the tamoxifen but not the aspirin. Polly becomes nauseated again, but eventually begins to feel well and gains weight while taking a reduced dose of tamoxifen. In the future, Ms. Steward handles Polly's medical problems, referring her to specialty physicians when needed, and making sure that the advice of one consultant does not interfere with the therapy of another specialist.

A concept that incorporates many of the elements of primary care is that of the primary care provider as gatekeeper. Gatekeeping took on pejorative connotations in the heyday of managed care, when, as described in Chapter 4, some types of financial arrangements with PCPs provided incentives for them to "shut the gate" in order to limit specialist referrals, diagnostic tests, and other services (Grumbach et al, 1998). A more accurate designation of the role of the PCP in helping patients navigate the complexities of the health care system is that of coordinator of care (Franks et al, 1992). Stories such as Polly's demonstrate the importance of having a generalist care coordinator who can advocate on behalf of his or her patients and work in partnership with patients to integrate an array of services involving multiple providers to avoid duplication of services, enhance patient safety, and care for the whole person.

▶ The Patient-Centered Medical Home

Dr. Retro is counting the days until he can retire from his solo practice of family medicine. He feels overwhelmed most days. The next available appointment in his office is in 10 weeks, and patients call every day frustrated about not being able to get appointments. A health plan just sent him a quality report card indicating that many diabetic patients in his practice have not achieved the targeted levels of control of their blood sugar, blood pressure, and lipids. He is also behind in keeping his patients up to date on their mammograms and colorectal cancer screening. Many days he has trouble finding information in the thick paper medical records about when his patients last received their preventive care services or diabetic tests. He was hoping to recruit a new family medicine residency graduate to take over his practice, but most young physicians in his region are pursuing more highly paid careers in non-primary care specialties.

Dr. Avantgard has always embraced innovation. When she read a series of articles in the Journal of the American Medical Association about new primary care practice models (Bodenheimer and Grumbach, 2007), she proposed to her 3 physician and 2 nurse practitioner partners that their primary care practice become a Patient Centered Medical Home. Dr. Avantgard starts by identifying a consultant to help the practice completely revamp their scheduling system to a "same-day" appointment system, where 50% of appointment slots are to be left unbooked until the day prior so that patients can call and be guaranteed a same day or next day appointment. Despite her partners' concerns about being overrun with patient appointments, the new scheduling system results in the same number of patients being seen each day, but with happier patients who are delighted to be able to get prompt access to care. The practice buys an electronic medical record system and uses the EMR to develop registries of all the patients in the practice due for preventive and chronic care services. Dr. Avantgard and her associates train their medical assistants to use the EMR, along with standing orders, to proactively order mammograms and blood lipid tests when due and to administer vaccinations and screen for depression during patient intake at medical visits. Now that many of the routine preventive and chronic care tasks are being capably handled by other staff, Dr. Avantgard and her clinician colleagues have more time during office visits to focus on the problems patients want to talk with them about and to work through complex medical problems. With the quality indicators and patient satisfaction scores for the practice rising to the top decile of scores for practitioners in the region, Dr. Avantgard plans to start negotiations with several health plans to add a monthly care coordination payment to the current fee-for-service payments they pay, so that the practice can be compensated for all the work they perform in care coordination outside of office visits.

By the turn of the 21st century, primary care in the US had reached a critical juncture (Bodenheimer, 2006). In 2006, the American College of Physicians sounded the alarm about an "impending collapse of primary care medicine" (American College of Physicians, 2006). Primary care clinicians like Dr. Retro struggled to meet patient demands for accessible, comprehensive, well-coordinated care. Many gaps in quality existed, and care often fell short of being patient centered. PCPs were demoralized by outmoded practice models ill-equipped to meet the demands of modern-day primary care and an ever-widening gap between their take-home pay and the escalating earnings of specialists. In response to this crisis, the 4 major professional organizations representing the nation's primary care physicians—the American Academy of Family Physicians, American College of Physicians, American Academy of Pediatrics, and American Osteopathic Association—came together in 2007 and issued a report on a shared vision for reform of primary care. The *Joint Principles of a Patient-Centered Medical Home* has served as a rallying point for building a broad movement to revitalize primary care in the US (Grundy et al, 2010).

The term "medical home" dates back to 1967, when it was first used by the American Academy of Pediatrics to describe the notion of a primary care practice that would coordinate care for children with complex needs. While the *Joint Principles* have several specific elements, Rittenhouse and Shortell (2009) have provided a straightforward conceptualization of the patient-centered medical home as consisting of four basic cornerstones: primary care, patient-centered care, new-model practice, and payment reform. This framework begins by reaffirming the fundamental functions of primary care and the goal of delivering accessible, comprehensive, longitudinal, and coordinated care. The concept then builds on those foundational principles by calling for greater attention to patient-centeredness, such as the type of same-day scheduling methods adopted by Dr. Avantgard; implementation of innovative practice models, such as Dr. Avantgard's development of team-care models that reengineer workflows and tasks; and changes in physician payment, such as blending fee-for-service with partial capitation and quality incentives. Another perspective on the patient-centered medical home is shown in Table 5–2.

The primary care reform movement in the United States has gathered momentum, with many large employers and consumer groups joining the physician organizations authoring the *Joint Principles* and other health professional groups to form the Patient Centered Primary Care Collaborative (Grundy et al, 2010). The Collaborative advocates and provides technical assistance for policy reforms to support primary care and transformation of practices into patient-centered medical homes. The push to enact the Affordable Care Act in 2010 focused lawmakers' attention on primary care. President Obama and many members of Congress recognized that expanding insurance coverage requires an adequate primary care workforce to provide first contact care for millions of newly insured people. The Affordable Care Act includes several measures to strengthen primary care, including increases in Medicare fees for primary care and support of patient-centered medical home reforms. Evaluation of the first wave of practices and systems implementing the types of practice innovations called for under patient-centered medical home reforms have demonstrated improvements in patient satisfaction and quality of care and reductions in use of costly emergency department and hospital services (Grumbach and Grundy, 2010). Whether the newfound enthusiasm for reform and renewal of primary care can be sustained and lead to a fundamental reorientation of the health system in the United States remains to be determined.

Table 5–2. "Old" and "new" model primary care: some elements of transforming a practice into a patient-centered medical home

Traditional Model		Patient-Centered Medical Home
My patients are those who make appointments to see me	→	Our patients are those who are registered in our medical home
Care is determined by today's problem and time available today	→	Care is determined by a proactive plan to meet health needs, with or without visits
Care varies by scheduled time and memory or skill of the doctor	→	Care is standardized according to evidence-based guidelines
I know I deliver high-quality care because I'm well trained	→	We measure our quality and make rapid changes to improve it
Patients are responsible for coordinating their own care	→	A prepared team of professionals works with all patients to coordinate care
It's up to the patients to tell us what happened to them	→	We track tests and consultations, and follow-up after ED and hospital care
Clinic operations center on meeting the doctor's needs	→	An interdisciplinary team works at the top of our licenses to serve patients

Source: Adapted with permission from F. Daniel Duffy, MD, MACP, Senior Associate Dean for Academics, University of Oklahoma School of Community Medicine.

FORCES DRIVING THE ORGANIZATION OF HEALTH CARE IN THE UNITED STATES

▶ The Biomedical Model

The growth of the dispersed mode of health care delivery in the United States was shaped by several forces. One factor was the preeminence of the biomedical model among medical educators and young physicians throughout the 20th century. The combination of stricter state licensing laws and an influential national study, the Flexner report of 1906, led to consolidation of medical training in academically oriented medical schools (Starr, 1982). These academic centers embraced the biomedical paradigm that was the legacy of such renowned 19th-century European microbiologists as Pasteur and Koch. The antimicrobial model engendered the faith that every illness has a discrete, ultimately knowable cause and that "magic bullets" can be crafted to eradicate these sources of disease. Physicians were trained to master pathophysiologic changes within a particular organ system, leading to the development of specialization (Luce and Byyny, 1979).

Advocates of a larger role for generalism and primary care in US health care have not so much rejected the concepts of scientific medicine and professional specialism as they have attempted to broaden the interpretation of these terms. They have called for a more integrated scientific approach to understanding health and illness that incorporates information about the individual's psychosocial experiences and family, cultural, and environmental context as well as physiologic and anatomic constitution (Engel, 1977). The attempt to more rigorously define the scientific and clinical basis of generalism contributed to the emergence of family medicine in the 1970s as a specialty discipline in its own right, and the 1-year general practice internship was replaced by a 3-year residency program and specialty board certification.

▶ Financial Incentives

A second and related factor influencing the structure of health care was the financial incentive for physician specialization and hospital expansion, which played out in a number of ways.

1. Insurance benefits first offered by Blue Cross covered hospital costs but not physician visits and other outpatient services.

2. As physician services came to be covered later under Blue Shield and other plans, a growing differential

in reimbursement between generalist and specialist physicians developed. New technologic and other procedures often required considerable physician time when first introduced, and higher fees were justified for these procedures. But as the procedures became routine, fees remained high, while the time and effort required to perform them declined (Starr, 1982); this resulted in an increasing disparity in income between PCPs and specialists (Bodenheimer et al, 2007). In the mid-1980s, the average PCP's income was 75% of the average specialist's income; by 2006, PCP income had dropped to only 50% of specialists' income (Council of Graduate Medical Education, 2010). As Figure 5–2 shows, the percentage of graduating medical students planning to enter careers in primary care tracks the PCP-specialist income gap closely, with the proportion of students entering primary care decreasing as the earnings of PCPs relative to specialists declines.

3. Federal involvement in health care financing further fueled the expansion of hospital care and specialization. The Hill–Burton Hospital Construction Act of 1946 allocated nearly $4 billion between 1946 and 1971 for expansion of hospital capacity rather than development of ambulatory services (Starr, 1982). The enactment of Medicare and Medicaid in 1965 perpetuated the private insurance tradition of higher reimbursement for procedurally oriented specialists than for generalists. Medicare further encouraged specialization through its policy

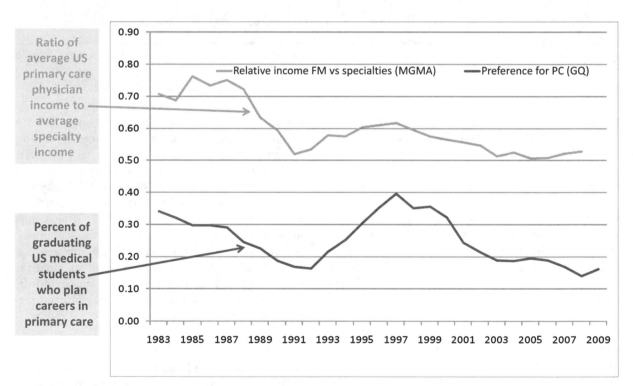

▲ **Figure 5–2.** Proportion of US medical students entering primary care strongly tracks relative incomes of primary care physicians. The figure shows trends over time in the average income of primary care physicians relative to specialist physicians in the United States, and in the percentage of graduating medical students in the United States planning on entering careers in primary care. In 1990, when the average primary care physician income was about half that of specialists, fewer than 20% of graduating students planned to enter primary care fields. By 1997, when primary care physician incomes had risen to more than 60% that of specialists, the proportion of graduating students entering primary care had increased in a parallel direction with 40% of graduates planning to enter primary care fields in 1997. Both relative incomes and intentions to enter primary care decreased after 1997. (From the Council on Graduate Medical Education. *Twentieth Report: Advancing Primary Care,* December 2010).

of extra payments to hospitals to cover costs associated with residency training. Linking Medicare teaching payments to the hospital sector added yet another bias against community-based primary care training.

The growth of hospitals and medical specialization was intertwined. As medical practice became more specialized and dependent on technology, the site of care increasingly shifted from the patient's home or physician's office to the hospital. The emphasis on acute hospital care had an effect on the nursing profession comparable to that on physicians. World War I was a watershed period in the transition of nursing from a community-based to a hospital-based orientation. During the war, US military hospitals overseas were much heralded for their success in treating acute war injuries. At the war's conclusion, the nation rallied behind a policy of boosting the civilian hospital sector. According to Rosemary Stevens (1989),

> Before the war, public-health nursing was the elite area; nurses had been instrumental in the campaigns against tuberculosis and for infant welfare. In contrast, the war emphasized the supremacy and glamour of hospitals. . . . nurses, like physicians, were trained—and ready—to perform in an increasingly specialized, acute-care medical environment rather than to expand their interests in social medicine and public health (Stevens, 1989).

▶ Professionalism

The final factor accounting for the organizational evolution of US health care delivery was the nature of control over health planning. The United States is unique in its relative laxity of public regulation of health care resources. In most industrialized nations, governments wield considerable control over health planning through measures such as regulation of hospital capacity and technology, allocation of the number of residency training positions in generalist and specialist fields, and coordination of public health with medical care services. In the United States, the government has provided much of the financing for health care, but without an attendant degree of administrative control. The Hill–Burton program, for example, did not make grants for hospital construction contingent upon any rigorous community-wide plan for regionalized

hospital services. Medicare funding for physician training did not stipulate any particular distribution of residency positions according to specialty.

With government controls kept largely at bay, the professional "sovereignty" of physicians emerged as the preeminent authority in health care (Starr, 1982). Societies grant certain occupations special status as "professions" because of the unique knowledge and skill required of members of the profession, and the expectation that this knowledge and skill will be applied beneficially (Friedson, 1970; Light and Levine, 1988). Professionalism thus involves a social contract; in return for the privilege of autonomy, physicians bear the responsibility for acting as the patient's agent, and the profession must regulate itself to preserve the public trust.

Their professional status vested physicians with special authority to guide the development of the US health care system. As described in Chapter 2, third-party payment for physician services was established with physician control of the initial Blue Shield insurance plans. Physician judgment about the need for technology and greater inpatient capacity drove the expansion of hospital facilities.

What was the nature of the profession that so heavily influenced the development of the US health care organization? It was a profession that, because of the primacy of the biomedical paradigm and the nature of financial incentives, was weighted toward hospital and specialty care. Small wonder that US health care has emphasized its tertiary care apex over its primary care base. In Chapter 16, we discuss the shifting power relationships in health care that are challenging the professional dominance of physicians.

CONCLUSION

Jeff leaves a town forum at the local medical center feeling confused. It featured two speakers, one of whom criticized the medical center as being out of touch with the community's needs, and the other of whom defended the center's contributions to society. Jeff found the first speaker very convincing about the need to pay more attention to primary care, prevention, and public health. He had never had a regular primary care physician, and the idea of having a family physician appealed to him. He was equally impressed by the second speaker, whose account of how research at the medical center had led to life-saving treatment of children with a hereditary blood disorder was very moving, and whose description of the hospital's plan for a new imaging center was spellbinding. Jeff felt that if he ever became seriously ill, he would certainly want all the specialized services the medical center had to offer.

The professional model and the biomedical paradigm are responsible for many of the attractive characteristics of the US health care system. The biomedical model has instilled respect for the scientific method and has helped to curtail medical quackery. Professionalism has directed physicians to serve as agents acting in their patients' best interests and has made the practice of medicine more than just another business. Expansion of hospital facilities has meant that people with health insurance have had convenient access to tertiary care services and new technology. Patients have been able to take advantage of the expertise and availability of a wide variety of specialists. In many circumstances, the system is well organized to deliver the "right care." For a patient in cardiogenic shock, the right place to be is an intensive care unit; for a patient with a detached retina, an ophthalmologist's office is the right place to be.

However, there is widespread concern that despite the benefits of biomedical science and medical professionalism, the US health care system is precariously off balance. A model of excellence focused on specialization, technology, and curative medicine has led to relative inattention to basic primary care services, including such needs as disease prevention and supportive care for patients with chronic and incurable ailments. The value placed on individualism and autonomy for health care professionals and institutions has contributed to a pluralistic delivery system in which care is often fragmented and lacking coordination. A system that prizes specialists who focus on organ systems and researchers who concentrate on splitting genes has bred apprehension that health care has somehow lost sight of the whole person and the whole community. The net result is a system structured to perform miraculous feats for individuals who are ill, but at great expense and often without satisfactorily attending to the full spectrum of health care needs of the entire population. During the 2009 debate in Congress leading up to the passage of the Affordable Care Act, one of the harshest critiques of the status quo in US health care came not from a Congressional Democrat, but from Senator Orrin Hatch, the senior Republican Senator from Utah. At a hearing on health reform, Senator Hatch said, "The US is first in providing rescue care, but this care has little or no impact on the general population. We must put more focus on primary care and preventive medicine. How do we transform the system to do this?" (Grundy et al, 2010).

REFERENCES

Akinbami LJ et al. Status of childhood asthma in the United States, 1980–2007. *Pediatrics.* 2009;123(Suppl 3):S131-45.

American College of Physicians. *The Impending Collapse of Primary Care Medicine and Its Implications for the State of the Nation's Health Care.* January 30, 2006. http://www.acponline.org/advocacy/events/state_of_healthcare/statehc06_1.pdf.

Baicker K, Chandra A. Medicare spending, the physician workforce, and beneficiaries' quality of care. *Health Aff (Millwood).* 2004:W4-184.

Bindman AB et al. Primary care and receipt of preventive services. *J Gen Intern Med.* 1996;11:269.

Bodenheimer T. Regional medical programs: No road to regionalization. *Med Care Rev.* 1969;26:1125.

Bodenheimer T. Primary care—will it survive? *N Engl J Med.* 2006;355:861.

Bodenheimer T et al. The primary care-specialty income gap: Why it matters. *Ann Intern Med.* 2007;146:301.

Bodenheimer T, Grumbach K. *Improving Primary Care. Strategies and Tools for a Better Practice.* New York, NY: McGraw-Hill; 2007.

Council on Graduate Medical Education. *Twentieth Report: Advancing Primary Care*, December 2010.

Dawson W. Interim report on the future provision of medical and allied services. In: Saward EW, ed. *The Regionalization of Personal Health Services.* London, England: Prodist; 1975.

Engel GL. The need for a new medical model: A challenge for biomedicine. *Science.* 1977;196:129.

Franks P et al. Gatekeeping revisited: Protecting patients from overtreatment. *N Engl J Med.* 1992;327:424.

Friedson E. *Professional Dominance: The Social Structure of Medicine.* Atherton, CA: Atherton Publishing; 1970.

Fry J. Primary care. In: Fry J, ed. *Primary Care.* London, England: William Heinemann; 1980.

Green LA et al. The ecology of medical care revisited. *N Engl J Med.* 2001;344:2021.

Grumbach K, Grundy P. *Outcomes of Implementing Patient Centered Medical Home Interventions: A Review of Evidence*

From Prospective Evaluation Studies in the United States. Washington, DC: Patient Centered Primary Care Collaborative, 2010. http://www.pcpcc.net/files/evidence_outcomes_in_pcmh.pdf.

Grumbach K et al. Primary care physicians' experience of financial incentives in managed care systems. N Engl J Med. 1998;339:1516.

Grumbach K et al. Regionalization of cardiac surgery in the United States and Canada: Geographic access, choice, and outcomes. JAMA. 1995;274:1282.

Grundy P et al. The multi-stakeholder movement for primary care renewal and reform. Health Affairs. 2010;29:791.

Halvorson GC, Isham GJ. Epidemic of Care. San Francisco, CA: Jossey-Bass; 2003.

Horrocks S et al. Systematic review of whether nurse practitioners working in primary care can provide equivalent care to doctors. BMJ. 2002;324:819.

Institute of Medicine. Primary Care: America's Health in a New Era. Washington, DC: National Academies Press; 1996.

Light D, Levine S. The changing character of the medical profession: A theoretical overview. Milbank Mem Fund Q. 1988;66:10.

Luce JM, Byyny RL. The evolution of medical specialism. Perspect Biol Med. 1979;22:377.

Rivo ML et al. Defining the generalist physician's training. JAMA. 1994;271:1499.

Rodwin VG. The Health Planning Predicament. Berkeley, CA: University of California Press; 1984.

Roos N. Who should do the surgery? Tonsillectomy-adenoidectomy in one Canadian province. Inquiry. 1979;16:73.

Rosenblatt RA et al. The generalist role of specialty physicians: is there a hidden system of primary care? JAMA. 1998;279:1364.

Safran DG et al. Linking primary care performance to outcomes of care. J Fam Pract. 1998;47:213.

Saultz JW, Albedaiwi W. Interpersonal continuity of care and patient satisfaction: A critical review. Ann Fam Med. 2004;2:445.

Saultz JW, Lochner J. Interpersonal continuity of care and care outcomes: a critical review. Ann Fam Med. 2005;3:159.

Shea S et al. Predisposing factors for severe, uncontrolled hypertension in an inner-city minority population. N Engl J Med. 1992;327:776.

Somers AR. Who's in charge here? Alice searches for a king in Mediland. N Engl J Med. 1972;287:849.

Starfield B. Primary Care. New York, NY: Oxford University Press; 1998.

Starfield B et al. Contribution of primary care to health systems and health. Milbank Q. 2005;83:457.

Starr P. The Social Transformation of American Medicine. New York, NY: Basic Books; 1982.

Stevens R. In Sickness and in Wealth: American Hospitals in the Twentieth Century. New York, NY: Basic Books; 1989.

Stewart AL et al. Primary care and patient perceptions of access to care. J Fam Pract. 1997;44:177.

Wachter RM, Goldman L. The emerging role of "hospitalists" in the American health care system. N Engl J Med. 1996;335:514.

White KL et al. The ecology of medical care. N Engl J Med. 19; 265:885.

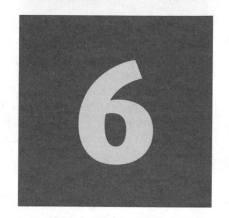

How Health Care Is Organized—II: Health Delivery Systems

The last chapter explored some general principles of health care organization, including levels of care, regionalization, physician and other practitioner roles, and patient flow through the system. This chapter looks more closely at actual structures of medical practice.

The traditional dispersed model of the US medical practice has been referred to as a "cottage industry" of independent private physicians working as solo practitioners or in small groups. A number of alternative organizational forms have existed in the United States, ranging from community health centers to prepaid group practices. The traditional model is in competition with a system of larger practice organizations and networks structured along a more integrated model of health care delivery.

THE TRADITIONAL STRUCTURE OF MEDICAL CARE

▶ Physicians and Hospitals

Dr. Harvey Commoner finished his residency in general surgery in 1956. For the next 30 years, he and another surgeon practiced medicine together in a middle-class suburb near St. Peter's Hospital, a nonprofit church-affiliated institution. Dr. Commoner received most of his cases from general practitioners and internists on the St. Peter's medical staff. By 1965, the number of surgeons operating at St. Peter's had grown. Because Dr. Commoner was not getting enough cases, he and his partner joined the medical staff of Top Dollar Hospital, a for-profit facility 3 miles away, and University Hospital downtown. On an average morning, Dr. Commoner drove to all three hospitals to perform operations or to do postoperative rounds on his patients. The afternoon was spent seeing patients in his office. He was on call every other night and weekend.

Dr. Commoner was active on the St. Peter's medical staff executive committee, where he frequently proposed that the hospital purchase new radiology and operating room equipment needed to keep up with advances in surgery. Because the hospital received hundreds of thousands of dollars each year for providing care to Dr. Commoner's patients, and because Dr. Commoner had the option of admitting his patients to Top Dollar or University, the St. Peter's administration usually purchased the items that Dr. Commoner recommended. The Top Dollar Hospital administrator did likewise.

During the period when Dr. Commoner was practicing, most medical care was delivered by fee-for-service private physicians in solo or small group practices. Most hospitals were private nonprofit institutions, sometimes affiliated with a religious organization, occasionally with a medical school, often run by an independent board of trustees composed of prominent people in the community. Most physicians in traditional fee-for-service practice were not employees of any hospital, but joined one or several hospital medical staffs, thereby gaining the privilege of admitting patients to the hospital and at times acquiring the responsibility to assist the hospital through work on medical staff committees or by caring for emergency department patients who have no physician.

For many years, the physicians were the dominant power in the hospital, because physicians admit the patients, and hospitals without patients have no income. Because physicians were free to admit their patients to more than one hospital, the implicit threat to take their patients elsewhere gave them influence. Under traditional fee-for-service medicine, physicians used informal referral networks, often involving other physicians on the same hospital medical staff. In metropolitan areas with a high ratio of physician specialists to population, referrals could become a critical economic issue. Most surgeons obtained their cases by referral from primary care physicians (PCPs) or medical specialists; surgeons like Dr. Commoner who were not readily available when called soon found their case load drying up.

THE SEEDS OF NEW MEDICAL CARE STRUCTURES

The dispersed structure of independent fee-for-service private practice was not always the dominant model in the United States. When modern medical care took root in the first half of the twentieth century, a variety of structures blossomed. Among these were multispecialty group practices, community health centers, and prepaid group practices. Some of these flourished but then wilted, while others became the seeds from which the future health care system of the twenty-first century may germinate.

▶ Multispecialty Group Practice

In 1905, Dr. Geraldine Giemsa joined the department of pathology at the Mayo Clinic. The clinic, led by the brothers William and Charles Mayo, was becoming a nationally renowned referral center for surgery and was recruiting pathologists, microbiologists, and other specialized diagnosticians to support the work of the clinic's group of surgeons. Dr. Giemsa received a salary and became an employee of the group practice. With time, she became a senior partner and part owner of the Mayo Clinic.

Together with their father, the Mayo brothers, who were general practitioners skilled at surgical techniques, formed a group practice in the small town of Rochester, MN, in the 1890s. As the brothers' reputation for clinical excellence grew, the practice added

several surgeons and physicians in laboratory-oriented specialties. By 1929, the Mayo Clinic had more than 375 physicians and 900 support staff and eventually went on to open its own hospitals (Starr, 1982). Although the clinic paid its physician staff by salary, the clinic itself billed patients, and later third-party insurance plans, on a fee-for-service basis. The Mayo Clinic was the inspiration for other group practices that developed in the United States, such as the Menninger Clinic in Topeka, KS, and the Palo Alto Medical Foundation in California. These clinics were owned and administered by physicians and featured physicians working in various specialties—hence the common use of the term *multispecialty group practice* to describe this organizational model. As in the case of the Mayo Clinic, these multispecialty group practices were innovative in the manner in which they brought a large number of physicians together under one roof to deliver care.

By formally integrating specialists into a single clinic structure, group practice attempted to promote a collaborative style of care. Lacking a strong role for the PCP as coordinator of services, the specialty-oriented group practice model attempted to use the structure of the practice organization itself as a means of creating an environment for coordinated care among specialist physicians. Enhancement of quality of care was also expected from the greater opportunity for formal and informal peer review and continuing education when colleagues worked together and shared responsibility for the care of patients. Critics of group practice warned that large practice structures would jeopardize the intimate patient–physician relationship possible in a solo or small group setting, arguing that large groups would subject patients to an impersonal style of care with no single physician clearly accountable for the patient's welfare.

In 1932, the blue ribbon Committee on the Costs of Medical Care recommended that the delivery of care be organized around large group practices (Starr, 1982). The eight physicians in private practice who were members of the committee dissented from the recommendations, roundly criticizing the sections on group practice. An editorial in the *Journal of the American Medical Association* was even more scathing in its attack on the committee's majority report:

The physicians of this country must not be misled by utopian fantasies of a form of medical practice, which would equalize all physicians by placing them in groups under one administration. The public will find to its cost, as it has elsewhere, that such schemes do not answer that hidden desire in each human breast for human kindliness, human forbearance, and human understanding. It is better for the American people that most of their illnesses be treated by their own physicians rather than by industries, corporations, or clinics. (The Committee on the Costs of Medical Care, 1932)

Several multispecialty group practices flourished during the period between the world wars, and to this day remain among the most highly regarded systems of care in the United States. Yet multispecialty group practice did not become the dominant organizational structure. In part, resistance to this model by professional societies blunted the potential for growth. In addition, as hospitals assumed a central role in medical care, group practice lost some of its unique attractions. Hospitals could provide the ancillary services physicians needed for the increasingly specialized and technology-dependent work of medicine. Hospitals also served as an organizational focus for the informal referral networks that developed among private physicians in independent practice.

▶ Community Health Centers

One of the most far-reaching alternatives to fee-for-service medical practice is the community health center, emphasizing primary and preventive care and also striving to take responsibility for the health status of the community served by the health center. An early twentieth-century example of such an institution was the Greater Community Association at Creston, IA. The association brought together civic, religious, education, and health care groups in a coordinated system centered on the community hospital serving a six-county area with 100,000 residents. The plan placed its greatest emphasis on preventive care and public health measures administered by public health nurses. In describing the association, Kepford (1919) wrote:

The motto of the Greater Community Association is "Service." Among the principles of the hospital management are the precept that it shall be a long way from the threshold of the hospital to the operating room. . . . We have a hospital that makes no attempt to pattern after the great city institutions, but is organized to meet the needs of a rural neighborhood. The Greater Community Association has been taught to regard the hospital as a repair shop, necessary only where preventive medicine has failed. (Kepford, 1919)

In 1928, Sherry Kidd joined the Frontier Nursing Service in Appalachia as a nurse midwife. For $5 per year, families could enroll in the service and receive pregnancy-related care. Sherry was responsible for all enrolled families within a 100-mile radius. She referred patients with complications to an obstetrician in Lexington, KY, who was the service's physician consultant.

Another pioneering model, the Frontier Nursing Service was established by Mary Breckinridge, an English-trained midwife, in 1925 (Dye, 1983). Breckinridge designed the service to meet the needs of a poor rural area in Kentucky that lacked basic medical and obstetric care and suffered from high rates of maternal and infant mortality. The Frontier Nursing Service shared many of the features of the Creston, IA, model: regionalized services planned on a geographic basis to serve rural populations with an emphasis on primary care and health education. Like the Creston system, the service relied on nurses to provide primary care, with physicians reserved for secondary medical services on a referral basis.

These rural programs had their urban counterparts in health centers that focused on maternal and child health services during the early 1900s (Rothman, 1978; Stoeckle and Candib, 1969). The clinics primarily served populations in low-income districts in large cities and were often involved with large immigrant populations. As in the rural systems, public health nurses played a central role in an organizational model geared toward health education, nutrition, and sanitation. Both the urban and rural models of community health centers waned during the middle years of this century. Public health nursing declined in prestige as hospitals became the center of activity for nursing education and practice (Stevens, 1989). A team model of nurses working in collaboration with physicians withered under a system of hierarchical professional roles.

The community health center model was revived in 1965, when the federal Office of Economic Opportunity, the agency created to implement the "War on

Poverty," initiated its program of community health centers. The program's goals included the combining of comprehensive medical care and public health to improve the health status of defined low-income communities, the building of multidisciplinary teams to provide health services, and participation in the governance of the health centers by community members.

> *Dr. Franklin Jefferson was professor of hematology at a prestigious medical school. His distinguished career was based on laboratory research, teaching, and subspecialty medical practice, with a focus on sickle cell anemia. Dr. Jefferson felt that his work was serving his community, but that he would like to do more. In 1965, with the advent of the federal neighborhood health center program, he left his laboratory in the hands of a well-trained assistant and began to talk with community leaders in the poor neighborhood that surrounded the medical school. After a year, the trust that was developed between Dr. Jefferson and members of the neighborhood bore fruit in a decision to approach the medical school dean about a joint medical school–community application for funds to create a neighborhood health center. Two years later, the center opened its doors, with Dr. Jefferson as its first medical director.*

By the early 1980s, 800 federally funded community health centers were in operation in the United States, administered by governing boards that included patients enrolled in the health center. Many of the centers trained community members as outreach workers, who became members of health care teams that included public health nurses, physicians, mental health workers, and health educators. Some of the health centers made a serious attempt to meld clinical services with public health activities in programs of community-oriented primary care. For example, the rural health center in Mound Bayou, MS, helped organize a cooperative farm to improve nutrition in the county, dig wells to supply safe drinking water, and train community residents to become health care professionals. By improving the care of low-income ambulatory patients, the centers were able to reduce hospitalization and emergency department visits by their patients. Community health centers also had some success in improving community health status,

particularly by reducing infant and neonatal mortality rates among African Americans (Geiger, 1984). In the past decade, the federal government invested in a new period of expansion of community health centers, and these health centers are viewed as a critical access point for the reforms enacted in the Affordable Care Act of 2010. In 2008, more than 1000 community health centers at 7500 sites were serving 17 million people, three-quarters of them uninsured or covered by Medicaid (Kaiser Commission, 2010).

▶ Prepaid Group Practice and Health Maintenance Organizations

Historically, one alternative to small office-based, fee-for-service practice became the major challenge to that traditional model: prepaid group practice, one of the models upon which the modern HMO is based.

In 1929, the Ross–Loos Clinic began to provide medical services for employees of the Los Angeles Department of Water and Power on a prepaid basis. By 1935, the clinic had enrolled 37,000 employees and their dependents, who each paid $2 per month for a specified list of services. Also in 1929, an idealistic physician, Dr. Michael Shadid, organized a medical cooperative in Elk City, OK, based on four principles: group practice, prepayment, preventive medicine, and control by the patients, who were members of the cooperative. In the late forties, more than a hundred rural health cooperatives were founded, many in Texas, but they tended to fade away, partly from the stiff opposition of organized medicine. In the 1950s, another version of the consumer-managed prepaid group practice sprang up in Appalachia, where the United Mine Workers established union-run group practice clinics, each receiving a budget from the union-controlled, coal industry–financed medical care fund. Meanwhile, the Group Health Association of Washington, DC, had been organized in 1937 as a prepaid group practice whose board was elected by the cooperative's membership. A few years later in Seattle, Group Health Cooperative of Puget Sound acquired its own hospital, began to grow, and by the mid-1970s had 200,000 subscribers, a fifth of the Seattle-area population. In 1947, the Health Insurance Plan of New York opened its doors, operating 22 group practices; within 10 years, Health Insurance Plan's enrollment approached 500,000 (Starr, 1982).

The most successful of the prepaid group practices that emerged in the 1930s and 1940s was the Kaiser Health Plan. In 1938, a surgeon named Sidney Garfield began providing prepaid medical services for industrialist Henry J. Kaiser's employees working at the Grand Coulee Dam in Washington State. Rather than receiving a salary from Kaiser, Garfield was prepaid a fixed sum per employee, a precursor to modern capitation payment. Kaiser transported this concept to 200,000 workers in his shipyards and steel mills on the West Coast during World War II (Garfield, 1970; Starr, 1982). In this way, company-sponsored medical care in a remote area gave birth to today's largest alternative to fee-for-service practice. Kaiser opened its doors to the general public after World War II. Kaiser now operates in nine states and Washington, DC, with nearly 9 million patients enrolled.

The contemporary systems that grew out of the Kaiser and consumer cooperative models share several important features. Rather than preserving a separation between insurance plans and the providers of care, these models attempt to meld the financing and delivery of care into a single organizational structure. Paying a premium for health insurance coverage in this approach does not just mean that a third-party payer will reimburse some or all the costs of care delivered by independent practitioners. Rather, the premium serves to directly purchase, in advance, health services from a particular system of care. This is the notion of "prepaid" care that is one component of the prepaid group practice model. (As discussed in Chapter 2, the Baylor Hospital plan in the 1930s was a parallel attempt to develop a model of prepaid hospital care.) The second component is care delivered by a large group of practitioners working under a common administrative structure—the "group practice" aspect of prepaid group practice.

Systems such as Kaiser and Group Health Cooperative of Puget Sound were commonly referred to as *prepaid group practices* until the 1970s, when terminology underwent a transformation as part of a political effort to sell the public and Congress on this model of care as a centerpiece of health care reform under the Nixon administration. Paul Ellwood, a Minnesota physician and advisor to President Nixon, suggested that prepaid group practices be referred to as "health maintenance organizations" (Ellwood et al, 1971; Starr, 1982). This change in name was intended in part to break from the political legacy of the prepaid group practice

movement, a legacy colored with populist tones from the cooperative plans and tainted by organized medicine's common criticism of prepaid group practice as a socialist threat. The term *health maintenance* was also designed to suggest that these systems would place more emphasis on preventive care than had the traditional medical model. Although HMOs were initially synonymous with prepaid group practice, by the 1980s, several varieties of HMO plans emerged that departed from the prepaid group practice organizational form. We describe the Kaiser model to fully illustrate the first-generation HMO model, and then proceed to discuss the second-generation HMOs known as independent practice associations (IPAs) or network HMOs.

FIRST-GENERATION HEALTH MAINTENANCE ORGANIZATIONS AND VERTICAL INTEGRATION: THE KAISER–PERMANENTE MEDICAL CARE PROGRAM

Mario Fuentes was a professor at the University of California. He and his family belonged to the Kaiser Health Plan, and the university paid his family's premium. Professor Fuentes had once fractured his clavicle, for which he went to the urgent care clinic at Kaiser Hospital in Oakland; otherwise, he had not used Kaiser's facilities. Mrs. Fuentes suffered from rheumatoid arthritis; her regular physician was a salaried rheumatologist at the Permanente Medical Clinic, the group practice in which Kaiser physicians work. One of the Fuentes' sons, Juanito, had been in an automobile accident a year earlier near a town 90 miles away from home. He had been taken to a local emergency department and released; Kaiser had paid the bill because no Kaiser facility was available in the town. Three days after returning home, Juanito developed a severe headache and became drowsy; he was taken to the urgent care clinic, received a CT scan, and was found to have a subdural hematoma. He was immediately transported to Kaiser's regional neurosurgery center in Redwood City, CA, where he underwent surgery to evacuate the hematoma.

Dr. Roberta Short had mixed feelings about working at Kaiser. She liked the hours, the salary, and the paucity of administrative tasks. She particularly liked working in the same building with other general internists and specialists, providing the opportunity for frequent discussions on diagnostic and therapeutic problems. However, she was not happy about seeing 4 or 5 patients per hour. Such a pace left little time to talk to the patients or to make important phone calls to patients or specialists. It was tough for Dr. Short's patients to get appointments with her, and it was even harder to arrange prompt appointments with specialists, who were as busy as she was. Moreover, the rules for ordering magnetic resonance imaging scans and other expensive tests were strict, though by and large reasonable. Overall, Dr. Short felt that the Kaiser system worked well but needed more physicians per enrolled patient.

The Kaiser–Permanente Medical Care Program is the largest of the nation's prepaid group practice HMOs, consisting of three interlocking administrative units:

1. The Kaiser Foundation Health Plan, which performs the functions of health insurer, such as administering enrollment and other aspects of the financing of care.

2. The Kaiser Foundation Hospitals Corporation, which owns and administers Kaiser hospitals (the same individuals sit on the boards of directors for the Health Plan and the Hospitals Corporation).

3. Permanente medical groups, the physician organizations that administer the group practices and provide medical services to Kaiser plan members under a capitated contract with the Kaiser plan.

The organizational model typified in the Kaiser–Permanente HMO has come to be known as vertical integration. *Vertical integration* refers to consolidating under one organizational roof and common ownership all levels of care, from primary to tertiary care, and the facilities and staff necessary to provide this full spectrum of care (Figure 6–1). Although structures differ somewhat across Kaiser's regional health plans, most Kaiser–Permanente regional units own their hospitals and clinics, hire the nurses and other personnel staffing these facilities, and contract with a single large group practice (Permanente) to exclusively serve patients covered by the Kaiser health plan.

The Kaiser form of HMO differs from traditional fee-for-service models in how it pays physicians (salary) and hospitals (global budget). It also differs in how health services are organized. Most obvious is the

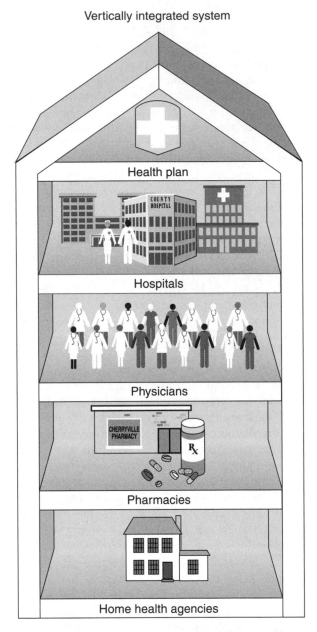

▲ **Figure 6–1.** Vertical integration consolidates health services under one organizational roof.

prepaid group practice structure that contrasts with the traditional US style of solo, independent private practice. In addition, Kaiser has typically regionalized tertiary care services at a select number of specialized centers. For example, Northern California Kaiser has centralized all neurosurgical care at only two hospitals; patients with spinal cord injuries, brain tumors, and other neurosurgical conditions are referred to these centers from other Northern California Kaiser hospitals. The distribution of specialties within the physician staff in The Permanente Medical Group is approximately half generalists and half specialists. Most regions have also integrated nonphysicians, such as nurse practitioners and physician assistants, into the primary care team.

Many observers consider this ability to coherently plan and regionalize services to be a major strength of vertically integrated systems (Figure 6–1). Unlike a public district health authority in the United Kingdom, an HMO such as Kaiser–Permanente is not responsible for the entire population of a region, but these private, vertically integrated systems in the United States do assume responsibility for organizing and delivering services to a population of plan enrollees. The prepaid nature of enrollment in the Kaiser plan permits Kaiser to orient its care more toward a population health model.

SECOND-GENERATION HEALTH MAINTENANCE ORGANIZATIONS AND "VIRTUAL INTEGRATION": NETWORK MODEL HMOs, INDEPENDENT PRACTICE ASSOCIATIONS, AND INTEGRATED MEDICAL GROUPS

As more and more of her patients switched from fee-for-service health plans to the new HMO plans run by commercial insurers that were capturing a growing share of the private health insurance market in California, Dr. Westcoast figured she had no choice but to start contracting with these HMOs if she wanted to retain her patients. She joined the Good Health Independent Practice Association (IPA), an organization that helped solo practitioners like Dr. Westcoast contract with different HMOs. Within 3 years, 30% of the patients in her internal medicine practice were covered by 4 HMO plans that contracted with the Good Health IPA.

Although having HMO contracts was clearly proving to be important for the viability of her practice, Dr. Westcoast found much of the new arrangements frustrating. Each HMO sent her annual reports on various quality-of-care measures for the diabetic patients that the HMO showed as having Dr. Westcoast as their PCP. The trouble was that,

many of the patients were not actually patients in her practice, and it was hard to reconcile the reports for a few diabetic patients from each of the 4 HMOs with all the diabetic patients she saw, including many not enrolled in HMOs, to understand how she really was doing in meeting quality standards for all the diabetic patients in her practice. Good Health IPA sent her its own quality report about the diabetic patients that Good Health thought had Dr. Westcoast as a PCP, and the information in that report didn't match the data sent by the HMOs. To make matters worse, each HMO had a different formulary of the diabetic medications that were covered by the health plan, and Dr. Westcoast spent a lot of time helping exasperated patients who needed their prescriptions changed to a different medication. She wondered about giving up her practice to join Kaiser, where she would be less independent but at least she wouldn't have to deal with so many different HMOs, each with their different set of rules.

In 1954, the medical society in San Joaquin County, CA, fretted about the possibility of Kaiser moving into the county. Private fee-for-service patients might go to the lower cost Kaiser, and physicians' incomes would fall. An idea was born: To compete with Kaiser, the San Joaquin Foundation for Medical Care was set up as a network of physicians in independent private practice to contract as a group with employers for a monthly payment per enrollee; the foundation would then pay the physicians on a discounted fee-for-service basis and conduct utilization review to discourage overtreatment (Starr, 1982). It was hoped that the plan would reduce the costs to employers, who would choose the foundation rather than Kaiser.

When the Health Maintenance Organization Act of 1973 was enacted into law as the outcome of President Nixon's health care reform strategy, network model HMOs were included along with prepaid group practice as legitimate HMOs. The HMO law stimulated HMO development by requiring large- and medium-sized businesses that provided health insurance to their employees to offer at least one federally qualified HMO as an alternative to traditional fee-for-service insurance if such an HMO existed in the vicinity (Starr, 1982). Network-model HMOs were far easier to organize than prepaid group practices; a county or state medical society, a hospital, or an insurance company could simply recruit the office-based, fee-for-service physicians practicing in the community into network, and thereby create the basis for an HMO. The physicians could continue to see their non-HMO patients as well. The inclusion of the network form of HMO in the 1973 legislation ensured that the HMO movement would not produce rapid alterations in the traditional mode of delivering medical care.

Some of the initial network-model HMOs were organized on the two-tiered payment model described in Chapter 4. Under this model, an HMO contracts with many individual physicians to care for HMO enrollees. Some network-model HMOs have evolved into models that use a three-tiered payment structure whereby the HMO does not contract directly with individual physicians but rather with a large group of physicians. These groups may take several forms. The San Joaquin Foundation for Medical Care was an early example of the Independent Practice Association (IPA) model, consisting of a network of physicians who agree to participate in an association for purposes of contracting with HMOs and other managed care plans. Physicians maintain ownership of their practices and administer their own offices. The IPA serves as a vehicle for negotiating and administering HMO contracts.

Unlike the "monogamous" arrangement between each Kaiser region and its respective Permanente medical group, in network models physicians can establish contractual relationships with numerous HMOs and IPAs. A physician may participate in more than one IPA, and each IPA may in turn have contracts with many HMO and managed care plans. The result of this more open HMO–physician relationship is a series of physician panels in the same community that overlap partially, but not completely, for patients covered by different HMOs. While this more open-ended network approach may have some appeal to physicians and patients in contrast to more tightly integrated HMO models like Kaiser, it can also produce the types of frustrations experienced by Dr. Westcoast. A PCP, who may see patients from several HMOs and participate in more than one IPA, often finds that a specialist or hospital participates in the network for one HMO or IPA but not another, causing disruption and confusion when it comes to figuring out which specialist or hospital is eligible to accept a referral (Bodenheimer, 2000). Patients may find that

their PCP is in one IPA but their preferred specialist is not in the same network—with physicians often moving in and out of various networks as contracts are renegotiated.

IPAs initially did little more than to act as brokers between physicians and HMOs, replacing the need for physicians to negotiate contracts on an individual basis. As IPAs took on a larger portion of financial risk for care (see Chapter 4), they became more active in attempting to control costs and assumed responsibility for authorizing utilization of services, profiling physicians' practice patterns, and administering other cost control strategies. Some IPAs have attempted to fashion themselves into more than simply contractual and financial intermediaries by facilitating quality improvement efforts and adoption of electronic medical records among participating practices.

Another structure related to second-generation HMOs is the integrated medical group. Integrated medical groups have a tighter organizational structure than IPAs, consisting of groups in which physicians no longer own their practices and office assets, but become employees of an organization that owns and manages their practice. Some modern-day integrated groups are survivors of the original breed of multispecialty group practices, such as the Mayo Clinic and Palo Alto Medical Foundation described earlier. Others lack these clinics' historical genesis and consist of new organizations created in the managed care era. Some of these newer organizations were created by large, for-profit companies buying up the practices of formerly independent physicians and hiring these same physicians to work as employees of the medical group (Robinson and Casalino, 1996). Others are owned by hospitals or medical schools or are privately held companies with physician partners as owners. Similar to IPAs, integrated medical groups contract with multiple managed care plans and also typically care for patients in fee-for-service private insurance plans and Medicare.

Yet another organizational structure to have emerged is the Physician Hospital Organization (PHO). PHOs developed in the 1980s as an alternative to the IPA model. Instead of creating a physician association to negotiate health plan contracts, physicians partnered with a hospital to jointly contract with health plans for both physician and hospital payment rates. The physicians participating in PHOs often consisted of both private practitioners on the hospital's medical

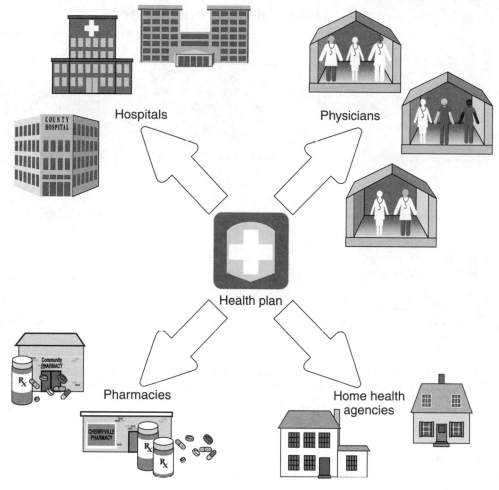

▲ **Figure 6–2.** Virtual integration involves contractual links between HMOs and physician groups, hospitals, and other provider units.

staff and physicians directly employed by the hospital. Formation of PHOs received a setback in the 1990s when the Federal Trade Commission deemed that some PHO arrangements constituted collusion in price setting between physicians and hospitals to an extent that violated anti-trust laws.

The network model HMO represents an alternative to the vertically integrated HMO. As shown in Figure 6–2, managed care relationships involving IPAs and medical groups consist of a network of contractual links between HMOs and autonomous physician groups, hospitals, and other provider units, rather than the "everything-under-one-roof" model of vertical integration.

Observers have dubbed the network forms of managed care organization "virtual integration," signifying an integration of services based on contractual relationships rather than unitary ownership (Robinson and Casalino, 1996). In these virtually integrated systems, HMOs do not directly provide health services through their own hospitals and physician organizations.

COMPARING VERTICALLY AND VIRTUALLY INTEGRATED MODELS

In 2009, about one in four people in the United States was enrolled in some type of HMO, including Medicare and Medicaid beneficiaries participating in HMOs

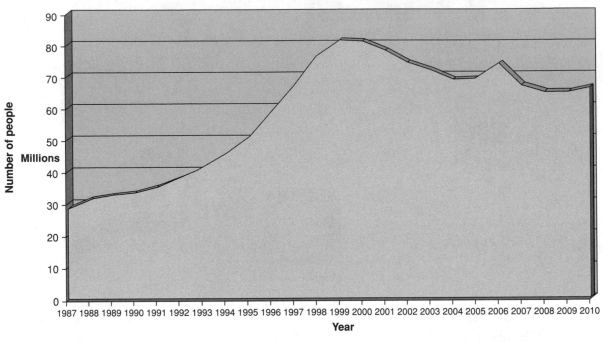

National HMO enrollment

▲ **Figure 6–3.** Trends in HMO enrollment in the United States. Enrollment includes individuals enrolled through Medicare and Medicaid HMO options, as well as through employment-based and other privately insured HMO plans. (MCOL Managed Care Fact Sheets, 2011; http://www.mcareol.com/factshts/factnati.htm.)

(Kaiser Family Foundation, 2011) (Figure 6–3). There is wide variation across states in HMO enrollment, ranging from more than half of insured people in California to under 10% in many other states. For many years, policy analysts predicted that the organizational efficiency and coherence of vertically integrated, first-generation HMOs would position these systems of care to prevail as health care entered a more competitive era. These predictions have not come true, as enrollment in virtually integrated systems has surpassed that of traditional HMOs. Whereas most vertically integrated HMOs are regionally based, non-profit health plans, national for-profit commercial insurers operate the plans enrolling the majority of patients in virtual HMO models.

In response to the reluctance of many patients to be locked into a limited panel of physicians and hospitals in conventional HMO plans, insurers have developed a variety of other products, such as the Preferred Provider Organization (PPO), which allow patients to see physicians not in the insurer's physician network, with the stipulation that patients pay a higher share of the cost out of pocket when they use non-network physicians and hospitals. Physicians joining the PPO network agree to accept discounted fees from the health plan with the hope that being listed as a "preferred" provider will attract more patients to their practice. PPO enrollment was about 50 million in 2009, compared with HMO enrollment of 70 million. Although both HMOs and PPOs are considered forms of "managed care," PPOs are essentially a variation on insurance product benefit structure and, unlike HMOs, involve very little in the way of change in the organization of the delivery of care.

Vertically integrated HMOs clearly represent a significantly different organizational model than the traditional dispersed cottage industry model. Are IPAs and PHOs and the other organizational forms that predominate under network model HMOs a meaningful break from the dispersed model, offering a better framework for the delivery of health care? Or, are these virtual organizations just that—loose confederacies of providers organized primarily for contracting and business objectives that offer little in the way of tangible gains in organizational coherence in the actual provision of health care?

Research suggests that more integrated organizational models have their advantages. Vertically integrated HMOs of the traditional prepaid group practice model tend to rank higher than network model HMOs on various measures quality of care, such as evidence-based care of chronic illnesses (Himmelstein et al, 1999). Integrated medical groups have been shown to perform better than IPAs in delivering up-to-date preventive care such as mammograms and Pap tests (Mehrotra et al, 2006). On general health plan satisfaction ratings, patients tend to rate integrated HMOs such as Kaiser ahead of network-model HMOs. Compared with physicians in IPAs or those not affiliated with any network, physicians in prepaid group practices report greater adoption of tools for quality improvement, such as more structured systems for planning and following through on care of patients with diabetes and other chronic illnesses (Rittenhouse et al, 2004). Size also seems to matter when it comes to the ability of medical groups to adopt the infrastructure for creating patient-centered medical homes; larger medical groups are more likely than small groups to have systems in place for care coordination, enhanced patient access, and related processes (Rittenhouse et al, 2008).

There is also evidence that moving from a completely dispersed model to a somewhat more organized model, even if only of a virtual network variety, can yield improvements in the delivery of care, especially when the network emphasizes linking patients with primary care clinicians and supports better coordination of care. An example is Community Care of North Carolina. Community Care linked North Carolina Medicaid and State Children's Health Insurance Program recipients with a primary care medical home at more than 1000 small private offices and community health centers and provided technical assistance to practices to improve chronic care services including a cadre of nurses to collaborate with practices in care management of high-risk patients. This model resulted in both better patient outcomes, such as reductions in emergency hospitalizations for children with asthma, and reductions in health care costs (Steiner et al, 2008).

The dispersed model does appear to have one important strength from the patient perspective, which is the satisfaction that comes from receiving care from a small practice where patients have a sense that clinicians and staff know them personally and the patient–clinician relationship is less encumbered by organizational bureaucracy. Studies of patient preferences have found that satisfaction is highest when care is received in small offices rather than larger clinic structures (Rubin et al, 1993). People value having a familiar receptionist at the end of the line when they call about a child with a fever rather than experiencing the frustration of navigating impersonal HMO and clinic switchboard operators and voicemail systems—what has been described as the "chain store" persona of some HMOs and large delivery systems (Mechanic, 1976). The computer era may be allowing many large medical groups and vertically integrated HMOs to jump ahead of small practices in providing the means for patients to communicate personally with their clinicians. Many large groups have implemented electronic medical records systems that allow patients to securely e-mail their clinicians and to promptly receive diagnostic test results through web-based "patient portals" providing patients direct access to their personal medical record.

ACCOUNTABLE CARE ORGANIZATIONS

As discussed in Chapter 5, the Affordable Care Act of 2010 is propelling not only an expansion of health insurance coverage, but also reform in how health care is organized and delivered. During the policy debates leading up to passage of the Affordable Care Act, the concept of Accountable Care Organizations (ACOs) emerged as a centerpiece of delivery system reform. ACOs have been defined as "a provider-led organization whose mission is to manage the full continuum of care and be accountable for the overall costs and quality of care for a defined population" (Rittenhouse et al, 2009). The Affordable Care Act authorized Medicare to initiate an ACO program beginning in 2012 (Health Policy Brief, 2010)

ACOs are envisioned as spanning a spectrum of organizational structures. On one end of this spectrum lie vertically integrated HMOs, with their medical groups and facilities well suited to provide comprehensive care to a defined population of enrolled patients under capitated payment. At the other end of the ACO spectrum lie loosely knit affiliations of providers in the traditional dispersed structure discussed at the beginning of this chapter, consisting of a hospital and the collection of private practice physicians who admit their patients to that hospital and maintain informal referral networks. Proponents of the ACO concept have proposed that Medicare could encourage such an informal hospital-physician network to function in a more cohesive and efficient manner by creating a "shared savings" program. Under the shared savings program, Medicare would still pay physicians by fee-for-service and hospitals by DRG, and patients would be allowed free choice of physician and hospital. However, Medicare would compare the costs and quality for the Medicare patients cared for by this virtual network; if the physicians were able to achieve certain targeted quality goals and keep costs below the predicted expenditures for these patients, Medicare would share a portion of the cost savings with the physicians and hospitals in this loosely affiliated ACO network. To qualify for such a shared-savings program, physicians and hospitals would have to create a formal ACO entity to accept shared savings payments. The variety of other organizational models discussed in this chapter, such as IPAs and PHOs, that fall between the poles of the hospital staff model and vertically integrated HMO would be other candidates for ACOs (Shortell et al, 2010).

One key difference between the proposed ACO program and the existing Medicare Advantage Program, discussed in Chapter 2, is the role of insurance companies. Medicare Advantage involves Medicare contracting with insurance plans that operate as HMOs, including both network and traditional prepaid group practice model HMOs. The Medicare ACO program is envisioned as a more direct financial relationship between Medicare and provider organizations. Prepaid group practice model HMOs could qualify as ACOs because they consist of an integrated delivery organization attached to a single insurance plan. However, network model HMO insurers would not, and, under the ACO program, Medicare would look to establish financial arrangements directly with IPAs, PHOs, and other provider-led organizations.

Whether the Medicare ACO program will succeed in moving the US further along the road to more organized, integrated care structures that can improve quality and "bend the cost curve" remains to be determined. Regardless of whether the ACO program as articulated by its proponents will be fully realized, the ACO concept has stimulated considerable attention in the United States on reforming the delivery system to focus more on proactive care of a defined population of patients rather than just reactive care for individual patients, and on holding providers accountable for the quality and costs of care delivered.

FROM MEDICAL HOMES TO MEDICAL NEIGHBORHOODS

In Chapter 5, we discussed the concept of medical homes. Much of what has been discussed in this chapter on delivery system organization could aptly be described as the attempt to create well-functioning medical neighborhoods. The medical *neighborhood* is a term coined by Fisher to describe the constellation of services, providers, and organizations in a health system that contributes to the care of a population of patients (Fisher, 2008). The primary care medical home resides in the medical neighborhood, but the medical neighborhood consists of much more than just medical homes and includes the secondary, tertiary, community, and related services needed by different patients at different times to meet their comprehensive health care needs. High-performing health care requires both excellent medical homes and excellent medical neighborhoods (Rittenhouse et al, 2009). The distinguishing feature of a hospitable medical neighborhood is care that is functionally integrated, but not necessarily structurally integrated along the lines of traditional HMOs. According to one definition, "Integrated health care starts with good primary care and refers to the delivery of comprehensive health care services that are well coordinated with good communication among providers; includes informed and involved patients; and leads to high-quality, cost-effective care. At the center of integrated health care delivery is a high-performing primary care provider who can serve as a medical home for patients" (Aetna Foundation, 2010).

Organizations that are structurally integrated have an advantage in being able to provide care that is functionally integrated. These organizations have assets such as multispecialty groups, a unified electronic medical record, interdisciplinary health care teams, and a quality improvement infrastructure equipped to promote care coordination and the free flow of information among all providers involved in a patient's care. One of the ongoing challenges in the United States is whether organizations that are less structurally integrated than traditional prepaid group practice HMOs will be able to achieve the

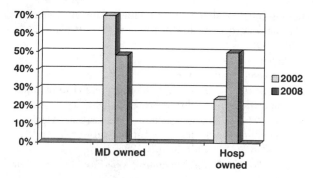

▲ **Figure 6–4.** Ownership of medical practices. (Harris G. *More doctors giving up private practices. New York Times*, March 25, 2010.)

degree of functional integration needed to deliver more effective and efficient care and overcome what we cited in Chapter 5 as the "fragmentation, chaos, and disarray" that has long plagued the US health system.

Despite the admonitions of the dissenting *JAMA* editorialists in 1932 who warned physicians not to be "misled by utopian fantasies" of group practice, it appears that in the early part of the twenty-first century a tipping point has occurred in the United States and the health care cottage industry is rapidly giving way to larger organizations for delivering care. From 2002 to 2008, the percentage of medical practices that are doctor-owned fell from 70% to 48% while the percentage owned by hospitals grew from 24% to 50% (Figure 6–4). Most new residency graduates are eschewing the tradition of becoming autonomous proprietors of their own private practices and seeking employed positions, seeking what the *New York Times* has described as "regular paychecks instead of shopkeeper risks" (Harris, 2011). Hospitals are merging with one another and with physician organizations and creating large, regional delivery systems.

Will the rapid organizational changes occurring in health care in the United States result in a higher-quality, more affordable health system? Will patients be cared for at the proper level of care—primary, secondary, and tertiary? Will the flow of patients among these levels be constructed in an orderly way within each geographic region—a regionalized structure? Will a sufficient number of primary care providers—generalist physicians, physician assistants, and nurse practitioners—be available so that everyone in the United States can have a

regular source of primary care that allows for continuity and coordination of care? Will HMOs, ACOs, and other organizations require their physicians to take responsibility for the health of their enrollee population, or will physicians be content to care only for whoever walks in the door? What is an ideal health delivery system? Different people would have different answers. One vision is a system in which people choose their own primary care clinicians in modest-sized, decentralized, prepaid group practices that would be linked to community hospitals, including specialists' offices providing secondary care. Difficult cases could be referred to the academic tertiary care center in the region. In the primary care practices, teams of health caregivers would endeavor to provide medical care to those people seeking attention, and would also concern themselves with the health status of the entire population served by the practice.

REFERENCES

Aetna Foundation. Program Areas: Specifics, 2010. http://www.aetna.com/about-aetna-insurance/aetna-foundation/aetna-grants/program-area-specifics.html.

Bodenheimer T. Selective chaos. *Health Aff (Millwood)*. 2000;19(4):200.

The Committee on the Costs of Medical Care. Editorial. *JAMA*. 1932;99:1950.

Dye NS. Mary Breckinridge, the Frontier Nursing Service and the introduction of nurse-midwifery in the United States. *Bull Hist Med*. 1983;57:485.

Ellwood PM et al. Health maintenance strategy. *Med Care*. 1971;9:291.

Fisher ES. Building a medical neighborhood for the medical home. *N Engl J Med*. 2008;359:1202.

Garfield SR. The delivery of medical care. *Sci Am*. 1970;222:15.

Geiger HJ. Community health centers: Health care as an instrument of social change. In: Sidel VW, Sidel R, eds. *Reforming Medicine*. New York: Pantheon Books; 1984.

Harris G. More Doctors Giving up Private Practice, and Family Physicians Can't Give Away Solo Practice. *New York Times*. March 25 and April 22, 2011.

Health Policy Brief: Accountable care organizations. *Health Affairs*. July 27, 2010.

Himmelstein DU et al. Quality of care in investor-owned vs not-for-profit HMOs. *JAMA*. 1999;282:159.

Kaiser Commission on Medicaid and the Uninsured. Issue Brief. *Community Health Centers: Opportunities and Challenges of Health Reform*. Washington, DC: The Kaiser Commission on Medicaid and the Uninsured; 2010. http://www.kff.org/uninsured/upload/8098.pdf.

Kaiser Family Foundation. Total HMO Enrollment, July 2009. State Health Facts, 2011. http://www.statehealthfacts.org/comparetable.jsp?ind=348&cat=7&sub=85&yr=194&typ=1&sort=a.

Kepford AE. The Greater Community Association at Creston, Iowa. *Mod Hosp.* 1919;12:342.

Mechanic D. *The Growth of Bureaucratic Medicine.* New York: John Wiley & Sons; 1976.

Mehrotra A et al. Do integrated medical groups provide higher-quality medical care than individual practice associations? *Ann Intern Med.* 2006;145:826.

Rittenhouse DR et al. Physician organization and care management in California: From cottage to Kaiser. *Health Aff (Millwood).* 2004;23(6):51.

Rittenhouse DR et al. Measuring the medical home infrastructure in large medical groups. *Health Aff (Millwood).* 2008;27:1246.

Rittenhouse DR et al. Primary care and accountable care—two essential elements of delivery-system reform. *N Engl J Med.* 2009;361:2301.

Robinson JC, Casalino LP. Vertical integration and organizational networks in health care. *Health Aff (Millwood).* 1996;15:7.

Rothman SM. *Woman's Proper Place: A History of Changing Ideals and Practices.* New York: Basic Books; 1978.

Rubin HR et al. Patients' ratings of outpatient visits in different practice settings. *JAMA.* 1993;270:835.

Shortell SM et al. How the Center for Medicare and Medicaid innovation should test accountable care organizations. *Health Aff (Millwood).* 2010;29:1293.

Starr P. *The Social Transformation of American Medicine.* New York: Basic Books; 1982.

Steiner BD et al. Community care of North Carolina: Improving care through community health networks. *Ann Fam Med.* 2008;6:361.

Stevens R. *In Sickness and in Wealth: American Hospitals in the Twentieth Century.* New York: Basic Books; 1989.

Stoeckle JD, Candib LM. The neighborhood health center: Reform ideas of yesterday and today. *N Engl J Med.* 1969;280:1385.

The Health Care Workforce and the Education of Health Professionals

A health care system is only as good as the people working in it. The most valuable resource in health care is not the latest technology or the most state-of-the-art facility, but the health care professionals and other workers who are the human resources of the health care system.

In this chapter, we discuss the nation's three largest health professions—nurses, physicians, and pharmacists, as well as a closely linked profession, physician assistants (Table 7–1). What are the educational pathways and licensing processes that produce the nation's practicing physicians, nurses (including nurse practitioners), pharmacists, and physician assistants? How many of these health care professionals are working in the United States, and where do they practice? Do we have the right number? Too many? Too few? How would we know if we had too many or too few? Are more women becoming physicians? Are more men becoming nurses? Is the growing racial and ethnic diversity of the nation's population mirrored in the racial and ethnic composition of the health professions? To answer these questions, we begin by providing an overview of each of these professions, describing the overall supply and educational pathways. We then discuss several crosscutting issues pertinent to all these professions.

PHYSICIANS

Susan Gasser entered medical school in 1997. During college, she had worked in the laboratory of an anesthesiologist, which made her seriously consider a career in that specialty. During her first year of medical school, the buzz among the fourth-year students was that practice opportunities were drying up fast in anesthesiology. Health maintenance organizations (HMOs) wanted more primary care physicians, not more specialists. Almost none of the fourth-year students applied to anesthesiology residency programs that year. Susan started to think more about becoming a primary care physician. In her third year of school, she had a gratifying experience during her family practice rotation working in a community health center and started to plan to apply for family practice residencies.

At the beginning of her fourth year of school, Susan spent a month in the office of a suburban family physician, Dr. Woe. Dr. Woe frequently remarked to Susan about the pressures he felt to see more patients and about how his income had fallen because of low reimbursement and higher practice expenses. He mentioned that the local anesthesiology group was having difficulty finding a new anesthesiologist to join the group to help keep up with all the surgery being performed in the area. The group was guaranteeing a first-year salary that was twice what Dr. Woe earned as an experienced family physician. Susan quickly began to reconsider applying to anesthesiology residency programs.

Approximately 873,000 physicians are professionally active in the United States. One-third are in primary care fields, and two-thirds in non–primary care fields. Of physicians who have completed residency training, more than 90% have patient care as their principal activity, with the remainder primarily active in teaching, research, or administration (US

Table 7-1. Number of active practitioners in selected health professions in the United States, by profession and year

Registered nurses (2008)	2,596,400
Nurse practitioners (2008)	141,200
Physicians (2010)	872,900
Pharmacists (2010)	251,100
Dentists (2004)	170,000
Physical therapists (2004)	145,000
Psychologists (2004)	98,000
Chiropractors (2004)	86,600
Physician assistants (2010)	60,000
Optometrists (2004)	23,000

Source: New York Center for Health Workforce Studies. The United States Health Workforce Profile. Health Resources and Services Administration; 2006. US Department of Health and Human Services. The Physician Workforce: Projections and Research Into Current Issues Affecting Supply and Demand. Health Resources and Services Administration, Bureau of Health Professions, 2008a. US Department of Health and Human Services. The Adequacy of Pharmacist Supply, 2004–2030. Health Resources and Services Administration, Bureau of Health Professions, 2008b. US Department of Health and Human Services. The Registered Nurse Population. Findings From the 2008 National Sample Survey of Registered Nurses. Health Resources and Services Administration, Bureau of Health Professions, 2010.
Note: Nurse practitioners are a subset of registered nurses.

Department of Health and Human Services, 2008a). Licensing of all types of health care professionals, including physicians, is a state jurisdiction. State medical boards require that physicians applying for licensure document a passing grade on national licensing examinations, certification of graduation from medical school, and (in most states) completion of at least one year of residency training after medical school.

▶ Medical Education

The University of Pennsylvania opened the first medical school in the colonies in 1765, promoting a curriculum that emphasized the therapeutic powers of blood letting and intestinal purging. Many other medical sects coexisted in this era, including the botanics, "natural bonesetters," midwives, and homeopaths, without any one group winning dominance. Few regulations impeded entry into a medical career; physicians were as likely to have completed informal apprenticeships as to have graduated from medical schools. Most medical schools operated as small, proprietary establishments profiting their physician owner rather than as university-centered academic institutions (Starr, 1982).

The modern era of the US medical profession dates to the 1890–1910 period. In 1893, the opening of the Johns Hopkins University School of Medicine ushered in a new tradition of medical education. Johns Hopkins University implemented many features that remain the standard of medical education in the United States: a 4-year course of study at the graduate school level, competitive selection of students, emphasis on the scientific paradigms of clinical and laboratory science, close linkage between a medical school and a medical center hospital, and cultivation of academically renowned faculty.

The second key event in the creation of a reformed twentieth-century medical profession was the publication of the Flexner Report in 1910. At the behest of the American Medical Association, the Carnegie Foundation for the Advancement in Teaching commissioned Abraham Flexner to perform an evaluation of medical education in the United States. Flexner's report indicted conventional medical education as conducted by most proprietary, nonuniversity medical schools. Flexner held up the example of Johns Hopkins as the standard by which the nation's institutions of medical education should be judged. Flexner's report was extremely influential. More than 30 medical schools closed in the decades following the Flexner Report, and academic standards at the surviving schools became much more stringent (Starr, 1982). More vigorous regulatory activities in respect to credentialing of medical schools and licensure for medical practice soon enforced the standards promoted in the Flexner Report, and only schools meeting the standards of the Licensing Council on Medical Education (LCME) were allowed to award MD degrees. Unlike the state boards licensing practice entry, which are government agencies, the LCME was a private agency operating under the authority of medical professional organizations. LCME-accredited schools became known as "allopathic" medical schools to distinguish themselves from homeopathic schools and practitioners. Although homeopaths still practice in the United States (there is now a resurgence of homeopathic practitioners), homeopaths are not officially sanctioned as "physicians" by licensing agencies in the United States. However, one alternative medical tradition has survived in the United States that carries the official imprimatur of the physician rank—osteopathy. Osteopathy originated as a medical practice developed by a Missouri physician, Andrew Still, in the 1890s, emphasizing mechanical manipulation of the body as a therapeutic maneuver (Starr, 1982). Schools of osteopathy award DO degrees and have their own accrediting organization. Much of the educational content of modern-day osteopathic medical schools has converged with that of allopathic schools. Most state licensing boards grant physicians with MD and DO degrees equivalent scopes of practice, such as prescriptive authority. By the middle of the twentieth century, regulatory restrictions on practice entry, institutionalization of a rigorous standard of academic training, and the rapid growth of medical science and technology solidified the prestige and authority of licensed physicians in the United States.

In 2010, allopathic schools had 16,838 graduates, and osteopathic schools 3631. The annual number of allopathic school graduates changed little between 1980 and 2008, and only started to increase in 2009 in response to a new surge of medical school expansion starting in the first decade of the twenty-first century. In contrast, the annual number of osteopathic graduates has grown steadily over past decades, increasing threefold between 1980 and 2010.

▶ Postdoctoral Education

At least one year of formal education after medical school is required for licensure in most states, and most physicians complete additional training to become certified in a particular specialty. Traditionally, the first year of postdoctoral training was referred to as an "internship," with subsequent years referred to as "residency." Before the advent of specialization, many physicians completed only a single year of a general "rotating" internship. Physicians aspiring to full specialty training became residents (with trainees often literally "residing" in the hospital because of endless hours of on-call duty). Now, almost all physicians in the United States complete a full residency training experience.

Residency training is much more decentralized than medical school education. Although some residency training programs are integrated into the same large academic medical centers that are home to the nation's allopathic medical schools, many smaller community hospitals sponsor residency-training programs, often in only one or two specialties. The Accreditation Council for Graduate Medical Education (ACGME), a private agency, accredits allopathic residency training programs. Residency training ranges from 3 years for generalist fields, such as family medicine and pediatrics, through 4 to 5 years for specialty training in fields such as surgery and obstetrics–gynecology, to 6 years or longer for physicians pursuing highly subspecialized training. Some osteopathic schools sponsor osteopathic residency programs.

Once physicians have completed residency training, another private consortium, the American Board of Medical Specialties, certifies physicians for board certification in their particular specialty field. Criteria for board certification usually consist of completion of training in an ACGME-accredited program and passing of an examination administered by the specific specialty board (eg, the American Board of Pediatrics). Board certification is not required for state licensure. Physicians may advertise to patients their status as specialty board-certified to promote their expertise and qualifications, and board certification may be a factor considered by hospitals when deciding whether to allow a physician to have "privileges" to care for patients in the hospital or for managed care organizations deciding whether to include a physician in the organization's physician network. Many specialty boards now require periodic reexamination to maintain certification.

Each year, approximately 25% more physicians enter ACGME residency programs than the number of students graduating from US allopathic medical schools. Who fills these extra residency positions? Approximately 7% are filled by graduates of schools of osteopathy; half of DO graduates enter allopathic residencies rather than residency programs sponsored by schools of osteopathy. The remainder of the ACGME residency positions are filled by physicians who graduated from medical schools outside the United States. A complex regulatory structure exists to govern which international medical graduates are eligible to enter residency training in the United States, involving state licensing board sanctioning of the graduate's foreign medical school and graduates completing US medical licensing examinations. There is almost no opportunity for international graduates to become licensed to practice in the United States without first undergoing residency training in the United States, even if the physician has been fully trained abroad and has years of practice experience. Some international medical graduates are US citizens who decided to train abroad, often because they were not admitted to a US medical school. However, the majority are not US residents, and most of these physicians come from India, the Philippines, sub-Saharan Africa, and other developing nations (Mullan, 2005). International medical graduates who are not US citizens receive only a temporary educational visa while in residency training, and in principle there is an expectation that these individuals will return to their nations of origin once they have completed training. However, various visa-waiver programs exist to allow these physicians to remain in the United States after completing training, usually linked to a period of service in a US community with a physician shortage. Controversy exists about this reliance on international medical graduates to meet US physician workforce needs, with critics arguing that the United States fosters a "brain drain," depleting developing nations of vital human resources (Mullan, 2005).

▶ Financing Medical Education

Who pays the cost of medical education in the United States? Unlike the case in most developed nations, where medical schools levy no or only nominal tuition, students pay high amounts of tuition and fees to attend US medical schools. Approximately half of US medical schools are public state institutions, with state tax revenues helping to subsidize medical school education. The Federal Government plays a minor role in financing medical student education, but is a major source of funds to support residency training. Medicare allocates "graduate medical education" funding to hospitals that sponsor residency programs. These funds are considerable, amounting to $9.5 billion annually, and include "direct" education payments for resident stipends and faculty salaries plus indirect education payments to defray other costs associated with being a teaching hospital. The joint federal–state Medicaid programs contribute an additional $3 billion annually to residency education (Iglehart, 2010). Although in 1997, Medicare capped the number of residency program slots it would

pay for, Medicare gives hospitals considerable latitude in how to spend their Medicare medical education dollars. Hospitals can decide which specialties, and how many slots in each specialty, they wish to sponsor for residency training, and can qualify for Medicare education payments as long as the positions are ACGME accredited. Hospitals may also invest non-Medicare revenues in their residency education programs and are not beholden to a prescriptive national workforce planning policy. Hospitals have tended to preferentially add new residency positions in non–primary care fields, guided more by the value of residents as low-cost labor to staff hospital-based specialty services than by an assessment of regional physician workforce needs and priorities. Between 2002 and 2007, hospitals added nearly 8000 new residency positions despite the cap on Medicare-funded positions, with virtually all the gains occurring in specialist positions and family medicine residency positions losing ground during the same period (Salsberg et al, 2008).

PHYSICIAN ASSISTANTS

Jillian Boca was a speech therapist at a community hospital. She liked her work but wanted to advance in her career. She was talking to some of her colleagues who were physical therapists and x-ray technicians; they were thinking of going back to school to become physician assistants. One of the registered nurses at the hospital was also planning to go back to school to become a nurse practitioner. A local medical school sponsored a program with physician assistant and nurse practitioner students receiving their training together. Jillian and two of her colleagues were admitted to the program.

As the name suggests, physician assistants (PAs) are closely linked with physicians. The profession of PA originated in the United States in 1965 with the establishment of the first PA training program at Duke University School of Medicine. The PA profession developed to fill the niche of a broadly skilled clinician who could be trained without the many years of medical school and residency education required to produce a physician, and who would work in close collaboration with physicians to augment the effective medical workforce, especially in primary care fields and underserved communities. The first wave of PAs trained in the United States included many veterans who had acquired considerable clinical skills working as medical corpsmen in the Vietnam War. PA training programs served as an efficient means to allow these veterans to "retool" their skills for civilian practice.

The American Academy of Physician Assistants defines PAs as "health professionals licensed to practice medicine with physician supervision" (Jones, 2007). PAs are usually licensed by the same state boards that license physicians, with the requirement that PAs work under the delegated authority of a physician. In practical terms, "delegated authority" means that PAs are permitted to perform many of the tasks performed by physicians as long as the tasks are performed under physician supervision. Studies of PAs in primary care settings have found that their scope overlaps with approximately 80% of the scope of work of primary care physicians. To be eligible for licensure in most states, PAs must have graduated from an accredited training program and pass the Physician Assistant National Certifying Examination, administered by the National Commission on Certification of Physician Assistants. Approximately 60,000 PAs are professionally active in the United States. Traditionally, the majority of PAs worked in primary care fields. However, currently only one-third of PAs now practice in primary care, with many finding employment opportunities in surgical and medical specialty fields (Jones, 2007). PAs work in diverse settings, including private physician offices, community clinics, HMOs, and hospitals.

▶ Physician Assistant Education

PA training has been described as a "condensed version of medical school" (Jones, 2007). The duration of training ranges from 20 to 36 months, with an average of 27 months (Hooker, 2006). Many of the initial training programs did not award degrees and accepted applicants with varying levels of prior formal education. Currently, of the 136 accredited PA training programs in the United States, 79% award a master's degree and require applicants to have attained a baccalaureate degree (Jones, 2007). Approximately half of PA training programs are based at academic health centers and are directly affiliated with medical schools. Several PA programs have established postgraduate training programs, typically one year in duration and focused on subspecialty training.

PA programs produce about 5,600 graduates annually, compared with the 20,500 graduates of allopathic and osteopathic medical schools. Enrollment in PA programs has grown steadily over the past decades, with the number of PA graduates more than doubling between 1990 and 2010.

REGISTERED NURSES

Felicia Comfort has worked for 20 years as a registered nurse on hospital medical–surgical wards. Although the work has always been hard, Felicia has found it gratifying to care for patients when they are acutely ill and need the clinical skills and compassion of a good nurse. But lately the work seems even more difficult. The pressure to get patients in and out of the hospital as soon as possible has meant that the only patients occupying hospital beds are those who are severely ill and require a tremendous amount of nursing care. At age 45, Felicia finds that her back has problems tolerating the physical labor of moving patients around in bed. Making matters worse, the hospital recently decided to "re-engineer" its staffing as a cost containment strategy and has hired more nursing aides and fewer registered nurses, adding to Felicia's work responsibilities. Felicia decides that it is time for a change. She takes a job as a visiting nurse with a home health care agency, providing services to patients after their discharge from a hospital. She likes the pace of her new job and finds the greater clinical independence refreshing after her years of dealing with rigid hospital regimentation of nurses and physicians.

Registered nurses represent the single largest health profession in the United States. In 2008, approximately 3,000,000 registered nurses were licensed in the United States (US Department of Health and Human Services, 2010). Approximately 80% of licensed registered nurses are actively employed in nursing jobs, with most of these nurses working full-time. In 2008, hospitals were the primary employment setting for 62% of nurses. Approximately 25% work in ambulatory care or other community-based settings, and 5% in long-term care facilities. The national licensing examination for registered nurses is administered by the National Council of

State Boards of Nursing, a nonprofit organization comprising representatives of each of the state boards of nursing.

Registered Nurse Education

Historically, many nurses received their education in vocational programs administered by hospitals not integrated into colleges and universities. These programs awarded diplomas of nursing rather than college degrees and tended to have the least demanding curricula. Over time, nursing education shifted into academic institutions. Most nurses are now educated either in 2- to 3-year associate degree programs administered by community colleges, or in baccalaureate programs administered by 4-year colleges. Of nurses active in 2008, 20% received their basic nursing training in diploma programs, 45% in associate degree programs, and 34% in baccalaureate degree programs (US Department of Health and Human Services, 2010). Many nursing leaders have called for nursing education to move almost completely to baccalaureate-level programs. At least one study has found that patient outcomes are better when hospitals are staffed with baccalaureate, trained nurses (Aiken et al, 2003). Of the nurses sitting for the national licensing examination in 2005, only 4% attended diploma programs. However, associate degree programs have remained a more affordable and accessible option than baccalaureate programs for many students, with nearly twice as many new registered nurses coming from community college programs as from baccalaureate programs.

Enrollment in registered nurse training programs has had a cyclical pattern over recent decades, corresponding to perceptions of surpluses and shortages in the labor market for nurses. The number of US-educated nurses taking the national licensing examination for the first time (a proxy for new nurse graduates) increased by approximately 50% between 1990 and 1995, reaching 96,610 in 1995, and then fell back to 1990 levels by 2000 (National Council of State Boards of Nursing, 2006). Graduation numbers have recently rebounded in response to aggressive advertising campaigns promoting nursing as a career, such as the Campaign for Nursing's Future led by the Johnson & Johnson Company, and large increases in starting salaries for nurses. In 2006, nearly 110,000 nurses graduated from US programs (National Council of State Boards of Nursing, 2006).

Historically, most registered nurses in the United States were educated at US schools. However, as the numbers of US nursing graduates decreased in the late 1990s and hospital demand for nurse labor increased, growing numbers of foreign-educated nurses began entering the US health workforce. Unlike the situation for physicians, international nursing school graduates do not have to undergo training in the United States to become eligible for licensure. They may sit for the US registered nurse licensing examination, and upon passing the examination may apply for an occupational visa to work as a nurse. According to Dr. Linda Aiken, the United States has now become the "world's largest importer of nurses," with approximately 15,000 internationally trained nurses passing the US licensing examination in 2005 (Aiken, 2007). Approximately one-third of internationally educated nurses in the United States immigrated from a single nation, the Philippines. This recent upswing in nurse immigration has raised the same concerns about a brain drain from developing nations that has been voiced about physician immigration.

NURSE PRACTITIONERS

Felicia Comfort has now been working as a home care nurse for 2 years. She has taken on growing responsibility as a case manager for many home care patients with chronic, debilitating illnesses, coordinating services among the physicians, physical therapists, social workers, and other personnel involved in caring for each patient. She decides that she would like to become the primary caregiver for these types of patients, and applies to a nurse practitioner training program in her area. After completing her 2 years of nurse practitioner education, she finds a job as a primary care clinician at a geriatric clinic.

Eight percent of registered nurses in the United States have obtained advanced practice education in addition to their basic nursing training (US Department of Health and Human Services, 2010). Advanced practice nurses include clinical nurse specialists, nurse anesthetists, clinical nurse midwives, and nurse practitioners. The approximately 140,000 professionally active nurse practitioners represent the largest single group of advanced practice nurses.

Nurse practitioner education typically involves a 2-year master's degree program for individuals who previously attained a baccalaureate degree in nursing. Education emphasizes primary care, prevention, and health promotion, preparing nurse practitioners for a broad scope of clinical practice, although some training programs also prepare nurse practitioners for work in non–primary care fields. Approximately 50% to 60% of nurse practitioners work in primary care settings.

Many nurse practitioner programs were established in the 1970s with federal funding as part of the same national effort to boost the number of primary care clinicians that gave rise to PA training programs. Enrollment in nurse practitioner programs grew slowly in the 1980s and exploded in the 1990s, with the number of nurse practitioner training programs more than doubling between 1992 and 1997. Whereas 1500 nurse practitioners graduated in 1992, more than 8000 graduated in 1997 (Hooker and Berlin, 2002). Unlike the trend for PAs, the number of annual nurse practitioner graduates has decreased in recent years, falling to approximately 6500 graduates in 2005 (Hooker, 2006); the number of graduates is projected to decrease further to 4000 annually by 2015 (Robert Graham Center, 2005). The causes of this decrease are multifactorial, including an initial pent-up demand for advanced practice training among the existing pool of registered nurses that was met by the expansion of programs in the 1990s, leaving a lower "steady state" demand once the initial demand was met, and increases in salaries for registered nurses that has lessened the additional earnings that may be gained by advanced practice training.

Licensing and related regulations for nurse practitioners are less uniform across states than those for physicians, physician assistants, and registered nurses. Slightly more than half of state nursing boards require nurse practitioners to have attained a master's degree, but other states accept less extensive training (Christian et al, 2007). Rather than a single national licensing examination for all nurse practitioners, certification examinations are administered by different organizations and are specialty-specific, akin to medical specialty board certification. State boards of nursing also vary in the scope of practice they allow nurse practitioners. Most states require that nurse practitioners work in collaboration with a physician, usually with written practice protocols in place. Eleven states have more liberal regulations permitting nurse practitioners to practice with complete independence from physicians, while at the other extreme, 10 states require physicians to directly supervise nurse practitioners (Christian et al, 2007).

Similar to physician assistants, nurse practitioners working in primary care settings typically perform approximately 80% of the types of tasks performed by physicians. Two meta-analyses provide evidence that nurse practitioners can deliver care of equivalent quality to that delivered by primary care physicians (Brown and Grimes, 1995; Horrocks et al, 2002), with the caveat that most studies reviewed included small numbers of clinicians and few examined long-term outcomes for patients with chronic illness or complex conditions.

Much of the initial impetus for developing training programs for both nurse practitioners and PAs in the 1960s was to create substitutes for physicians in an era when there was a perceived shortage of physicians, especially in primary care fields. As concerns about a physician shortage waned in subsequent decades and the era of cost containment arrived, substitution came to mean less a matter of filling shortages than of finding a less expensive type of clinician to substitute for physician labor. A different view of nurse practitioners and PAs sees them less as physician substitutes than as complements in a health care team that includes a variety of personnel. In this view, each profession brings its own unique training and skills to create a health care team in which the whole is more than the sum of its parts (Wagner, 2000). For example, care of patients with chronic diseases such as diabetes is enhanced by multidisciplinary teams (Grumbach and Bodenheimer, 2004). In these types of teams, nurse practitioners often play a leading role by providing care management, health promotion, and instruction in patient self-care, while physicians focus more on medication management and treatment of acute complications.

The boldest effort to promote advance practice nurses as substitutes for physicians comes from proponents of doctoral-level professional degrees for nurses, known as doctor of nursing practice (DrNP) degrees. A few DrNP training programs have been established in the United States, involving a 4-year graduate education experience following the initial baccalaureate nursing training. Leaders of these programs have articulated the vision of producing nursing graduates carrying the title of "doctor" who will be able to practice autonomously with a scope equivalent to that of physicians, including independent practice in acute care hospital settings. Whether there will be ample numbers of registered nurses interested in pursuing this level of training, along with sufficient liberalization of state scope of practice regulations, to actualize this vision for DrNPs in the health workforce in the United States remains to be determined.

PHARMACISTS

Rex Hall has worked for 5 years as a pharmacist at a chain drug store. He is not sure that his extensive professional education and skills as a pharmacist are being fully utilized in his current job. Some of his time is spent discussing possible drug interactions with physicians and suggesting alternative drug regimens, as well as counseling patients about side effects and proper use of their medications. But too much of his time is taken up answering calls from physicians and patients who are ordering prescription refills, counting out pills, filling pill bottles, and figuring out which medications are covered by which health plan. He sees a job posting for a new pharmacist position at a local hospital. The job description states that the pharmacist will review drug use in the hospital and develop strategies to work with physicians, nurses, and other staff to minimize drug errors and inappropriate prescribing practices. Rex decides to apply for the job.

Pharmacists constitute the nation's third largest health care profession. About 250,000 pharmacists were actively practicing in 2010 (US Department of Health and Human Services, 2008b). Although historically most pharmacists were educated in baccalaureate degree programs, in 2004 all programs were required to extend the training period by 1 to 2 years and award Doctorate of Pharmacy degrees. Pharmacy education is in a period of expansion, with the number of accredited schools increasing from 82 in 2000 to 119 in 2011, and the number of graduates growing from 7300 in 2000 to 11,500 in 2010 (US Department of Health and Human Services, 2008b). Approximately 60% of pharmacists work in retail pharmacies, mostly as employees rather than as owners. Over the past decades, drug store chains such as Walgreens and Longs have largely displaced the independently owned pharmacy. Hospitals are the second largest employer of pharmacists, with HMOs and other managed care organizations, long-term care facilities, and clinics

also offering practice settings for pharmacists. The content of pharmacists' work is changing, as noted in the vignette above and in a further discussion later in this chapter.

SOCIAL WORKERS

Social work is a growing profession, with the number of social workers projected to increase from 642,000 in 2008 to 745,000 in 2018; 43% of social workers are dedicated to health care, with about half of these in the fields of mental health and substance abuse. Social workers are trained in assessment skills, diagnostic impressions, psychosocial support to patients and families; and assistance with navigation of the health and social service systems including transitions between hospital, extended care facilities, and home. Some specific tasks carried out by social workers include assessing patients' personal, behavioral, and family/home/job situation for the health care team, connecting patients to durable medical equipment and in-home services, finding placements for hospital in-patients unable to go home, helping patients to get health insurance and other community services, investigating possible neglect or abuse, and counseling patients on healthy behavior change (Kitchen and Brook, 2005).

The minimum educational requirement is a bachelor's degree, but most social work positions in the health care field require a masters in social work plus state licensure. Licensed clinical social workers (LCSWs) must have at least a master's degree plus 2 years of academic and practical experience in the field, during which they serve as members of care teams in hospital, primary care, and behavioral health settings. LCSWs may be generalists or be specialized in the management of geriatric patients, children, or persons with developmental disabilities, mental health, and substance abuse diagnoses.

SUPPLY, DEMAND, AND NEED

Justin Case began his premed studies in college in 1993. He was taken aback one morning to read an article in the newspaper reporting that a prestigious national commission had just issued a report declaring that the United States was training too many physicians and that medical schools should reduce their enrollment by 25%. Nonetheless, he

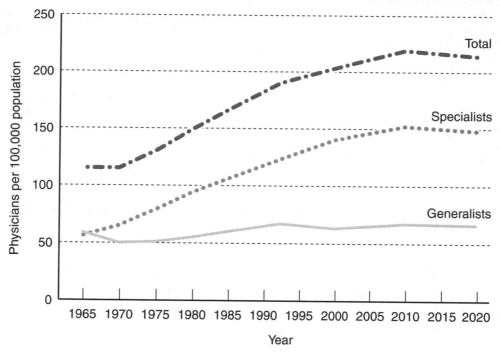

▲ **Figure 7–1.** Supply of practicing physicians in the United States. Note: Includes patient care physicians who have completed training, and excludes physicians employed by the federal government (Council on Graduate Medical Education (COGME). *Patient Care Physician Supply and Requirements: Testing COGME Recommendations.* US Department of Health and Human Services; 1996 [HRSA-P-DM 95–3].)

pressed on in his studies, medical schools did not decrease the number of first-year positions, and Justin succeeded in gaining admission to medical school. By the time he finished his residency training in internal medicine in 2004, he was hearing reports that the United States was facing a shortage of physicians and he received many offers to join medical practices as a primary care internist. However, he opted to do a fellowship in cardiology at a prominent cardiac center in Miami, FL. One of his classmates warned him that Miami already had more cardiologists than most cities of comparable size. Justin told his friend, "I'm not worried about finding a good job in Miami when I finish my fellowship. Everyone tells me that there will always be more than enough work for interventional cardiologists in Florida."

The supply of health workers in all the professions discussed in this chapter has been growing over past decades (Figures 7–1 to 7–3). Between 1975 and 2005, the number of active registered nurses per capita in the United States nearly doubled, the number of physicians per capita grew by approximately 75%, and the number of pharmacists per capita increased by approximately 50%. Increases in the supply of PAs and nurse practitioners have been even more dramatic. For physicians, virtually all the growth in supply is accounted for by increasing numbers of non–primary care specialists. Interestingly, although supply has steadily increased during these years, health workforce analysts have alternated between sounding alarms about shortages and surpluses of physicians and nurses. For example, in the 1980s and 1990s, several commissions warned of a surplus of physicians in the United States (Graduate Medical Education National Advisory Committee, 1981; Pew Health Professions Commission, 1995; Council on Graduate Medical Education, 1996). By the early years of the twenty-first century, some policy analysts were declaring a physician shortage (Council on

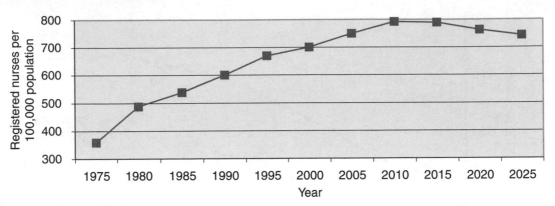

▲ **Figure 7–2.** Supply of active registered nurses per 100,000 population in the United States. (Peter I. Buerhaus, PhD, RN, FAAN, Douglas O. Staiger, PhD, and David I. Auerbach, PhD, *The Future of the Nursing Workforce in the United States: Data, Trends and Implications,* 2009: Jones & Bartlett Publishers, Sudbury, MA. www.jbpub.com. Reprinted with permission.)

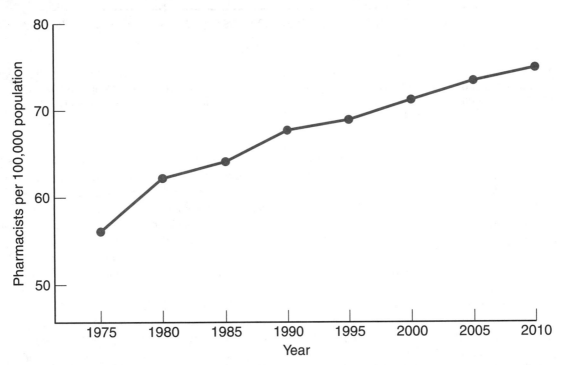

▲ **Figure 7–3.** Supply of active pharmacists per 100,000 population in the United States. (Bureau of Health Professions. *The Pharmacist Workforce. A Study of the Supply and Demand for Pharmacists.* Rockville, MD: Health Resources and Services Administration; 2000.)

Graduate Medical Education, 2005). Similarly, concerns about an oversupply of nurses in the mid-1990s were supplanted in 1998 by declarations of a nursing shortage (Buerhaus et al, 2000).

What explains why perceptions turned from surplus to shortage when supply was continuing to increase? One concern was that overall supply trends might present a misleading picture of the actual labor participation of health care professionals. For example, female physicians work on average fewer hours per week than male physicians. Women constitute a growing share of the physician workforce, and therefore head counts of the number of practicing physicians may overstate the full-time equivalent supply of physicians. In nursing, concerns were voiced that overly stressful working conditions on hospital wards were driving licensed nurses out of the workforce. This concern was magnified by the fear that the sudden plummeting of enrollment in nursing schools portended a major downturn in entry of newly trained nurses into the workforce.

However, the supply of health care professionals is only one part of the equation for determining the adequacy of the workforce. The other part of the equation is a judgment about how many physicians, nurses, or pharmacists are actually required. Even when the supply of health care professionals per capita is growing, there may be a perception of a workforce shortage if the requirements for these workers are judged to be increasing more rapidly than supply. There are two general schools of thought about how to define health workforce requirements (Grumbach, 2002). One view considers market demand as the arbiter of workforce requirements. According to this view, if there is unmet market demand for, let us say, nurses, as indicated by many vacant nursing positions at hospitals, then a shortage exists. Or, to the contrary, if many nurses are unemployed or underemployed, a surplus exists. An alternative approach defines workforce requirements on the basis of population need rather than market demand. For example, a need-based approach for nursing would attempt to evaluate whether a certain level of nursing supply optimizes patient outcomes, such as by determining whether higher registered nurse staffing levels for a given volume and acuity of hospital inpatients result in fewer medication errors and hospital-acquired infections and better overall patient outcomes.

In the case of registered nursing, both demand and need perspectives converged to conclude that a shortage

existed in the late 1990s (Bureau of Health Professions, 2002). As the intensity of hospital care increased and hospitals sought more highly trained registered nurses to staff their facilities, vacancy rates increased for hospital nurses. In response, hospitals began to increase wages to attract nurses into the workforce. Researchers around this time also began to produce evidence that lower levels of registered nurse staffing in hospitals were associated with worse clinical outcomes for hospitalized patients (Aiken et al, 2002; Needleman et al, 2002), suggesting a true medical need for more registered nurses in hospitals. One state, California, proceeded to codify a need-based approach to nurse supply by enacting legislation requiring a minimum nurse staffing level per occupied hospital bed (Spetz, 2004). In response to concerns about a nurse shortage, comprehensive strategies have been implemented that appear to be succeeding in attracting more applicants to nursing programs, increasing enrollment in these programs, and increasing the proportion of licensed nurses who are working as nurses. These strategies include actions by private entities, such as hospitals increasing wages for nurses and the Johnson & Johnson–sponsored advertising campaign mentioned above, and actions by government agencies, such as appropriating more funds for expansion of community and state college nursing program capacity.

The case of the physician workforce has been less straightforward. While most nurses work as employees of hospitals or other employers, most physicians are self-employed or part-owners of a medical group that acts as their employer, making vacancy rates or other typical labor market metrics less reliable indicators of the demand for physicians. Moreover, physicians' authority and influence over medical care give them considerable market power and create opportunities for supplier-induced demand (see Chapter 9), particularly when costs are covered by third-party payers. In a health care environment like that in the United States, in which demand for physician labor may be almost limitless, physicians tend to keep busy even as supply continues to rise. Dr. Richard Cooper has been the most vocal advocate of the position that the United States currently faces a physician shortage, based on his view that the public's demand for physician services is increasing rapidly because of an aging population and the expanding national economy, while growth in physician supply per capita in the United States is beginning to level off

(Cooper et al, 2002). Countering this view has been research that raises questions about whether the public really needs and benefits from more physicians, particularly more specialists. Studies comparing patient outcomes across regions in the United States have found that while a very low supply of physicians is associated with higher mortality, once supply is even modestly greater, patients derive little further survival benefit (Goodman and Grumbach, 2008). For example, mortality rates for high-risk newborns are worse in regions with a very low supply of neonatologists than in regions with a somewhat greater supply, but above that level, further increases in the supply of neonatologists are not associated with better clinical outcomes for newborns (Goodman et al, 2002). At the other age extreme, Medicare beneficiaries residing in areas with high physician supply do not report better access to physicians or higher satisfaction with care and do not receive better quality of care (Goodman and Grumbach, 2008). One exception to these patterns is when studies focus on primary care physician supply, rather than on overall physician supply or the supply of specialists. These studies tend to find that patient outcomes and quality of care are better in regions with a more primary care-oriented physician workforce (Baicker and Chandra, 2004; Starfield et al, 2005). Proponents of a need-based approach to physician workforce planning argue that because much of physician training is supported by tax dollars, and because there is little true market restraint on demand for medical care, society should plan physician supply based on considerations of quality, affordability, and prioritization of health care services informed by the type of research evidence cited above (Grumbach, 2002).

In assessing the adequacy of health care professional supply, it is important not just to count the number of workers, but to examine how these workers are deployed. The quest for effective deployment of the workforce has been characterized using the following analogy: "Before adding another spoonful of sugar to your tea, first stir up the sugar already in your tea cup." In other words, does the health system make the most of its existing supply of highly trained health care professionals? The case of the pharmacist workforce highlights this issue. As has been the case for nurses and physicians, concerns have recently been raised about a shortage of pharmacists. One of the factors cited is the steep rise in the prescribing of medications, which may be considered an indicator of the demand for pharmacists. Approximately 3.6 billion prescriptions were dispensed in 2005, 70% more than in 1994 (US Health and Human Services, 2008b). The estimated number of prescriptions filled per pharmacist in retail pharmacies grew from 17,400 in 1992 to 22,900 in 1999 (Bureau of Health Professions, 2000). In response, pharmacies sought to hire more pharmacists, and between 1998 and 2000, the number of unfilled pharmacist positions in chain store pharmacies more than doubled (Bureau of Health Professions, 2000; Cooksey et al, 2002). Partly in response to increased output from pharmacy schools, the percentage of pharmacist employment positions unfilled dropped from 9% to 5% between 2000 and 2004 (US Department of Health and Human Services, 2008b).

Although these trends would suggest a shortage of pharmacists based on a traditional demand model, some observers have questioned whether the existing supply of pharmacists is optimally deployed. Many pharmacists still spend a great deal of time performing the basic "pill counting" tasks of drug dispensing. Should pharmacists continue to perform most dispensing functions, or would their extensive training be better utilized in more clinically challenging activities—especially now that all newly graduated pharmacists in the United States are required to have doctoral-level training? The occupation of pharmacy technician has been developed in the United States to assist pharmacists with drug dispensing (Cooksey et al, 2002). An estimated 69% of pharmacists' time is spent on activities that properly trained technicians could perform—counting, packaging, and labeling prescriptions, and resolving third-party insurance issues. Greater use of properly supervised pharmacy technicians might increase the productivity of the existing pharmacists. In addition, innovations in automation of pill dispensing could reduce pharmacist workload. Delegating more tasks to pharmacy assistants and automated systems would allow pharmacists to optimize their clinical training and skills for patient counseling about medications, collaborating on patient safety programs to reduce the epidemic of medication errors, monitoring drug use for chronic disease management programs, and participating in multidisciplinary clinical teams in both hospitals and ambulatory settings. These same types of concerns have been raised about whether other health care professionals are being deployed with maximum efficiency and productivity and working at their highest level of skill. For example, new models of primary care are emphasizing that many preventive and chronic care tasks traditionally performed by physicians could be delegated to medical assistants and assisted by electronic technologies (Bodenheimer and Grumbach, 2007), allowing more productive use of the work effort of primary care clinicians.

WOMEN IN THE HEALTH PROFESSIONS

Dr. Jenny Wong works as a general internist for the Suburbia Medical Group. She never has to check her schedule in advance, because she knows that every appointment is always booked, not to mention the last minute add-ons. As one of only two women in a group of eleven primary care physicians, she is in demand. In particular, female patients in the practice have sought her out to become their primary care physician. While gratified to be responding to this demand, Dr. Wong also finds it a bit daunting. She senses that her patients expect her to spend more time with them to explain

diagnoses and treatments and discuss their overall well-being. But Dr. Wong has the same 15-minute appointment times as every other physician in the practice and continually finds herself falling behind in her schedule. Today Dr. Wong is feeling especially stressed. She is scheduled to meet at lunchtime with the director of Suburbia Medical Group to discuss plans for her impending maternity leave. She knows he will not take kindly to her intention of taking 4 months off after the birth of her child.

Historically, most physicians and pharmacists in the United States have been men, and most nurses women. For physicians and pharmacists, this demographic pattern is in the midst of a dramatic change. In 1970, 13% of pharmacists were women, but by 2010, more than half of pharmacists were women. The proportion of women among physicians increased from 8% in 1970 to more than 30% in 2010 (Figure 7–4). The figures are

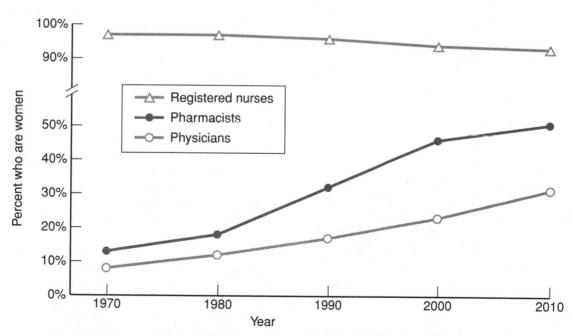

▲ **Figure 7–4.** Women as a percentage of physicians, nurses, and pharmacists in the United States. (US Department of Health and Human Services. The Physician Workforce: Projections and Research into Current Issues Affecting Supply and Demand. Health Resources and Services Administration, Bureau of Health Professions, 2008a. US Department of Health and Human Services. The Adequacy of Pharmacist Supply, 2004–2030. Health Resources and Services Administration, Bureau of Health Professions, 2008b. US Department of Health and Human Services. The Registered Nurse Population. Findings from the 2008 National Sample Survey of Registered Nurses. Health Resources and Services Administration, Bureau of Health Professions, 2010.)

even more dramatic when examining the makeup of current students in training: women constituted 47% of medical students and 61% of pharmacy students in 2010. In contrast, nursing has long been a profession mainly comprising women, and this is changing very slowly. In 2008, only 10% of registered nurses were men, up slightly from 5% in 1996.

As noted above, women, on average, work fewer hours per week than men and are more likely to work on a part-time basis. However, the practices of male and female health care professionals differ in ways other than simply the number of hours worked. Female physicians attract more female patients, in part because female patients highly value more time spent and clearer explanations from their physicians than do male patients, and female physicians spend more time with their patients than do male physicians. Several studies have shown that female physicians deliver more preventive services than male physicians, especially for their female patients (Lurie et al, 1993). Female physicians appear to communicate differently with their patients, with both adults and children, being more likely to discuss lifestyle and social concerns, and to give more information and explanations during a visit (Elderkin-Thompson and Waitzkin, 1999; Roter et al, 2002). Female physicians are more likely to involve patients in medical decision-making than male physicians (Cooper-Patrick et al, 1999).

UNDERREPRESENTED MINORITIES IN THE HEALTH PROFESSIONS

Cynthia Cuidado is the first person in her family to go to college, much less the first to become a health professional. A large contingent of her extended family celebrates her graduation from her master's degree family nurse practitioner training program. Although HMOs in the city where Cynthia trained had several open positions for nurse practitioners, she has decided to take a job at a migrant farm worker clinic in a rural community near where she grew up.

The United States is a nation of growing racial and ethnic diversity. According to the 2010 US census, African Americans, Latinos, and Native Americans now account for nearly one-third of the population, yet the health professions fail to reflect the rich racial and ethnic diversity of the US population. Only about 10% of pharmacists, 9% of physicians, 8% of physician

assistants, 10% of nurses, and 5% of dentists are from these three underrepresented racial and ethnic groups (Grumbach and Mendoza, 2008).

Health professions have made efforts to increase the number of underrepresented minorities enrolling in their training programs. In nursing, these efforts appear to be paying dividends (Figure 7–5). Underrepresented minorities as a proportion of students in baccalaureate nursing programs increased from 12.2% in 1991 to 18.1% in 2005. Medical schools have experienced a different trend. Underrepresented minorities as a percentage of medical students increased in the early 1990s, from 12.2% in 1991 to 15.5% in 1997. However, the percentage of underrepresented minority medical students dropped after 1997, falling to 13.9% in 2005. The decrease in underrepresented minority student enrollment in medical schools beginning in the mid-1990s coincided with the onset of a wave of antiaffirmative action policies, such as Proposition 209 in California and the Hopwood vs. Texas federal court ruling that curtailed the ability of university admissions committees to give special consideration to applicants' race and ethnicity (Grumbach and Mendoza, 2008). Pharmacy schools also showed little net increase in underrepresented minority enrollment, with 11% of pharmacy students in 1990 and 2010 being from underrepresented minority groups.

The problem of underrepresented minorities in the health professions is an especially compelling policy concern. As discussed in Chapter 3, minority communities experience poorer health and access to health care compared with communities populated primarily by non-Latino whites. Minority health care professionals are more likely to practice in underserved minority communities and serve disadvantaged patients, such as the uninsured and those covered by Medicaid (Moy and Bartman, 1995; Cantor et al, 1996; Komaromy et al, 1996; Mertz and Grumbach, 2001). Research has also found salutary effects of ethnically concordant relationships between minority patients and health care professionals on the use of preventive services, patient satisfaction, and ratings of the physician's participatory decision-making style (Saha et al, 2000; Cooper et al, 2003; US Department of Health and Human Services, 2006). Some studies focusing specifically on language concordance when patients have limited English proficiency have also found that access to language concordant clinicians is associated with better patient experiences and outcomes such as reductions in

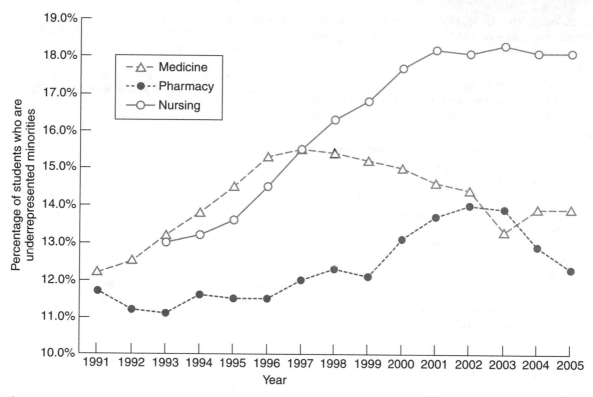

▲ **Figure 7–5.** Underrepresented minorities as a percentage of students in selected health professions in the United States. Note: Medical schools include only allopathic schools. (American Association of Colleges of Nursing, Enrollment and Graduations in Baccalaureate & Graduate Programs in Nursing; Association of American Medical Colleges, Data Warehouse. *Applicant Matriculant File.* Association of Colleges of Pharmacy, Profile of Pharmacy Students Application Trends; 2007.)

patient reports of medication errors (Wilson et al, 2005). Thus, the underrepresentation of minorities is not just a matter of equality of opportunity; it has profound implications for racial and ethnic disparities in access to care and in health status.

CONCLUSION

An intricate array of educational pathways, accreditation of teaching institutions, and credentialing of individuals to legally practice a healing profession defines the composition of the health workforce. Access, cost, and quality—the three overriding issues in health care—are all inextricably linked to trends in the health care workforce. An inadequate supply of health care professionals may impede patients' access to care or

compromise the quality of care. But increases in the supply of health care professionals may fuel intolerable escalation of health care costs. It is not surprising, then, to find disagreement about whether a health system has enough, too few, or too many of a particular class of health care professionals. The recent consensus in the United States about a shortage of registered nurses is one of the rare instances in which analyses based on demand models and on need models arrived at similar conclusions. The current debate over the adequacy of the physician workforce in the United States is more typical of the challenges in coming to agreement about the adequacy of supply, revealing how different frames of reference for judging the nation's requirement for health care professionals lead to different policy conclusions. In addition to the overall supply of health professionals, the demographic composition of the workforce in terms of gender and race–ethnicity also has important policy implications.

Although making definitive determinations about the "right" number of health care professionals often proves elusive, two conclusions may be made with more confidence. First, all health systems should deploy their workers in a manner that makes the best use of their training and skills, creating practice structures that allow each health care professional to operate at his or her highest level of capability and ensuring that those patients most in need benefit from the clinical expertise of the health care professionals working in the system. Most systems fall short of this goal and have not fully "stirred the sugar in the cup of tea," failing to continually reassess and adapt the roles and responsibilities of the members of the health care team to the changing needs of modern-day health systems. Second, all systems need to ensure that their health professionals are highly qualified and embrace a culture of continuous quality improvement (discussed in Chapter 10). To echo the opening of this chapter, a health care system is only as good as the people working in it.

REFERENCES

Aiken LH. U.S. nurse labor market dynamics are key to global nurse sufficiency. *Health Serv Res*. 2007;42:1299.

Aiken LH et al. Hospital nurse staffing and patient mortality, nurse burnout, and job dissatisfaction. *JAMA*. 2002;288:1987.

Aiken LH et al. Educational levels of hospital nurses and surgical patient mortality. *JAMA*. 2003;290:1617.

Baicker K, Chandra A. Medicare spending, the physician workforce, and beneficiaries' quality of care. *Health Affairs Web Exclusive*. 2004;(suppl):W184–W197.

Bodenheimer T, Grumbach K. *Improving Primary Care: Strategies and Tools for a Better Practice*. New York: McGraw-Hill; 2007.

Brown SA, Grimes DE. A meta-analysis of nurse practitioners and nurse midwives in primary care. *Nurs Res*. 1995;44:332.

Buerhaus PI et al. Implications of an aging registered nurse workforce. *JAMA*. 2000;283:2948.

Buerhaus PI et al. The Future of the *Nursing Workforce in the United States: Data, Trends and Implications, 2009*. Sudbury, MA: Jones & Bartlett Publishers; 2008.

Bureau of Health Professions. *The Pharmacist Workforce. A Study of the Supply and Demand for Pharmacists*. Rockville, MD: Health Resources and Services Administration; 2000.

Bureau of Health Professions. *Projected Supply, Demand, and Shortages of Registered Nurses, 2000–2020*. Rockville, MD: Health Resources and Services Administration; 2002.

Cantor JC et al. Physician service to the underserved: Implications for affirmative action in medical education. *Inquiry*. 1996;33:167.

Christian S et al. *Overview of Nurse Practitioner Scopes of Practice in the United States*. University of California, San Francisco, Center for the Health Professions; 2007. http://www.acnpweb.org/files/public/UCSF_Discussion_2007.pdf. Accessed November 14, 2011.

Cooksey JA et al. Challenges to the pharmacist profession from escalating pharmaceutical demand. *Health Aff (Millwood)*. 2002;21(5):182.

Cooper RA et al. Economic and demographic trends signal an impending physician shortage. *Health Aff (Millwood)*. 2002;21:140.

Cooper LA et al. Patient-centered communication, ratings of care and concordance of patient and physician race. *Ann Intern Med*. 2003:139:907.

Cooper-Patrick L et al. Race, gender and partnership in the patient-physician relationship. *JAMA*. 1999;282:583.

Council on Graduate Medical Education (COGME). *Eighth Report: Patient Care Physician Supply and Requirements: Testing COGME Recommendations*. Rockville, MD: Council on Graduate Medical Education; 1996.

Council on Graduate Medical Education (COGME). *Sixteenth Report: Physician Workforce Policy Guidelines for the United States, 2000–2020*. Rockville, MD: Council on Graduate Medical Education; 2005.

Elderkin-Thompson B, Waitzkin H. Differences in clinical communication by gender. *J Gen Intern Med*. 1999;14:112.

Goodman D et al. The relation between the availability of neonatal intensive care and neonatal mortality. *N Engl J Med*. 2002;346:1538–1544.

Goodman D, Grumbach K. Does having more physicians lead to better health system performance? *JAMA*. 2008;299:335.

Graduate Medical Education National Advisory Committee. *Summary Report*. DHHS Pub. No. (HRA) 81–651. Washington, DC; 1981.

Grumbach K. Fighting hand to hand over physician workforce policy. *Health Aff (Millwood)*. 2002;21(5):13.

Grumbach K, Bodenheimer T. Can health care teams improve primary care practice? *JAMA*. 2004;291:1246.

Grumbach K, Mendoza R. Disparities in human resources: Addressing the lack of diversity in the health professions. *Health Aff (Millwood)*. 2008;27(2):413.

Hooker RS. Physician assistants and nurse practitioners: the United States experience. *Med J Aust*. 2006;185:4.

Hooker RS, Berlin LE. Trends in the supply of physician assistants and nurse practitioners in the United States. *Health Aff (Millwood)*. 2002;21(5):174.

Horrocks S et al. Systematic review of whether nurse practitioners working in primary care can provide equivalent care to doctors. *BMJ*. 2002;324:819.

Iglehart J. Health reform, primary care, and graduate medical education. *N Engl J Med* 2010;363:584.

Jones PE. Physician assistant education in the United States. *Acad Med*. 2007;82:882.

Kitchen A, Brook J. Social work at the heart of the medical team. *Soc Work Health Care*. 2005;40:1

Komaromy M et al. The role of black and Hispanic physicians in providing health care for underserved populations. *N Engl J Med*. 1996;334:1305.

Lurie N et al. Preventive care for women: Does the sex of the physician matter? *N Engl J Med*. 1993;329:478.

Mertz EA, Grumbach K. Identifying communities with low dentist supply in California. *J Public Health Dent*. 2001;61:172.

Moy E, Bartman BA. Physician race and care of minority and medically indigent patients. *JAMA*. 1995;273:1515.

Mullan F. The metrics of the physician brain drain. *N Engl J Med*. 2005;353:1850.

National Council of State Boards of Nursing. *Nurse Licensure and NLCEX Examination Statistics*. 2006. https://www.ncsbn.org/1236.htm.

Needleman J et al. Nurse-staffing levels and the quality of care in hospitals. *N Engl J Med*. 2002;346:1715.

Pew Health Professions Commission. *Critical Challenges. Revitalizing the Health Professions for the Twenty-First Century*. San Francisco: UCSF Center for the Health Professions; December 1995.

Robert Graham Center Policy Studies in Family Medicine and Primary Care. *Physician Assistant and Nurse Practitioner Workforce Trends*. One-pagers, 37, 2005. http://www.aafp.org/afp/2005/1001/p1176.html. Accessed November 14, 2011.

Roter D et al. Physician gender effects in medical communication: a meta-analytic review. *JAMA*. 2002;288:756.

Salsberg E et al. US residency training before and after the 1997 Balanced Budget Act. *JAMA*. 2008;300:1174.

Saha S et al. Do patients choose physicians of their own race? *Health Aff (Millwood)*. 2000;19(4):76.

Spetz J. California's minimum nurse-to-patient ratios: The first few months. *J Nurs Adm*. 2004;34:571.

Starfield B et al. The effects of specialist supply on populations' health: assessing the evidence. *Health Aff Web Exclusives*. 2005;(suppl):W5-97—W5-107.

Starr P. *The Social Transformation of American Medicine*. New York: Basic Books; 1982.

US Department of Health and Human Services. The Rationale for Diversity in the Health Professions: A Review of the Evidence. Health Resources and Services Administration; 2006. http://bhpr.hrsa.gov/healthworkforce/reports/diversityreviewevidence.pdf.

US Department of Health and Human Services. The Physician Workforce: Projections and Research into Current Issues Affecting Supply and Demand. Health Resources and Services Administration, Bureau of Health Professions, 2008a. http://bhpr.hrsa.gov/healthworkforce/reports/physwfissues.pdf

US Department of Health and Human Services. The Adequacy of Pharmacist Supply, 2004–2030. Health Resources and Services Administration, Bureau of Health Professions, 2008b. http://bhpr.hrsa.gov/healthworkforce/reports/pharmsupply20042030.pdf

US Department of Health and Human Services. The Registered Nurse Population. Findings From the 2008 National Sample Survey of Registered Nurses. Health Resources and Services Administration, Bureau of Health Professions, 2010. http://bhpr.hrsa.gov/healthworkforce/rnsurveys/rnsurveyfinal.pdf

Wagner EH. The role of patient care teams in chronic disease management. *Br Med J*. 2000;320:569.

Wilson E et al. Effects of limited English proficiency and physician language on health care comprehension. *J Gen Intern Med*. 2005;20(9):800-806.

Painful Versus Painless Cost Control

Dr. Joshua Worthy is chief of neurology at a large staff model health maintenance organization (HMO) and serves as the physician representative to the HMO's executive committee. A national health plan has just been enacted that imposes mandatory cost controls. The HMO's budget for the coming year will be frozen at the current year's level. In past years, the annual growth in the HMO's budget has averaged 12%.

The health plan CEO begins the committee meeting by groaning, "These cuts are draconian! To meet these new budget limits we'll have to cut staff and ration life-saving technologies. Patients will suffer." A consumer member responds, "We all know there's fat in the system. Why, in the newspaper just the other day there was an article about how rates of back surgery in our city are twice the national average. And if we're going to talk about cuts, maybe we should start by looking at your salary and the number of administrators working here. I'm not so sure patients have to suffer just because we're adopting the kind of reasonable spending limits that they have in most countries."

Dr. Worthy remains silent for much of the meeting. He wonders to himself, "Is the CEO right? Is cost containment inevitably a painful process that will deprive our patients of valuable health services? Or, could we be doing a better job with the resources we're already spending? Is there a way that our HMO could implement these cost controls in a relatively painless fashion as far as our patients' health

is concerned?" Interpreting Dr. Worthy's silence as an indication of great wisdom and judgment, the committee assigns him to chair the HMO's task force charged with developing a cost control strategy to meet the new budgetary realities.

Concerns about the rise of health care costs dominate the health policy agenda in the United States. Another pressing health policy concern—lack of adequate insurance and access to care for tens of millions of people—is in part attributable to the problem of rising costs. Health care inflation has made health insurance and health services unaffordable to many families and employers.

Private and public payers in the United States have taken aim at health care inflation and discharged volleys of innovative strategies attempting to curb expenditure growth, such as creating new approaches to utilization review, encouraging HMO enrollment, making patients pay more out-of-pocket for care, and a multitude of other measures. These approaches had little noticeable impact on the rate of growth of health care costs in the United States. National health expenditures per capita increased over sevenfold between 1980 and 2009, rising from $1110 to $8086 per capita (Figure 8–1). Viewed as a percentage of gross domestic product (GDP), US health expenditures increased from 9.2% in 1980 to 17.6% in 2009 (Figure 8–2). Health expenditures as a percentage of GDP are projected to rise to 19.6% by 2019 (Sisko et al, 2010).

Health care providers are discovering that they have to adjust to the prospect of practicing in an era of

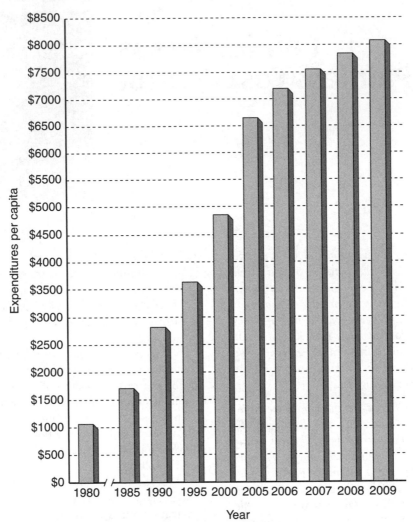

▲ **Figure 8–1.** US per capita health care expenditures. (Martin A et al. Recession contributes to slowest annual rate of increase in health spending in five decades. *Health Aff (Millwood)*. 2011;30:11.)

finite resources. Like Dr. Worthy, physicians and other health caregivers need to deliberate about how constraints on expenditure growth may affect patients' health. Must cost control necessarily be painful, leading to rationing of beneficial services? Or, is there a painless route to containing costs, reached by eliminating unnecessary medical treatments and administrative expenses?

In this chapter, the painful–painless cost control debate will be explored. First a model will be constructed describing the relationship between health care costs and benefits in terms of improved health outcomes. Then different general approaches to cost containment and their potential for achieving painless cost control will be discussed. Chapter 9 will describe specific cost control measures in more detail.

HEALTH CARE COSTS AND HEALTH OUTCOMES

Before entering medical school, Dr. Worthy worked in the Peace Corps in a remote area in Central America. At the time he first arrived in the region, the infant mortality rate was quite high, with

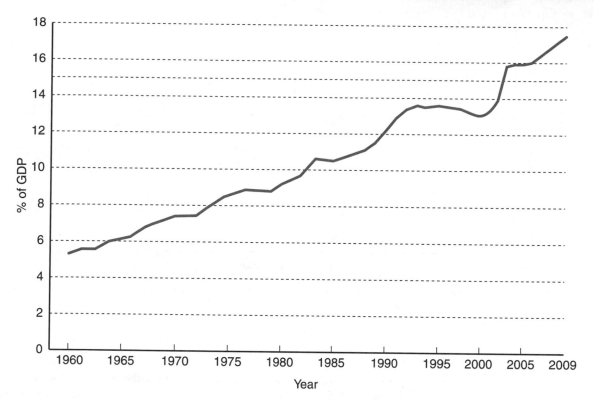

▲ **Figure 8–2.** US health care expenditures as a percentage of the gross domestic product. (Martin A et al. Recession contributes to slowest annual rate of increase in health spending in five decades. *Health Aff (Millwood).* 2011;30:11.)

many deaths due to infectious gastroenteritis. Dr. Worthy participated in the creation of a sewage treatment system and clean well-water sources for the region, as well as a program for implementing oral rehydration techniques for infants. By the end of Dr. Worthy's 2-year stay, the infant mortality rate had dropped by nearly 25%. The cost for the entire program amounted to 15 cents per capita, paid for by the World Health Organization.

Conditions have been very different for Dr. Worthy as a practicing neurologist in the United States. In the past 5 years, over a dozen new magnetic resonance imaging (MRI) scanners have been installed in the city in which his HMO is located, an urban area with a population of 800,000. Dr. Worthy has found that MRI scans provide images that are better than those of computed tomography (CT) scans,

allowing him to more accurately diagnose conditions such as multiple sclerosis in earlier stages. He is less certain about the extent to which these superior images allow superior health care for his patients.

From society's point of view, the value of health care expenditures lies in purchasing better health for the population. The concept of "better health" is a broad one, encompassing improved longevity and quality of life, reduced mortality and morbidity rates from specific diseases, relief of pain and suffering, enhanced ability to function independently for those with chronic illnesses, and reduction in fear of illness and death. Thus, it is important to know whether investing more resources in health care buys improved health outcomes for society, and if so, what magnitude of the improvement in outcomes may be relative to the amount of resources invested.

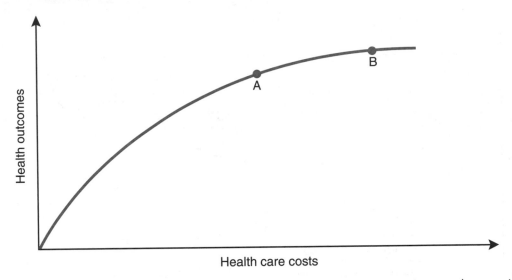

▲ Figure 8–3. A theoretic model of costs and health outcomes. Moving from point A to point B on the curve is associated with both higher costs and better health outcomes.

Figure 8–3, drawn from the work of Robert Evans (1984), illustrates a theoretic relationship between health care resource input and health care outcomes. Initially, as health care resources increase, these outcomes improve, but above a certain level, the slope of the curve diminishes, signifying that increasing investments in health care yield more marginal benefits. In terms of Dr. Worthy's experiences, the Central American region in which he worked lay on the steep slope of this cost–benefit curve: A small investment of resources to create more sanitary water supplies and to administer inexpensive rehydration therapy yielded dramatic improvements in health. On the other hand, purchasing MRI scanners to supplement CT scanners represents a health care system operating on the flatter portion of the curve: Large investments of resources in new technologies may produce more marginal and difficult-to-measure improvements in the overall health of a population.

Naturally, different medical interventions lie on steeper (eg, childhood immunizations) or on flatter (eg, the costly prolongation of life for an anencephalic infant) portions of the curve. The curve in Figure 8–3 may be viewed as an aggregate cost–benefit curve for the functioning of a health care system as a whole. The system may be an entire nation or a smaller entity such as an HMO, with its defined population of enrollees.

Overall, the US health care system currently operates somewhere along the flatter portion of the curve. Let us assume that Dr. Worthy's HMO system lies at point A on the curve in Figure 8–3, with average total health care expenditures per HMO enrollee being the same as the average overall per capita health care cost in the United States (roughly $8000 in 2009). If stringent new cost containment policies forced the HMO to virtually freeze spending at point A rather than increasing annual expenditures at their usual clip to move to point B, then Figure 8–3 implies that the HMO would sacrifice improving the health of its enrollees by an amount equal to the distance between points A and B on the vertical axis.

Such an analysis would confirm the opinion of those who argue that cost containment requires painful choices that affect the health of the population. Among the most forceful proponents of this view are Aaron and Schwartz (1984 and 1990), who have described cost containment as a "painful prescription" requiring rationing of beneficial care. In Figure 8–3, the distance between points A and B on the y axis measures how much health "pain" accompanies the decision to limit spending at point A instead of advancing to point B. Some degree of pain is inherent in the curve. As Evans (1984) observes, "if its slope is everywhere positive, then

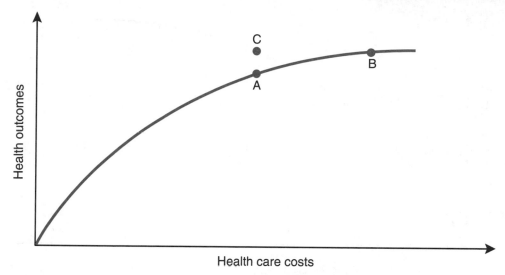

▲ **Figure 8–4.** Moving off the curve. Point C represents achievement of better health outcome without increased costs.

in a world of finite resources, unmet needs are inevitable." No matter where we sit on the curve, it will always be true that if we spent more we could do a little better.

In Figure 8–3, the distance between points A and B on the y axis is small, given the relatively flat slope of the curve at these points. But reassurances about relatively mild cost containment pain bring to mind the physician, scalpel in hand, hovering over a patient and declaring that "it will only hurt a little bit." A little pain, necessary as it may be, is not the same as no pain; or as Fuchs (1993) puts it, " 'low yield' medicine is not 'no yield' medicine."

Before allowing ourselves (and Dr. Worthy) to become overly chagrined at the inevitable painfulness of cost containment, let us add the new dimension of efficiency. We can picture a point C (Figure 8–4) at which spending is the same as that at point A, but outcomes improve. How does the model account for point C, a point off the curve?

The move to point C requires a shifting of the curve (Figure 8–5), signifying a new, more efficient (or productive) relationship between costs and health outcomes (Donabedian, 1988). There are numerous possible routes to greater efficiency. For example, diagnostic radiographic imaging services are a rapidly inflating expenditure in the United States. Research has concluded that 20% to 40% of imaging studies are not

clinically necessary, and that radiation exposure from diagnostic x-rays carries a risk of inducing malignant cancers (Brenner and Hricak, 2010). Eliminating unnecessary diagnostic radiographic procedures, such as head CT scans for patients with uncomplicated tension headaches, could simultaneously decrease health care costs and improve health. In the remainder of this chapter, we will examine in greater detail the various possible methods that Dr. Worthy's cost control task force could consider to achieve more health "bang" for the health care "buck." Before turning to this discussion, however, it is necessary to make explicit three assumptions about this model of costs and outcomes.

1. Implicit in the model is the notion that the relevant outcome of interest is the overall health of a population rather than of any one individual patient. A number of authors have emphasized the need for physicians to broaden their perspective to encompass the health of a general population, as well as their narrower traditional focus on providing the best possible care for each patient (Eddy, 1991; Greenlick, 1992). The population-oriented model of costs and outcomes depicted in Figures 8–3, 8–4, and 8–5 may not fit easily with many physicians' experiences of caring for a particular patient. At the level of the individual patient, the outcome may be

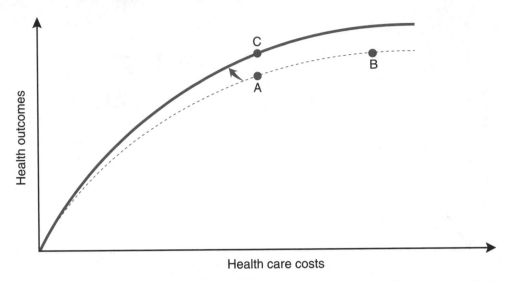

▲ **Figure 8–5.** Shifting the curve. The shift of the curve represents moving to a more efficient relationship between costs and health outcomes.

all or nothing (eg, the patient will almost certainly live if he or she receives an operation and die without it) and not easily thought about in terms of curves and slopes. Rather than focusing on any one particular intervention or patient, the curve attempts to represent the overall functioning of a health care system in the aggregate for the population under its care. (The ethical issues of the population health perspective are discussed in Chapter 13.)

2. The model assumes that it is possible to quantify health at a population level. Traditionally, health status at this level has been measured relatively crudely, using vital statistics such as life expectancy and infant mortality rates. While an index such as infant mortality rates may be a sensitive, meaningful way of evaluating the impact of health care and public health programs in rural Central America, many analysts have questioned whether such crude indicators accurately gauge the impact of health care services in wealthier industrialized nations. In these latter nations, much of health care focuses on "softer" health outcomes such as enhancement of functional status and quality of life in individuals with chronic diseases—aspects more difficult to monitor at the population level than death rates and related vital statistics. In other words, it may be

difficult to conceptualize a scale on the *y* axis of Figures 8–3, 8–4, and 8–5 that can register both the effects of managing gastroenteritis in a poor nation and the addition of MRI scanners in a US city.

3. When evaluating population health, it is difficult to disentangle the effects of health care on health from the effects of such basic social factors as poverty, education, lifestyle, and social cohesiveness (see Chapter 3). For the purpose of our discussion of cost control, we view the curves depicted in Figures 8–3, 8–4, and 8–5 as representing the workings of the health care system (including public health) per se rather than of the broader economic and social milieu. We therefore use the term *health outcomes* to describe the *y* axis, a term intended to suggest that we are evaluating those aspects of health status directly under the influence of health care. The *x* axis correspondingly represents expenditures for formal health care services.

▶ **Prices and Quantities**

We have shown that painless cost control is theoretically possible. But can efficiency be improved in the real world? What strategies could Dr. Worthy's task force propose to move the HMO from point A to point C on the curve? An answer to these questions requires further scrutiny of resource costs in the health care sector.

Costs may be described by the equation

$$\text{Cost} = \text{Price} \times \text{Quantity}$$

Price refers to such items as the hospital daily room charge or the physician fee for a routine office visit. *Quantity* represents the volume and intensity of health service use (eg, the length of stay in an intensive care unit, or the number and types of major diagnostic tests performed during a hospitalization). Lomas and colleagues (1989), noting this distinction between prices (Ps) and quantities (Qs), refer to cost containment as "minding the Ps and Qs" of health care costs.

Let us look at an example of the $C = P \times Q$ equation:

Blue Shield pays Dr. Morton $600 for 10 office visits at a fee of $60 per visit. The next year, the insurer pays Dr. Morton $720 for 10 visits at $72 per visit.

Prudential pays Dr. Norton $600 for 10 office visits, and the next year pays $720 for 12 visits at the same $60 fee. An identical cost increase is a price rise for Dr. Morton but an increase in quantity of care for Dr. Norton.

Changes in prices and quantities have different implications for patients and providers (Reinhardt, 1987). In the preceding example, both physicians increase their income (and both insurance plans increase their expenditures) by $120, though in the case of the price increase, the additional income does not require a higher volume of work. To the patient, however, only the additional $120 spent on a greater number of visits purchases more health care services. (For simplicity's sake, we assume that all visits are identical and that the price rise does not reflect increased quality of service, but simply a higher price for the same product.) A cost increase that merely represents higher prices without additional quantities of health care is an inefficient use of resources from the patient's point of view. Returning to the diagrams in Figures 8–3 and 8–4, if real costs in a health care system were rising only because medical price inflation was exceeding general price inflation while the quantity of care per capita remained static, then increased health costs would not bring about improved health outcomes, and the overall curve would become absolutely flat.

COST CONTROL STRATEGIES

▶ Controlling Price Inflation

After intense deliberation, Dr. Worthy's task force submits a plan for "painless cost containment" to the HMO executive committee. The first proposal calls for the HMO to aggressively seek discounts on the prices paid for supplies, equipment, and pharmaceuticals by having the HMO selectively contract with suppliers for bulk purchases and stock a more limited variety of product lines and drugs within the same therapeutic class. The proposal also calls for a 10% reduction in salaries for all HMO employees earning over $150,000 per year, as well as a 10% reduction in the capitation fee paid to the HMO's physician group. The executive committee never gets beyond this part of the plan, as furious argument erupts over the proposed income cuts.

Price inflation has been a major contributor to the rise of health care costs in recent decades. Between 1947 and 1987, US health care costs rose 2.5% per year faster than the growth in the overall economy. Two-thirds of this higher growth rate, or 1.6%, was due to health care prices rising more rapidly than prices in the overall economy. The remaining 0.9% differential was due to differences in the rate of increase of quantities of health care relative to increases in the overall quantity of goods and services (Fuchs, 1990).

The rapid rise of health care prices manifests itself in such ways as prices for prescription drugs in the United States often being over 50% higher than prices for the same products sold in other nations. Also, specialist physician incomes have increased rapidly. Higher prices explain much of the higher costs of health care in the United States compared with the costs in other industrialized nations (Peterson and Burton, 2007). Limiting this type of price inflation is one way to restrain expenditures without inflicting "pain" on the public's health (Table 8–1).

▶ Eliminating Ineffective and Inappropriate Care

After a brief hiatus to let the furor subside, the HMO executive committee reconvenes. Dr. Worthy introduces his task force's second recommendation— developing appropriateness of care guidelines—by recounting one of his own clinical experiences. When

Table 8–1. Examples of painless cost control

Controlling fees and provider incomes
Cutting the price of pharmaceuticals and other supplies
Reducing administrative waste
Eliminating medical interventions of no benefit
Substituting less costly technologies that are equally effective
Increasing the provision of those preventive services that cost less than the illnesses they prevent

Dr. Worthy first came to the HMO, the neurologists were keeping their stroke patients at bed rest for 1 week before initiating physical therapy. Dr. Worthy, in contrast, began physical therapy and discharge planning for stroke patients the moment their neurologic status was stable. The average length of stay in the acute hospital for his stroke patients was 3 days, compared with 9 days for other neurologists. Dr. Worthy gave a grand rounds presentation demonstrating that 4 days of exercise are required to regain the strength lost from each day of bed rest, meaning that stroke patients would have better outcomes and use fewer resources—shorter acute hospital stays and less rehabilitation—under his care than under the care of his colleagues. Dr. Worthy cites this as just one example of how the HMO may be devoting resources to ineffective, or even harmful, care.

If controlling prices is one approach to painless cost control, are there also ways to contain the "Q" (quantity) factor in a manner that does not sacrifice beneficial care? Earlier, we cited unnecessary diagnostic imaging studies as an example of a source of inefficient resource use in terms of quantities of services that add to costs without, in many cases, adding health benefits. A number of researchers have found convincing evidence of substantial amounts of unnecessary care in the United States (Brook and Lohr, 1986; Leape, 1992; Brownlee, 2007; Kilo and Larsen, 2009). Physicians in the United States perform large numbers of inappropriate procedures (Schuster et al, 1998; Deyo et al, 2009), and physicians may inappropriately and harmfully accept new technologies as a result of industry influence rather than proven efficacy (Grimes, 1993; Avorn, 2007).

Persuasive evidence comes from the work of Fisher, Wennberg and colleagues, who found that per capita Medicare costs are over twice as high in some cities (eg, Miami) than in other metropolitan areas (eg, Minneapolis). This difference is explained not by prices or degree of illness but is related to the quantity of services provided, which in turn is associated with the predominance of specialists in the higher-cost areas (Fisher et al, 2003). Moreover, residents of areas with a greater per capita supply of hospital beds are up to 30% more likely to be hospitalized than those in areas with fewer beds, after controlling for socioeconomic characteristics and disease burden (Fisher et al, 2000). As for the value of this spending, quality of care and health outcomes are, if anything, worse in the highest spending regions than in areas with less intensive use of services. These findings suggest that a great deal of unnecessary care is taking place in the high-cost areas.

The slope of the cost–benefit curve would become more favorable if a system could eliminate those components of rising expenditures that have flat slopes (no medical benefit) or negative slopes (harm exceeding benefit, as in the case of inappropriate surgical procedures or prolonged bed rest after strokes). However, inducing physicians and patients to selectively eliminate unnecessary care is no easy matter.

▶ **Administrative Waste**

The third item on Dr. Worthy's painless cost containment plan targets the HMO's administrative costs. The task force proposes eliminating the HMO's TV and radio advertising budget, laying off 25% of all HMO administrative personnel, and reassigning 25 of the 50 staff members in the department that handles contracts with employers to a new department designed to develop a program to ensure that the HMO provides up-to-date child immunizations and adult preventive care services for 100% of plan enrollees. The HMO's marketing director patiently explains to Dr. Worthy that although he, in principle, agrees with these recommendations, he does not consider it in the HMO's best interest to cut costs in a way that jeopardizes the plan's ability to maintain its market share of enrollees.

Not all quantities in the health care cost equation are clinical in nature. The tremendous administrative overhead of the US health care system has come under increasing scrutiny in recent years as a source of inefficiency in health care expenditures. Woolhandler and colleagues (2003) have estimated that as many as 31 cents of every dollar of US health care spending goes for such quantities of administrative services as insurance marketing, billing and claims processing, and utilization review, rather than for actual clinical services. US administrative costs are over twice as high proportionately as those in nations such as Canada and have been rising more rapidly than the rate of overall national health care inflation. While some level of administrative service is necessary for health care finance management and related activities such as quality assurance, few argue that the burgeoning administrative and marketing activities translate into meaningful improvement in patient health. Reducing administrative services is another route to painless cost containment.

Eliminating purely wasteful quantities of health care services, be they ineffective clinical services or unnecessary administrative activities, is a relatively straightforward approach to painless cost control. The motto of this approach is: Stop doing things of no clinical benefit. More complicated are approaches to efficiency that involve not simply ceasing completely unproductive activities, but doing things differently. Examples of this latter approach include innovations that substitute less costly care of equal benefit, preventive care, and redistribution of resources from services with some benefit to services with greater benefit relative to cost. Let us examine each of these examples in turn.

▶ Innovation and Cost Savings

Much of the process of innovation in health care involves the search for less costly ways of producing the same or better health outcomes. A new drug is developed that is less expensive but is equally efficacious and well tolerated as a conventional medication. Services provided by highly paid physicians can often be delivered with the same quality by nurses, nurse practitioners, or physician assistants. A clinical trial documents that infusion of chemotherapy for many cancer treatments may be done safely on an outpatient basis, averting the expense of hospitalization. Often new technologies are introduced in hopes that they will ultimately prove to be less costly than existing treatment methods.

However, new technologies often fail to live up to cost-saving expectations (Bodenheimer, 2005). A case

in point is that of laparoscopic cholecystectomy. Through the use of fiberoptic technology, the gallbladder may be surgically removed using a much smaller abdominal incision than that required for traditional open cholecystectomy, thereby significantly shortening the time required for postoperative recuperation in the hospital. The shorter length of hospital stay reduces the overall cost of the operation, with improved outcomes due to less postoperative pain and disability—seemingly a classic case of "efficient substitution" that lowers costs and improves health outcomes. There's a catch, however. The necessity of gallbladder surgery is not always clear-cut for patients with gallstones. Many patients have only occasional, mild symptoms, and prefer to tolerate these symptoms rather than undergo an operation. Rates of cholecystectomy increased dramatically following the advent of the laparoscopic technique, apparently because more patients with milder symptoms were undergoing gallbladder surgery. In one HMO, the cholecystectomy rate increased by 59% between 1988 and 1992 after the introduction of the laparoscopic technique. Even though the average cost per cholecystectomy declined by 25%, the total cost for all cholecystectomies in the HMO rose by 11% because of the increased number of procedures done (Legorreta et al, 1993).

▶ Ounces of Prevention

If an ounce of prevention is worth a pound of cure, then replacement of expensive end-stage treatment with low-cost prevention would appear to be an ideal candidate for the "painless cost controller award." Investing in prevention sometimes generates this type of efficiency in health care spending (eg, many childhood vaccinations cost less than caring for children with infections) (Armstrong, 2007). However, the prevention story is not always so simple. In many cases, the cost of implementing a widespread prevention program may exceed the cost of caring for the illness it aims to prevent. For example, screening the general population for elevated blood pressure and providing long-term treatment for those with mild-to-moderate hypertension to prevent strokes and other cardiovascular complications has been found to cost more than the expense of treating the eventual complications themselves (Russell, 2009). For some diseases, this is the case because the complications are rapidly and inexpensively fatal, while successful prevention leads to a long life with high medical costs, perhaps for a different illness, required at some point. Similarly a program of routine mammography screening and biopsy following abnormal test results costs more than it saves by detecting breast cancers at earlier stages. Blood pressure and breast cancer screening programs result in the improved health of the population but require a net investment in additional resources.

▶ Prioritization and Analysis of Cost Effectiveness

A fourth recommendation of Dr. Worthy's task force involves the diagnosis and treatment of colon cancer. Many HMO physicians suggest screening colonoscopy for their patients over age 50 for early detection of colon cancer. All the HMO's oncologists strongly recommend chemotherapy for patients who develop metastatic colon cancer. Analysis of cost-effectiveness has demonstrated that screening colonoscopy saves many more years of life per dollar spent than chemotherapy for metastatic colon cancer. Yet chemotherapy allows some patients with metastatic disease to enjoy an extra 6–12 months of life. The task force takes the position that the HMO's physicians should do screening colonoscopies, but that the HMO insurance plan should not cover chemotherapy for metastatic colon cancer.

The most controversial strategy for making health care more efficient is the redistribution of resources from services with some benefit to services with greater benefit relative to cost. This approach is commonly guided by cost-effectiveness analysis, which as defined by Eisenberg (1989).

> *. . . measures the net cost of providing a service (expenditures minus savings) as well as the outcomes obtained. Outcomes are reported in a single unit of measurement, either a conventional clinical outcome (eg, years of life saved) or a measure that combines several outcomes on a common scale. (Eisenberg, 1989)*

An example is a cost-effectiveness analysis of different strategies to prevent heart disease, showing that the cost per year of life saved (in 1984 dollars) was approximately $1000 for brief advice about smoking cessation during a routine office visit,

$24,000 for treating mild hypertension, and nearly $100,000 for treating elevated cholesterol levels with drugs (Cummings et al, 1989). In order to get the most "bang" for the health care "buck," this analysis suggests that a system operating under limited resources would do better by maximizing resources for smoking cessation before investing in cholesterol screening and treatment.

Cost-effectiveness analysis must be used with caution. If the data used are inaccurate, the conclusions may be incorrect. Moreover, cost-effectiveness analysis may discriminate against people with disabilities. Researchers are likely to assign less worth to a year of life of a disabled person than does the person himself or herself; thus, analyses using "quality-adjusted life years" may have a built-in bias against persons with less capacity to function independently (Menzel, 1992).

Dr. David Eddy (1991, 1992, 1993), in a series of provocative articles in the *Journal of the American Medical Association,* has discussed the practical and ethical challenges of applying cost-effectiveness analysis to medical practice. Two of the essays involve the case of an HMO trying to decide whether to adopt routine use of low-osmolar contrast agents, a type of dye for special x-ray studies that carries a lower risk of provoking allergic reactions than the cheaper conventional dye. With the use of this agent for all x-ray dye studies, 40 nonfatal allergic reactions would be avoided annually and the cost to the HMO would be $3.5 million more per year, compared with costs for use of the older agent in routine cases and use of the low-osmolar dye only for patients at high risk of allergy. The same $3.5 million dollars invested in an expanded cervical cancer screening program in the HMO would prevent approximately 100 deaths from cervical cancer per year.

In discussing how best to deploy these resources, Eddy highlights several points of particular relevance to clinicians:

1. It must be agreed upon that resources are truly limited. Although the cost-effectiveness of low-osmolar contrast dye and cervical cancer screening is quite different, both programs offer some benefit (ie, they are not flat-of-the-curve medicine). If no constraints on resources existed, the best policy would be to invest in both services.

2. If resources are limited and trade-offs based on cost-effectiveness considerations are to be made, these trade-offs will have professional legitimacy only if it is clear that resources saved from denying services of low cost-effectiveness will be reinvested in services with greater cost-effectiveness, rather than siphoned off for ineffective care or higher profits.

3. Ethical tensions exist between maximizing health outcomes for a group or population as opposed to the individual patient. The radiologist experiences the trauma of patients having severe allergic reactions to the injection of contrast dye. Preventing future deaths from cervical cancer in an unspecified group of patients not directly under the radiologist's care seems an abstract and remote benefit from his or her perspective—one that may be perceived as conflicting with the radiologist's obligation to provide the best care possible to his or her patients.

Many analysts, including those who question the methods of cost-effectiveness analysis, share Eddy's conclusion: Physicians must broaden their perspective to balance the needs of individual patients directly under their care with the overall needs of the population served by the health care system, whether the system is an HMO or the nation's health care system as a whole (see Chapter 13). Professional ethics will have to incorporate social accountability for resource use and population health, as well as clinical responsibility for the care of individual patients (Greenlick, 1992; Hiatt, 1975).

The final recommendation of Dr. Worthy's task force is for the HMO to hire a consultant to advise the HMO on the relative cost-effectiveness of different services offered by the HMO, in order to prioritize the most cost-effective activities. While waiting for the consultant's report, the task force suggests that the HMO begin implementing this strategy by allocating an extra 5 minutes to every routine medical appointment for patients who smoke, so that the physician, nurse practitioner, or physician assistant has time to counsel patients on smoking cessation, as well as by setting up two dozen new community-based group classes in smoking cessation for HMO members. The costs of these new activities are to be funded from the HMO's existing budget for coronary artery stenting, and the number of these stent procedures is to be restricted to 30 fewer than the number performed during the current year. The day following

the executive committee meeting, the HMO's health education director buys Dr. Worthy lunch and compliments him on his "enlightened" views. On the way back from lunch, the chief of cardiology accosts Dr. Worthy in the corridor and says, "Why don't you just take a few dozen of my patients with severe coronary artery disease out and shoot them? Get it over with quickly, instead of denying them the life-saving stents they need."

CONCLUSION

The relationship between health outcomes and health care costs is not a simple one. The cost–benefit curve has a diminishing slope as increasing investment of resources yields more marginal improvements in the health of the population. The curve itself may shift up or down, depending on the efficiency with which a given level of resources is deployed.

The ideal cost containment method is one that achieves progress in overall health outcomes through the "painless" route of making more efficient use of an existing level of resources. Examples of this approach include restricting price increases, reducing administrative waste, and eliminating inappropriate and ineffective services. "Painful" cost containment represents the other extreme, when controls on expenditures are accomplished only by sacrificing quantities of medically beneficial services. Making trade-offs in services based on relative cost-effectiveness may be felt as painless or painful, depending on one's point of view; some individuals may experience the pain of being denied potentially beneficial services, but at a net gain in health for the overall population through more efficient use of the resources at hand.

Cost containment in the real world tends to fall somewhere between the entirely painless paragon and the completely painful pariah (Ginzberg, 1983). As the experiences of Dr. Worthy reveal, putting painless cost control into practice may be impeded by political, organizational, and technical obstacles. Price controls may make economic sense but risk intense opposition from providers. Administrative savings may be largely beyond the control of any single HMO or group of providers and require an overhaul of the entire health care system. Identifying and modifying inappropriate clinical practices is a daunting task, as is prioritizing services on the basis of cost-effectiveness. But while painless cost control may be difficult to achieve, few would argue that the US health care system currently operates anywhere near a maximum level of efficiency. Regions in the nation with higher health care spending do not have better health outcomes (Fisher et al, 2003). The nation's lackluster performance on indices such as infant mortality and life expectancy rates suggests that the prolific degree of spending on health care in the United States has not been matched by a commensurate level of excellence in the health of the population (Davis et al, 2010). Making better use of existing resources must be the priority of cost control strategies in the United States.

REFERENCES

Aaron H, Schwartz WB. Rationing health care: The choice before us. *Science*. 1990;247:418.

Aaron H, Schwartz WB. *The Painful Prescription: Rationing Hospital Care*. Washington, DC: Brookings Institution; 1984.

Armstrong EP. Economic benefits and costs associated with target vaccinations. *J Manag Care Pharm*. 2007;13(Suppl S-b):S12.

Avorn J. Keeping science on top in drug evaluation. *N Engl J Med*. 2007;357:633.

Bodenheimer T. High and rising health care costs. Part 2: technologic innovation. *Ann Intern Med*. 2005;142:932.

Brenner DJ, Hricak H. Radiation exposure from medical imaging. *JAMA*. 2010;304:208.

Brook RH, Lohr KN. Will we need to ration effective health care? *Issues Sci Technol*. 1986;3:68.

Brownlee S. *Overtreated*. New York: Bloomsbury; 2007.

Cummings SR et al. The cost-effectiveness of counseling smokers to quit. *JAMA*. 1989;261:75.

Davis K et al. *Mirror, Mirror on the Wall*. New York: Commonwealth Fund; 2010.

Deyo RA et al. Overtreating chronic back pain: Time to back off. *J Am Board Fam Med*. 2009;22:62.

Donabedian A. Quality and cost: Choices and responsibilities. *Inquiry*. 1988;25:90.

Eddy DM. Applying cost-effectiveness analysis. *JAMA*. 1992;268:2575.

Eddy DM. Broadening the responsibilities of practitioners. *JAMA*. 1993;269:1849.

Eddy DM. The individual vs. society: Is there a conflict? *JAMA*. 1991;265:1446.

Eisenberg JM. Clinical economics. *JAMA*. 1989;262:2879.

Evans RG. *Strained Mercy: The Economics of Canadian Health Care*. Toronto, Ontario, Canada: Butterworths; 1984.

Fisher ES et al. The implications of regional variation in medicare spending. *Ann Intern Med*. 2003;138:273.

Fisher ES et al. Associations among hospital capacity, utilization, and mortality of US Medicare beneficiaries, controlling for sociodemographic factors. *Health Serv Res*. 2000;34:1351.

Fuchs VR. No pain, no gain: Perspectives on cost containment. *JAMA*. 1993;269:631.

Fuchs VR. The health sector's share of the gross national product. *Science*. 1990;247:534.

Ginzberg E. Cost-containment: Imaginary and real. *N Engl J Med*. 1983;308:1220.

Greenlick MR. Educating physicians for population-based clinical practice. *JAMA*. 1992;267:1645.

Grimes DA. Technology follies: The uncritical acceptance of medical innovation. *JAMA*. 1993;269:3030.

Hiatt HH. Protecting the medical commons: Who is responsible? *N Engl J Med*. 1975;293:235.

Kilo CM, Larsen EB. Exploring the harmful effects of health care. *JAMA*. 2009;302:89.

Leape LL. Unnecessary surgery. *Annu Rev Public Health*. 1992;13:363.

Legorreta AP et al. Increased cholecystectomy rate after the introduction of laparoscopic cholecystectomy. *JAMA*. 1993;270:1429.

Lomas J et al. Paying physicians in Canada: Minding our Ps and Qs. *Health Aff (Millwood)*. 1989;8(1):80.

Martin A et al. Recession contributes to slowest annual rate of increase in health spending in five decades. *Health Aff (Millwood)*. 2011;30:11.

Menzel PT. Oregon's denial: Disabilities and the quality of life. *Hastings Cent Rep*. 1992;22:21.

Peterson CL, Burton R. *U.S. Health Care Spending: Comparison with Other OECD Countries* (RL34175) [Electronic copy]. Washington, DC: Congressional Research Service; 2007. http://digitalcommons.ilr.cornell.edu/key_workplace/311/. Accessed November 14, 2011.

Reinhardt UE. Resource allocation in health care: The allocation of lifestyles to providers. *Milbank Mem Fund Q*. 1987;65:153.

Russell LB. Preventing chronic disease: An important investment, but don't count on cost savings. *Health Aff (Millwood)*. 2009;28:42.

Schuster M et al. How good is the quality of health care in the United States? *Milbank Q*. 1998;76:517.

Sisko AM et al. National health spending projections: The estimated impact of reform through 2019. *Health Aff (Millwood)*. 2010;29:1933.

Woolhandler S et al. Costs of health care administration in the United States and Canada. *N Engl J Med*. 2003;349:768.

Mechanisms for Controlling Costs

In Chapter 8, we discussed the general relationship between costs and health outcomes and explored the tension between painful and painless approaches to cost containment. In this chapter, we examine specific methods for controlling costs. Our emphasis is on distinguishing among the different types of cost control mechanisms and understanding their intent and rationale. We briefly cite evidence about how these mechanisms may affect cost and health outcomes.

Financial transactions under private or public health insurance (see Chapter 2, Figures 2–2, 2–3, and 2–4) may be divided into two components:

1. *Financing,* the flow of dollars (premiums or taxes) from individuals and employers to the health insurance plan (private health insurance or government programs), and

2. *Reimbursement,* the flow of dollars from insurance plans to physicians, hospitals, and other providers.

Cost-control strategies can be divided into those that target the financing side versus those that impact the reimbursement side of the funding stream (Figure 9–1 and Table 9–1).

FINANCING CONTROLS

Cost controls aimed at the financing of health insurance attempt to limit the flow of funds into health insurance plans, with the expectation that the plans will then be forced to modify the outflow of reimbursement. Financing controls come in two basic flavors— regulatory and competitive.

► Regulatory Strategies

Dieter Arbeiter, a carpenter in Berlin, Germany, is enrolled in one of his nation's health insurance plans, the "sick fund" operated by the Carpenter's Guild. Each month, Dieter pays 7.5% of his wages to the sick fund and his employer contributes an equal 7.5%. The German federal government regulates these payroll tax rates. When the government proposes raising the rate to 8.5%, Dieter and his coworkers march to the parliament building to protest the increase. The government backs down, and the rate remains at 7.5%. As a result, physician fees do not increase that year.

In nations with tax-financed health insurance, government regulation of taxes serves as a control over public expenditures for health care. This regulatory control is most evident when certain tax funds are earmarked for health insurance, as in the case of the German health insurance plans (see Chapter 14) or Medicare Part A in the United States. Under these types of social insurance systems, an increase in expenditures for health care requires explicit legislation to raise the rate of earmarked health insurance taxes. Public antipathy to tax hikes may serve as a political anchor against health care inflation.

A somewhat different model of financing regulation was offered by President Clinton's 1994 health care proposal (which never passed). This proposal called for government regulation of premiums paid to private health insurance plans.

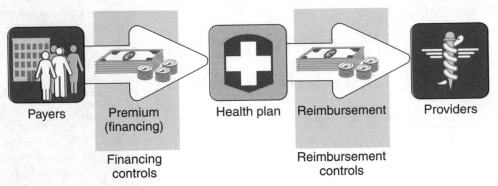

▲ **Figure 9–1.** Cost-control mechanisms may be applied to both the financing and reimbursement components of health care spending under a system of health insurance.

▶ Competitive Strategies

An alternative US proposal for containing health costs attempts to control the financing flow through a competitive strategy rather than through regulation. The basic premise of competitive financing strategies is to make employers, employees, and individuals more cost-conscious in their health insurance purchasing decisions. Health insurance plans would be encouraged to compete on the basis of price, with lower-cost plans being rewarded with a greater number of enrollees. Instead of having a government agency regulate financing, the competitive market would pressure plans to restrain their premium prices and overall costs.

Giovanni Costa works for General Auto (GA). It is 1985, and he and his family have Blue Cross health insurance that covers most services provided by the health care provider of his choice, with no deductible. Giovanni does not know how much his health plan costs, because GA pays the total premium. Once Giovanni asked his friend in the employee benefits department whether the company was worried about the costs of health insurance. "It's a problem," Giovanni was told, "but it's not too bad because our health insurance premiums are tax deductible for the company. Also, if we gave you higher wages you'd have to pay taxes on those wages, but if we give you better health care coverage, you don't pay taxes on the value of that coverage. So we're both better off by providing generous health care benefits. When it comes right down to it, the government's paying a portion of those premiums."

When considering competitive strategies that attempt to make purchasers more price sensitive, it is important to consider who the purchaser of health insurance really is. For employment-based health insurance, is the purchaser the employer selecting which health plans to offer employees, or is it the individual employee deciding to enroll in a specific plan? As in the case of Giovanni Costa and GA, the answer is often both: GA selects which plans to offer employees and what portion of the premium to subsidize, and

Table 9–1. Categories of cost controls

Financing controls
Regulatory: limits on taxes or premiums
Competitive
Reimbursement controls
Price controls
Regulatory
Competitive
Utilization (quantity) controls
Aggregate units of payment: capitation, diagnosis-related groups (DRGs), global budgets
Patient cost sharing
Utilization management
Supply limits
Mixed controls

Giovanni chooses a particular plan from those offered by GA.

Historically, several factors have blunted both employers' and employees' consideration of price in the purchase of health insurance (Enthoven, 1993). For employees, the fact that employers who provide health benefits usually pay a large share of the premium for their employees' private health insurance has insulated insured employees from the costs of insurance. Employees view health insurance premiums as an expense to the employer rather than as a cost borne by themselves. In fact, many employees might receive higher wages if the costs of health insurance were lower, but employees do not generally perceive health insurance benefits as foregone wages.

Moreover, the federal policy of treating health care benefits as nontaxable to both employee and employer makes it in the employee's financial interest to receive generous health care benefits and reduces the burden to the employer of paying for such benefits. A dollar contributed directly by the employer to a health plan goes farther toward the purchase of health insurance than a dollar in wages that is first taxed as income and then spent by the employee for health insurance. This dynamic, which cost the federal government about $260 billion in 2010 (Gruber, 2010), has shielded employees from the real price of health insurance and given employees less incentive to be cost-conscious consumers when selecting an insurance plan.

For employers, inflation of health insurance premiums in the 1950s and 1960s was an acceptable part of doing business when the economy was booming and health insurance costs consumed only a small portion of overall business expenses. However, as health insurance costs continued to spiral upward and economic growth slowed in recent decades, employers became more active in their approach to health insurance costs (see Chapter 16).

It is 2010, and GA now offers Giovanni Costa three choices of health insurance plans: The health maintenance organization (HMO) plan costs $1000 per month for family coverage, with GA paying 70% and Giovanni paying 30%; the preferred provider organization (PPO) plan is worth $1200 per month; and the fee-for-service plan runs $1400 a month. If Giovanni chooses the HMO plan, GA pays $700 (70%) and Giovanni pays

$300 (30%). If Giovanni signs up for the $1200 PPO plan, GA still pays $700 (70% of the lowest-cost plan) and Giovanni must pay the rest—$500. If Giovanni wants to choose the fee-for-service plan, GA pays $700 and Giovanni pays $700. GA negotiated with all three of its health plans that premium levels would be frozen at their 2008 rates for the next 3 years. A fourth plan previously offered by GA refused to agree to this stipulation, and GA dropped this plan from its portfolio of employee benefits. After 2011, however, the three health plans can demand yearly premium increases, increasing health insurance costs for both GA and Giovanni.

The competitive approach to health insurance financing encourages price-sensitive purchasing by both employer and employee. For employers, the competitive strategy calls for businesses to be more aggressive in their negotiations with health plans over premium rates. Employers bargain actively with health plans and offer employees only plans that keep their rates below a certain level. Moreover, employers make employees more cost-aware when selecting a health plan by limiting the amount of the insurance premium that the employer will pay. Rather than paying all or most of the premium, many employers offer a fixed amount of insurance subsidy—often indexed to the cost of the cheapest health plan—and compel employees selecting more costly plans to pay the extra amount. Economist Alain Enthoven, one of the chief proponents of the competitive approach, has called this strategy "managed competition" (Enthoven, 2003). The strategy is also known as the "defined contribution" approach.

Is the evolving competitive approach succeeding at controlling costs? From 2000 to 2010, employer-sponsored health insurance premiums rose by 114%, a major cost-control failure (Claxton et al, 2010). However, competition has never been truly instituted in the United States; 94% of metropolitan markets are controlled by one or two large commercial insurance companies that can extract increasing premiums from employers (Arnst, 2009). Moreover, insurance plans find it easier to compete by "gaming" the market through selection of low-cost enrollees rather than by disciplining providers to deliver a lower-cost, higher-quality product. Studies have shown that competing Medicare HMOs have utilized precisely that strategy (Mehrotra et al, 2006).

If competition could succeed at containing costs, would the outcome be painful or painless cost control? A fundamental concern about market-oriented reforms is that whatever pain may be produced would be experienced most acutely by individuals with lower incomes. Under competition, individuals with higher incomes would be the ones most likely to pay the extra premium costs to enroll in more expensive health plans, while individuals of lesser means could not afford the extra premiums and would be relegated to the lower-cost plans. If the differential in premium prices across plans were large, enrollees in low-cost plans might experience inferior quality of care and health outcomes.

▶ The Weaknesses of Financing Controls

For cost controls—whether regulatory or competitive—on the financing side of the health care equation to be successful, these strategies ultimately must produce reductions in the flow of funds on the reimbursement side. A government may try to limit the level of taxes earmarked for health care. However, if payments to physicians, hospitals, and other providers continue to grow at a rapid clip, the imbalance between the level of financing and level of reimbursement will produce budget deficits and ultimately force the government to raise taxes. Similarly, under competition, health insurers will attempt to hold down premium increases in order to gain more customers, but if these health plans cannot successfully control what they pay to hospitals, physicians, pharmacies, and other providers, then insurers will be forced to raise their premiums, and competitive relief from health care inflation will prove elusive. It is on the reimbursement side of the equation that the rubber meets the road in health care cost containment. Governments in nations with publicly financed insurance programs do not simply regulate health care financing, but are actively involved in controlling provider reimbursement. Competition would place the onus on private health insurance plans—rather than a public agency—to regulate reimbursement costs. We now turn to an examination of the options available to private insurers or government for controlling the flow of funds in the reimbursement transaction.

REIMBURSEMENT CONTROLS

In Chapter 8, we distinguished between the "Ps" and "Qs" of health care costs: prices and quantities. Cost equals price multiplied by quantity

$$C = P \times Q$$

Strategies to control costs on the reimbursement side can primarily target either prices or quantities (see Table 9–1).

▶ Price Controls

Under California's fee-for-service Medicaid program, Dr. Vincent Lo's reimbursement for a routine office visit has remained below $25 for the past 8 years.

The Medicare program reduced Dr. Ernesto Ojo's fee for cataract surgery from $1600 to $900.

Instead of paying all hospitals in the area the going rate for magnetic resonance imaging (MRI) brain scans ($1200), Apple a Day HMO contracts only with those hospitals who agree to perform scans for $800, and will not allow its patients to receive MRIs at any other hospital.

Metropolitan Hospital wants a contract with Apple a Day HMO at a per diem rate of $1750. Because Apple a Day can hospitalize its patients at Crosstown Hospital for $1400 a day, Metropolitan has no choice but to reduce its per diem rate to Apple a Day to $1400 in order to get the contract. In turn, to make up the $350 per day shortfall, Metropolitan increases its charges to several other private insurers.

In Canada and most European nations, a public or quasipublic agency regulates a uniform fee schedule for physician and hospital payments. Often, negotiations occur between the payers (payer is a general term that includes both purchasers and insurers—see Chapter 16) and professional organizations in establishing these fee schedules. In the United States, as discussed in Chapter 4, Medicare, Medicaid, and many private insurance plans have replaced "usual, customary, and reasonable" physician payment with predetermined prices for particular services. Competitive approaches to controlling prices have also been attempted in the United States. In the 1980s, California initiated competitive bidding among hospitals for Medicaid contracts, with contracts awarded to hospitals offering lower per diem charges. Private insurance plans have also used competitive bidding to bargain for reductions in physician and hospital fees.

Controlling prices has produced some limited success at restraining the growth of overall health care expenditures. However, two major problems limit the potency of price controls for containing overall costs, particularly when prices are regulated at the fee-for-service level.

1. The first problem occurs when price controls are implemented in a piecemeal fashion by different payers. Providers, like Metropolitan Hospital, often respond to price controls imposed by one payer by increasing charges to other payers with less restrictive policies on fees—a phenomenon known as *cost shifting*. The cost-shifting problem may be avoided when a uniform fee schedule is used by all payers (as in Germany) or by a single payer (as in Canada).

2. The quantity of services provided often surges when prices are strictly controlled, leading analysts to conclude that providers respond to fee controls by inducing higher use of services in order to maintain earnings (Bodenheimer, 2005).

Price controls have the appeal of being a relatively painless form of cost control insofar as they do not limit the quantity of services provided. However, variations in fee schedules may compromise access to care for certain populations; Medicaid fee-for-service rates to physicians are far below private insurance rates in most states, making it difficult for Medicaid patients to find private physicians who will accept Medicaid payment. In nations with uniform fee schedules, concerns have been voiced that ratcheting down of fees may result in "patient churning" (high volumes of brief visits), with a deterioration in quality of care and patient satisfaction.

▶ Utilization (Quantity) Controls

Because the effectiveness of price controls may be limited by increases in quantity, payers need to consider methods for containing the actual use of services. As indicated in Table 9–1, there are a variety of methods for attempting to control use. We begin by examining one strategy, changing the unit of payment, that we introduced in Chapter 4. We then describe additional mechanisms that attempt to restrain the quantity of services.

Changing the Unit of Payment

Dr. John Wiley is upset when the PPO reduces his fee from $75 to $60 per visit. In order to maintain his income, Dr. Wiley lengthens his day by half an hour so he can schedule more patient visits.

Dr. Jane Stuckey is angry when the HMO reduces her capitation payment from $20 to $15 per patient per month. She is unable to maintain her income by providing more visits because more patient visits do not bring her more money. She hopes that more HMO patients will enroll in her practice so that she can receive more capitation payments.

One simple way to get a handle on the quantity factor is by redefining the unit of payment. In Chapter 4, we discussed how services may be bundled into more aggregate units of payment, such as capitated physician payment and diagnosis-related group (DRG) episode-of-care hospital payment. The more bundled the unit of payment, the more predictable the quantity tends to be. For example, in the case of Dr. Wiley receiving fee-for-service payment, there is a great potential for costs to rise due to increases in the number of physician visits, surgical procedures, and diagnostic tests. When the unit of payment is capitation, as in the case of Dr. Stuckey, the quantity factor is not the number of visits but rather the number of individuals enrolled in a practice or plan. From a health plan's perspective, the $C = P \times Q$ formula still applies when paying physicians by capitation, but now the P is the capitation fee and the Q is the number of individuals covered. Other than by raising birth rates, physicians have little discretion in inducing a higher volume of "quantities" at the capitation level for the health care system as a whole. Similarly, under global budgeting of hospitals, P represents the average global budget per hospital and Q is the number of hospitals.

Shifting payment to a more aggregated unit has obvious appeal as a way for payers to counter cost inflation due to the quantity factor. Life is never so simple, however. In Chapter 4, we discussed how more aggregate units of payment shift financial risk to providers of care. Another way of describing this shifting of risk is that one person's solution to the quantity problem becomes another person's new quantity problem. A hospital paid by global budget instead of by fee-for-service now must monitor its own internal quantities of service lest these quantities drive hospital operating costs over budget. To the extent that providers are unsuccessful in managing resources under more global forms of payment, pressures mount to raise the prices paid at these more aggregated payment units.

Changes in policies for units of payment rarely occur independent of other reforms in cost-control strategies, making it difficult to isolate the specific effects of changing the unit of payment. For example, physician capitation usually occurs in the context of other organizational and cost-control features within a managed care plan. For example, group- and staff-model HMOs receiving capitation payments from employers and paying physicians by salary have been shown to reduce costs by reducing the quantity of services provided, in particular by reducing rates of hospitalization (Hellinger, 1996; Bodenheimer, 2005).

For hospitals, changing Medicare payments from a fee-for-service to an episode-of-care unit under the DRG-based system in 1983 resulted in a modest slowing of the rate of increase in Medicare Part A expenditures. However, hospitals were able to shift costs to private payers to make up for lower DRG revenues, and national health expenditures as a whole were not affected by Medicare's new payment mechanism (Rice, 1996). Global hospital budgeting in Canada has been a key element of that nation's relative success at containing hospital costs (Rice, 1996).

The health care system in Germany and in some Canadian provinces has countered the open-ended dynamic of fee-for-service payment by introducing global budgeting, called expenditure caps, for physician payment (Bodenheimer, 2005). Under Canadian expenditure caps, a budget is established for all physician services in a province. Although individual physicians continue to bill the provincial health plan on a fee-for-service basis, if increases in the use of services cause overall physician costs to exceed the budget, fees are reduced (or fee increases for the following year are sacrificed) to stay within the expenditure cap. Evidence from Canada suggests that implementation of expenditure caps was associated with stabilization of physician costs in the mid-1990s (Barer et al, 1996). In the United States, the Medicare program adopted a less-stringent version of an expenditure cap for physician fees, known as the "sustainable growth rate" (Vladeck, 2010). Expenditure caps for physician payments allow the payer to focus on the aggregate C part of the equation—in this case, the total physician budget. The shared savings program proposed under the new Medicare Accountable Care Organization initiative, discussed in Chapter 6, is a related strategy attempting to provide a global expenditure feedback loop to modulate fee-for-service payments.

Patient Cost Sharing

Randy Payton has an insurance policy with a $2000 deductible and 20% copayment for all services; if he incurs medical expenses of $6000, he pays the first $2000 plus 20% of $4000, for a total of $2800.

Joseph Mednick's health plan requires that he pay $20 each time he fills a prescription for a medication, with the health plan paying the cost above $20; because he suffers from diabetes, hypertension, and coronary artery disease, the copayments for his multiple medications cost him $1200 per year.

Cost sharing refers to making patients pay directly out of pocket for some portion of their health care. In managed competition, cost sharing occurs as part of the financing transaction *at the point of purchasing a health insurance plan.* In this section, we discuss the more traditional notion of cost sharing—using deductibles, copayments, and uncovered services as part of the reimbursement transaction to make patients pay a share of costs *at the point of receiving health care services.*

The primary intent of cost sharing at the point of service is to discourage patient demand for services. (Cost-sharing also shifts some of the overall bill for health care from third party payers to individuals in the form of greater out-of-pocket expenses.) As discussed in Chapter 3, when individuals have insurance coverage, they are more likely to use services than when they have no insurance. While protection against individual financial risk is one of the essential benefits of insurance, insurance coverage removes the market restraint on costs that occurs in a system of out-of-pocket payment.

Cost sharing at the point of service has been one of the few cost-containment devices subjected to the rigorous evaluation of a randomized controlled experiment. In the Rand Health Insurance Experiment, individuals were randomly assigned to health insurance plans with varying degrees of cost sharing. Individuals with cost-sharing plans made about one-third fewer visits and were hospitalized one-third less often than individuals randomized to the plan with no cost sharing (Newhouse et al, 1981).

Although the randomized controlled trial provides an excellent laboratory for scrutinizing the effect of a single cost-containment mechanism, some observers have cautioned that analyses based on controlled research designs may produce results that cannot be generalized to the real world of health policy. For example, the United States has a greater level of cost sharing than many industrialized nations, but also the highest overall costs. Studies have found that when cost sharing begins to produce lower use of services for a large population of patients rather than for a small number of patients in an experiment, physicians may increase the volume of services provided to patients with better insurance coverage (Beck and Horne, 1980; Fahs, 1992). Moreover, 70% of health care expenditures are incurred by 10% of the population—people who are extremely ill and generate huge costs through lengthy ICU stays and other major expenses. Cost sharing has little influence over this component of care. Compared to the micro-world of one not-very-sick patient deciding whether to spend some money on a physician visit, patient cost sharing in the macro-world may remove only a thin slice from a large, expanding pie (Bodenheimer, 2005).

The Rand experiment also evaluated the influence of cost sharing on appropriateness of care and health outcomes. Cost sharing did not reduce medically inappropriate use of services selectively, but equally discouraged use of appropriate and inappropriate services. Study patients (especially those with low incomes) with cost sharing received less preventive services and had poorer hypertension control than those without cost sharing (Brook et al, 1983). Patients are less likely to purchase needed medications under cost-sharing policies, for example Medicare Part D's "donut hole" (see Chapter 2), leading to worse control of chronic illnesses and more emergency hospitalizations (Hsu et al, 2006; Tamblyn et al, 2001; Goldman et al, 2007; Schneeweiss et al, 2009). These studies suggest that cost sharing is not a painless form of cost control.

Cost sharing for emergency department care may reduce inappropriate use of emergency services without adversely affecting appropriate use or patient health outcomes (Goodell et al, 2009). Cost sharing may be a painless form of cost control when used in modest amounts, not applied to low-income patients, and designed to encourage patients to use lower-cost alternative sources of care (eg, clinics instead of emergency departments) rather than to discourage use of services altogether.

Utilization Management

Thelma Graves suffers from a severe hyperthyroid condition; she and her physician agree that she will undergo thyroid surgery. Before scheduling the surgery, the physician has to call Ms. Graves' insurance company to obtain preauthorization, without which the insurer will not pay for the surgery.

Fred Brady is hospitalized for an acute myocardial infarction. The hospital contacts the utilization management firm for Mr. Brady's insurer, which authorizes 5 hospital days. On the fourth day, Mr. Brady develops a heart rate of 36 beats/min, requiring the insertion of a temporary pacemaker and prolonging the hospital stay for 10 extra days. After the fifth hospital day, Mr. Brady's physician has to call the utilization management (UM) firm every 2 days to justify why the insurer should continue to pay for the hospitalization.

Derek Jordan has juvenile-onset diabetes and at age 42 becomes eligible for Medicare due to his permanent disability from complications of his diabetes. He is admitted to the hospital for treatment of a gangrenous toe. Under Medicare's DRG method of payment, the hospital receives the same payment for Derek's hospitalization regardless of whether it lasts 2 days or 12 days. Therefore, the hospital wants Derek's physician to discharge Derek as soon as possible. Each day, a hospital UM nurse reviews Derek's chart and suggests to the physician that Derek no longer requires acute hospitalization.

Utilization management involves the surveillance of and intervention in the clinical activities of physicians for the purpose of controlling costs (Grumbach and Bodenheimer, 1990). In contrast to cost sharing, which attempts to restrict health care use by influencing patient behavior, UM seeks to influence physician behavior. The mechanism of influencing physician decisions is simple and direct: denial of payment for services deemed unnecessary.

UM is related to the unit of payment in the following way: Whoever is at financial risk (see Chapter 4) performs UM. Under fee-for-service reimbursement, insurance companies perform UM to reduce their payments to hospitals and physicians. The DRG system induces hospitals, at risk for losing money if their patients stay too long, to perform UM. Under an HMO capitation contract with a primary physician group, the physician group conducts UM so that it does not pay more to physicians than it receives in capitation payments. If an HMO pays a hospital a per diem rate, the HMO may send a UM nurse to the hospital each day to review whether the patient is ready to go home.

> *Micromanage, Inc., performs UM for several insurance companies. Each day, Rebecca Hasselbach reviews the charts of each patient hospitalized by these insurers to determine whether the patients might be ready for discharge. In some cases, Ms. Hasselbach discusses the case with her medical director and with the patient's attending physician. Usually, if the attending physician wants the patient to remain in the hospital, his or her opinion is honored. By pushing for early discharges, Ms. Hasselbach, her Micromanage colleagues around the country, and the medical director save their insurers about $1,000,000 each year. The annual cost of the UM operation is $900,000.*

Although a few case studies of UM have shown some short-term reduction in rates of hospitalization and surgery, there is little evidence that this approach yields substantial savings, particularly when the overhead of administering the UM program itself is taken into account (Wickizer, 1990). If successful at containing costs, UM would appear to be a painless form of cost control because it intends to selectively reduce inappropriate or unnecessary care. However, reviewers often make decisions on a case-by-case basis without explicit guidelines or criteria, with the result that decisions may be inconsistent both between different reviewers for the same case and among the same reviewer for different cases (Light, 1994).

UM has come under fire as a process of micromanagement of clinical decisions that intrudes into the physician–patient relationship and places an unwelcome administrative burden on physicians and other caregivers. Physicians in the United States have been called the most "second-guessed and paperwork-laden physicians in western industrialized democracies" (Lee and Etheredge, 1989). Substantial physician time goes into appealing denials and persuading insurers about the appropriateness of services delivered. A physician and public backlash to UM forced many health insurance plans to relax their UM activities in the late 1990s. However, many plans reintroduced UM around 2003 as costs escalated (Mays et al, 2004).

Several approaches to UM have been developed that attempt to avoid some of the onerous features of case-by-case utilization review. Practice profiling, rather than focusing on individual cases, uses summary data on practice patterns to identify physicians whose overall use of services significantly deviates from the standards set by other physicians in the community. Physician outliers identified by practice profiling are then subject to various interventions. In Canada and Germany, these interventions consist of educational and monitoring activities performed by regional medical societies. The questionable accuracy of some profile data and the need to account for underlying differences in patients' clinical needs that may in part explain practice variation have limited the utility of practice profiling as a cost-control tool (Bindman, 1999). Perhaps the most blunt form of utilization management is when a health plan simply refuses to cover an entire class of services, such as in vitro fertilization or experimental treatments for cancer. This approach is discussed in more detail in Chapter 13.

Supply Limits

> *Bob is a patient in the Canadian province of Alberta. He develops back pain, and after several visits to his family physician requests an MRI of his spine to rule out disk disease. His physician, who does not suspect a disk herniation, agrees to place him on the waiting list for an MRI, which for nonurgent cases is 5 months long.*

> *Rob lives in Alberta, and after lifting an 80-pound load at work, experiences severe lower back pain radiating down his right leg. Finding a positive*

straight-leg-raising test on the right with loss of the right ankle reflex, his family physician calls the radiologist and obtains an emergency MRI scan within 3 days.

Supply limits are controls on the number of physicians and other caregivers and on material resources such as the number of hospital beds or MRI scanners. Supply limits can take place within an organized delivery system such as an HMO in the United States, or for an entire geographic region such as a Canadian province.

The number of elective operations and invasive procedures, such as cardiac catheterization, performed per capita increases with the per-capita supply of surgeons and cardiologists, respectively (Bodenheimer, 2005). This phenomenon is sometimes called "supplier-induced demand" (Evans, 1984; Rice and Labelle, 1989; Phelps, 2003). Controlling physician supply may reduce the use of physician services and thereby contribute to cost containment.

Supplier-induced demand pertains to material capacity as well as to physician supply. Per-capita spending for fee-for-service Medicare patients is over twice as high in some regions of the United States than in others (Gawande, 2009, www.dartmouthatlas.org). This remarkable cost variation is not explained by differences in demographic characteristics of the population, prices of services, or levels of illness, but is due to the quantity of services provided. Residents of areas with a greater per-capita supply of hospital beds are up to 30% more likely to be hospitalized than those in areas with fewer beds (Fisher et al, 2000). The maxim that "empty beds tend to become filled" has been known as Roemer's law (Roemer and Shain, 1959). Conversely, strictly regulating the number of centers allowed to perform heart surgery establishes a limit for the total number of cardiac operations that can be performed. In situations of limited supply, physicians must determine which patients are most in need of the limited supply of services. Ideally, those truly in need gain access to appropriate services, with physicians possessing the wisdom to distinguish those patients truly in need (Rob) from those not requiring the service (Bob).

Although there may not always be a directly linear relationship between supply and use of services, there are clear instances in which limitations of capacity restrain use. For example, international comparisons demonstrate large variations in use of coronary revascularization procedures (coronary artery bypass surgery and angioplasty), with a relatively low rate of surgery in the United Kingdom, an intermediate rate in Canada, and the highest rate in the United States. These rates correspond to the degree to which these nations regulate (minimally in the case of the United States) the number of centers performing cardiac surgery. In spite of the large variations in the quantity of care, with the US performing almost four times the number of procedures per capita than the UK, there are minimal differences in heart disease mortality among these countries (OECD, 2009).

A "natural experiment" provides an illustration of how restricting the supply of a high cost resource may be implemented in a relatively painless manner for patients' clinical outcomes. A US hospital experiencing a nursing shortage abruptly reduced the number of staffed intensive care unit beds from 18 to 8 (Singer et al, 1983). For patients admitted to the hospital for chest pain, physicians became more selective in admitting to the intensive care unit only those patients who actually suffered heart attacks. Limiting the use of ICU beds did not result in any adverse health outcomes for patients admitted to nonintensive care unit beds, including those few nonintensive care unit patients who actually sustained heart attacks. This study suggests that when faced with supply limits, physicians may be able to prioritize patients on clinical grounds in a manner that selectively reduces unnecessary services. Establishing supply limits that require physicians to prioritize services based on the appropriateness and urgency of patient need represents a very different (and less intrusive) approach to containing costs than UM, which relies on external parties to authorize or deny individual services in a setting of relatively unconstrained capacity.

Controlling the Type of Supply

A specific form of supply control is regulation of the *types* (rather than the total number) of providers. Chapter 5 explored the balance between the number of generalist and specialist physicians in a health care system. Increasing the proportion of generalists may yield savings for two reasons. First, generalists earn lower incomes than specialists. Second, and of greater impact for overall costs, generalists appear to practice a less resource-intensive style of medicine and generate lower overall health care expenditures, including less use of hospital and laboratory services (Bodenheimer and Grumbach, 2007).

CONCLUSION

In the real world, cost containment strategies are applied not as isolated phenomena in a static system, but as an array of policies concerned with modes of financing, organization of health care delivery, and cost control all mixed together. Managed care is a strategy that utilizes mixture of cost control mechanisms: changing the unit of payment, utilization management, price discounts, and in some cases supply controls. The Canadian health care system (see Chapter 14) also relies on regulation of prices, global budgets and supply controls.

There is no perfect mechanism for controlling health care costs. Strategies must be judged by their relative success at containing costs and doing so in as painless a manner as possible—without compromising health outcomes. In the view of Dr. John Wennberg, the key to cost control in the United States

> is not in the micromanagement of the doctor-patient relationship but the management of capacity and budgets. The American problem is to find the will to set the supply thermostat somewhere within reason. (Wennberg, 1990)

Although US managed care plans and Canadian provincial health plans are often viewed as diametrically opposed paradigms for health care reform, both the Canadian plans and US group and staff model HMOs base their cost control approaches on what Wennberg terms "the management of capacity and budgets." In Canada, this management is under public control through regulation of physician supply, physician and hospital budgets, and technology. In the United States, private group and staff model HMOs adjust their own "thermostats" by setting their own budgets and numbers of physicians, hospital beds, and high-cost equipment.

If there is a lesson to be learned from attempts to control health care costs in the United States over the past decades, it is that cost-containment policies affecting provider reimbursement need to focus more on macromanagement and less on micromanagement.

Trying to manage costs at the level of individual patient encounters (ie, regulating fees for each service, reviewing daily practice decisions, or imposing cost sharing for every prescription and visit to the physician) is a cumbersome and largely ineffectual strategy for containing overall expenditures. Moreover, one payer lowering its costs by shifting expenses to another payer does not produce systemwide cost savings. Those systems that have been most successful in moderating the inexorable increase in health care costs have tended to emphasize global cost containment tools, such as paying by capitation or other aggregate units, limiting the size and specialty mix of the physician workforce, and concentrating high-technology services in regional centers. The future debate over cost containment in the United States will center on whether these cost-containment tools are best wielded by private health care plans operating in a price competitive market or by public regulation of health care providers and suppliers.

REFERENCES

Arnst C. In most markets, a few health insurers dominate. *Business Week.* July 23, 2009.

Barer ML et al. Re-minding our Ps and Qs: Cost controls in Canada. *Health Aff (Millwood).* 1996;15(2):216.

Bindman AB. Can physician profiles be trusted? *JAMA.* 1999;281:2142.

Bodenheimer T. High and rising health care costs. *Ann Intern Med.* 2005;142:847, 932, 996.

Bodenheimer T, Grumbach K. Improving primary care. *Strategies and Tools for a Better Practice.* New York: McGraw-Hill; 2007.

Brook RH et al. Does free care improve adults' health? *N Engl J Med.* 1983;309:1426.

Claxton G et al. Health benefits in 2010. *Health Aff (Millwood).* 2010;29:1942.

Enthoven AC. Employment-based health insurance is failing: now what? *Health Aff (Millwood).* 2003;(suppl web exclusives):W3–W237.

Enthoven AC. The history and principles of managed competition. *Health Aff (Millwood).* 1993;12(suppl): 24–48.

Evans RG. *Strained Mercy: The Economics of Canadian Health Care.* Toronto, Ontario, Canada: Butterworths; 1984.

Fisher ES et al. Associations among hospital capacity, utilization, and mortality of U.S. Medicare beneficiaries, controlling for sociodemographic factors. *Health Serv Res.* 2000; 34:1351.

Gawande A. The cost conundrum. *The New Yorker.* June 1, 2009.

Goldman DP et al. Prescription drug cost sharing: associations with medication and medical utilization and spending and health. *JAMA*. 2007;298:61.

Goodell S et al. *Emergency Department Utilization and Capacity*. Robert Wood Johnson Foundation Policy Brief. No. 17, July 2009. www.rwjf.org/files/research/45929.emergency utilization.brief.pdf. Accessed November 14, 2011.

Gruber J. *The Tax Exclusion for Employer-Sponsored Health Insurance*. National Bureau of Economic Research. February 2010. www.nber.org/papers/w15766. Accessed November 14, 2011.

Grumbach K, Bodenheimer T. Reins or fences: A physician's view of cost containment. *Health Aff (Millwood)*. 1990;9(3):120.

Hellinger FJ. The impact of financial incentives on physician behavior in managed care plans: A review of the evidence. *Med Care Res Rev*. 1996;53:294.

Hsu J et al. Unintended consequences of caps on Medicare drug benefits. *N Engl J Med*. 2006;354:2349.

Lee PR, Etheredge L. Clinical freedom: Two lessons for the UK from U.S. experience with privatisation of health care. *Lancet*. 1989;1:263.

Light DW. Life, death, and the insurance companies. *N Engl J Med*. 1994;330:498.

Mays GP et al. Managed care rebound? Recent changes in health plans' cost containment strategies. *Health Aff (Millwood)*. 2004;(suppl web exclusive):w4–427–36.

Mehrotra A et al. The relationship between health plan advertising and market incentives: Evidence of risk-selective behavior. *Health Aff (Millwood)*. 2006;25:759.

Newhouse JP et al. Some interim results from a controlled trial of cost sharing in health insurance. *N Engl J Med*. 1981;305:1501.

OECD. Health at a Glance. Organization for Economic Cooperation and Development, 2009. www.oecd.org/health.

Phelps CE. *Health Economics*. Boston, MA: Addison Wesley; 2003.

Rice TH. Containing health care costs. In: Andersen RM, Rice TH, Kominski GF, eds. *Changing the U.S. Health Care System*. San Francisco, CA: Jossey-Bass; 1996.

Rice TH, Labelle RJ. Do physicians induce demand for medical services? *J Health Polit Policy Law*. 1989;14:587.

Roemer MI, Shain M. *Hospital Utilization Under Insurance*. Chicago, IL: American Hospital Association; 1959.

Schneeweiss S et al. The effect of Medicare Part D coverage on drug use and cost sharing among seniors without prior drug benefits. *Health Aff (Millwood)*. 2009;28:w305.

Singer DE et al. Rationing intensive care: Physician responses to a resource shortage. *N Engl J Med*. 1983;309:1155.

Vladeck BC. Fixing Medicare's physician payment system. *N Engl J Med*. 2010;362:1955.

Wennberg JE. Outcomes research, cost containment, and the fear of health care rationing. *N Engl J Med*. 1990;323:1202.

Wickizer TM. The effect of utilization review on hospital use and expenditures: A review of the literature and an update on recent findings. *Med Care Rev*. 1990;47:327.

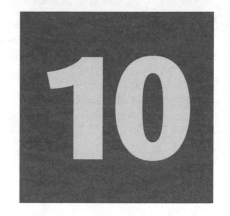

Quality of Health Care

Each year in the United States, millions of people visit hospitals, physicians, and other caregivers and receive medical care of superb quality. But that's not the whole story. Some patients' interactions with the health care system fall short (Institute of Medicine, 1999, 2001).

At the beginning of the twenty-first century, an estimated 32,000 people died in US hospitals each year as a result of preventable medical errors (Zahn and Miller, 2003). In addition, an estimated 57,000 people in the United States died because they were not receiving appropriate health care—in most cases, because common medical conditions such as high blood pressure or elevated cholesterol are not adequately controlled (National Committee for Quality Assurance, 2010). Hospitals vary greatly in their risk-adjusted mortality rates for Medicare patients; for 2000 to 2002, if hospitals with mortality rates higher than expected reduced deaths to the levels that were expected given their patient mix, 17,000 to 21,000 fewer deaths per year would have occurred (Schoen et al, 2006).

Fatal medication errors among outpatients doubled between 1983 and 1993 (Phillips et al, 1998). Prescribing errors occur in 7.6% of outpatient prescriptions (Gandhi et al, 2005), which amounts to 228 million errors in 2004. In 2007, about 25% of elderly patient received high-risk medications (Zhang et al, 2010). Diagnostic error rates are around 10% for a variety of medical conditions (Wachter, 2010). In some primary care practices, patients are not informed about abnormal laboratory results over 20% of the time (Casalino et al, 2009).

Forty-five percent of adults do not receive recommended chronic and preventive care, and 30% seeking care for acute problems receive treatment that is contra-indicated (Schuster et al, 1998; McGlynn et al, 2003). Only 50% of people with hypertension are adequately treated (Egan, 2010). Sixty-three percent of people with diabetes are inadequately controlled (Saydah et al, 2004). In many studies, racial and ethnic minority patients experience an inferior quality of care compared with white patients (Agency for Healthcare Research and Quality, 2010). The likelihood of patients being harmed by medical negligence is almost three times as great in hospitals serving largely low-income and minority patients than in hospitals with more affluent populations (Burstin et al, 1993a; Ayanian, 1994; Fiscella et al, 2000). A recent study of multiple quality measures found that the US continues to have serious quality problems and lags behind other developed nations (Schoen et al, 2006).

A prominent Institute of Medicine report (2001) concluded that between what we *know* and what we *do* lies not just a gap, but a chasm. Quality problems have been categorized as overuse, underuse, and misuse (Chassin et al, 1998). We will first examine the factors contributing to poor quality and then explore what can be done to elevate all health care to the highest possible level.

THE COMPONENTS OF HIGH-QUALITY CARE

What is high-quality health care? It is care that assists healthy people to stay healthy, cures acute illnesses, and allows chronically ill people to live as long and fulfilling a life as possible. What are the components of high-quality health care? (Table 10–1)

Table 10–1. Components of high-quality care

Access to care
Adequate scientific knowledge
Competent health care providers
Separation of financial and clinical decisions
Organization of health care institutions to maximize quality

Adequate Access to Care

Lydia and Laura were friends at a rural high school; both became pregnant. Lydia's middle-class parents took her to a nearby obstetrician, while Laura, from a family on welfare, could not find a physician who would take Medicaid. Lydia became the mother of a healthy infant, but Laura, going without prenatal care, delivered a low-birth-weight baby with severe lung problems.

To receive quality care, people must have access to care. People with reduced access to care suffer worse health outcomes in comparison to those enjoying full access—the quality problem of underuse (see Chapter 3). Quality requires equality (Schiff et al, 1994).

Adequate Scientific Knowledge

Brigitte Levy, a professor of family law, was started on estrogen replacement in 1960 when she reached menopause. Her physician prescribed the hormone pills for 10 years. In 1979, she was diagnosed with invasive cancer of the uterus, which spread to her entire abdominal cavity in spite of surgical treatment and radiation. She died in 1980 at age 68, at the height of her career.

A body of knowledge must exist that informs physicians what to do for the patient's problem. If clear scientific knowledge fails to distinguish between effective and ineffective or harmful care, quality may be compromised. During the 1960s, medical science taught that estrogen replacement, without the administration of progestins, was safe. Sadly, cases of uterine cancer caused by estrogen replacement did not show up until many years later. Brigitte Levy's physician followed the standard of care for his day, but the medical profession as a whole was relying on inadequate scientific knowledge. A great deal of what physicians do has never been evaluated by rigorous scientific experiment (Eddy, 1993), and many therapies have not been adequately tested for side effects. Treatments of uncertain safety and efficacy may cause harm and cost billions of dollars each year.

Competent Health Care Providers

Ceci Yu, age 77, was waking up at night with shortness of breath and wheezing. Her physician told her she had asthma and prescribed albuterol, a bronchodilator. Two days later, Ms. Yu was admitted to the coronary care unit with a heart attack. Writing to the chief of medicine, the cardiologist charged that Ms. Yu's physician had misdiagnosed the wheezing of congestive heart failure and had treated Ms. Yu incorrectly for asthma. The cardiologist charged that the treatment might have precipitated the heart attack.

The provider must have the skills to diagnose problems and choose appropriate treatments. An inadequate level of competence resulted in poor quality care for Ms. Yu.

The Harvard Medical Practice study reviewed 30,000 medical records in 51 hospitals in New York State in 1984 (Studdert et al, 2004). The study found that in approximately 4% of hospital admissions, the patient experienced a medical injury (ie, a medical problem caused by the management of a disease rather than by the disease itself); this is the quality problem of misuse. A more recent study placed the percent of hospital patients experiencing a medical injury at 13.8% (Meurer et al, 2006). Medical injuries can be classified as negligent or not negligent.

Jack was given a prescription for a sulfa drug. When he took the first pill, he turned beet red, began to wheeze, and fell to the floor. His friend called 911, and Jack was treated in the emergency department for anaphylactic shock, a potentially fatal allergic reaction. The emergency medicine physician learned that Jack had developed a rash the last time he took sulfa. Jack's physician had never asked him if he was allergic to sulfa, and Jack did not realize that the prescription contained sulfa.

Mack was prescribed a sulfa drug, following which he developed anaphylactic shock. Before writing the prescription, Mack's physician asked whether he had a sulfa allergy. Mack had said "No."

Medical negligence is defined as failure to meet the standard of practice of an average qualified physician practicing in the same specialty. Jack's drug reaction must be considered negligence, while Mack's was not. Of the medical injuries discovered in the Harvard study, 28% were because of negligence. In those injuries that led to death, 51% involved negligence. The most common injuries were drug reactions (19%) and wound infections (14%). Eight percent of injuries involved failure to diagnose a condition, of which 75% were negligent. Seventy percent of patients suffering all forms of medical injury recovered completely in 6 months or less, but 47% of patients in whom a diagnosis was missed suffered serious disabilities (Brennan et al, 1991; Leape et al, 1991).

Negligence cannot be equated with incompetence. Any good health care professional may have a mental lapse, may be overtired after a long night in the intensive care unit, or may have failed to learn an important new research finding.

▶ Money and Quality of Care

Nina Brown, a 56-year-old woman with diabetes, arrived at her primary care physician's office complaining of several bouts of chest pain over the past month. Her physician examined Ms. Brown, performed an electrocardiogram (ECG), which showed no abnormalities, diagnosed musculoskeletal pain, and recommended she take some ibuprofen. Five minutes later in the parking lot, Ms. Brown collapsed of a heart attack. The health plan insuring Ms. Brown had an incentive arrangement with primary care physicians whereby the physicians receive a bonus payment if the physicians reduce use of emergency department and referral services below the community average.

Completely healthy at age 45, Henry Fung reluctantly submitted to a treadmill exercise test at the local YMCA. The study was possibly abnormal, and Mr. Fung, who had fee-for-service insurance, sought the advice of a cardiologist. The cardiologist knew that treadmill tests are sometimes positive in healthy people. He ordered a coronary angiogram, which was perfectly normal. Three hours after the

study, a clot formed in the femoral artery at the site of the catheter insertion, and emergency surgery was required to save Mr. Fung's leg.

No one can know what motivated the physician to send Ms. Brown home instead of to an emergency department when unstable coronary heart disease was one possible diagnosis (underuse); nor can one guess what led the fee-for-service cardiologist to perform an invasive coronary angiogram of questionable appropriateness on Mr. Fung (overuse). One factor that bears close attention is the impact of financial considerations on the quantity (and thus the quality) of medical care (Relman, 2007). As noted in Chapter 4, fee-for-service reimbursement encourages physicians to perform more services, whereas capitation payment rewards those who perform fewer services.

More than 40 years ago, Bunker (1970) found that the United States performed twice the number of surgical procedures per capita than Great Britain. He postulated that this difference could be accounted for by the greater number of surgeons per capita in the United States and concluded that "the method of payment appears to play an important, if unmeasured, part." Most surgeons in the United States are compensated by fee-for-service, whereas most in Great Britain are paid a salary. From 8% to 86% of surgeries—depending on the type—have been found to be unnecessary and have caused substantial avoidable death and disability (Leape, 1992). As an example, spinal fusion surgery increased by 77% from 1996 to 2001, though little evidence supports this procedure in many cases. Complications are frequent and rates of reoperation (because of failure to relieve pain or worsening pain) are high. Reimbursement for this procedure is greater than that provided for most other procedures performed by orthopedists and neurosurgeons (Deyo et al, 2004).

It was a nice dinner, hosted by the hospital radiologist and paid for by the company manufacturing magnetic resonance imaging (MRI) scanners. After the meal came the pitch: "If you physicians invest money, we can get an MRI scanner near our hospital; if the MRI makes money, you all share in the profits." One internist explained later, "After I put in my $10,000, it was hard to resist ordering MRI scans. With headaches, back pain, and knee problems, the indications for MRIs are kind of fuzzy. You might order one or you might not. Now, I do."

Relman (2007) writes about the commercialization of medicine: "The introduction of new technology in the hands of specialists, expanded insurance coverage, and unregulated fee-for-service payments all combined to rapidly increase the flow of money into the health care system, and thus sowed the seeds of a new, profit-driven industry."

During the 1980s, many physicians formed partnerships and joint ventures, giving them part ownership in laboratories, MRI scanners, and outpatient surgicenters. Forty percent of practicing physicians in Florida owned services to which they referred patients. Ninety-three percent of diagnostic imaging facilities, 76% of ambulatory surgery centers, and 60% of clinical laboratories in the state were owned wholly or in part by physicians. The rates of use for MRI and CT scans were higher for physician-owned compared with non-physician-owned facilities (Mitchell and Scott, 1992). In a national study, physicians who received payment for performing x-rays and sonograms within their own offices obtained these examinations four times as often as physicians who referred the examinations to radiologists and received no reimbursement for the studies. The patients in the two groups were similar (Hillman et al, 1990).

After 2000, profitable diagnostic, imaging, and surgical procedures have rapidly migrated from the hospital to free-standing physician-owned ambulatory surgery centers, endoscopy centers, and imaging centers (Berenson et al, 2006). For example, the number of CT scans performed for Medicare patients increased by 65% from 2000 to 2005; during those years, the number of MRI scans jumped by 94% (Bodenheimer et al, 2007). The number of CT scans is growing by more than 10% per year, increasing patients' risk of radiation-related cancer (Smith-Bindman, 2010). A significant association exists between surgeon ownership of ambulatory surgery centers and a higher volume of surgeries; surgery volume increases immediately following surgeons' acquisition of the surgicenter (Hollingsworth et al, 2010).

Moving to the other side of the overuse–underuse spectrum, payment by capitation, or salaried employment by a for-profit business, may create a climate hostile to the provision of adequate services. In the 1970s, a series of HMOs called prepaid health plans (PHPs) sprang up to provide care to California Medicaid patients. The quality of care in several PHPs became a major scandal in California. At one PHP, administrators wrote a message to health care providers: "Do as little as you possibly can for the PHP patient," and charts audited by the California Health Department revealed many instances of undertreatment. The PHPs received a lump sum for each patient enrolled, meaning that the lower the cost of the services actually provided, the greater the PHP's profits (US Senate, 1975).

The quantity and quality of medical care are inextricably interrelated. Too much or too little can be injurious. The research of Fisher et al (2003) has shown that similar populations in different geographic areas have widely varying rates of surgeries and days in the hospital, with no consistent difference in clinical outcomes between those in high-use and low-use areas.

▶ Health Care Systems and Quality of Care

The personnel cutbacks were terrible; staffing had diminished from four RNs per shift to two, with only two aides to provide assistance. Shelley Rush, RN, was 2 hours behind in administering medications and had five insulin injections to give, with complicated dosing schedules. A family member rushed to the nursing station saying, "The lady in my mother's room looks bad." Shelley ran in and found the patient unconscious. She quickly checked the blood sugar, which was disastrously low at 20 mg/dL. Shelley gave 50% glucose, and the patient woke up. Then it hit her—she had injected the insulin into the wrong patient.

Health care institutions must be well organized, with an adequate, competent staff. Shelley Rush was a superb nurse, but understaffing caused her to make a serious error. The book *Curing Health Care* by Berwick et al (1990) opens with a heartbreaking case:

She died, but she didn't have to. The senior resident was sitting, near tears, in the drab office behind the nurses' station in the intensive care unit. It was 2:00 AM, and he had been battling for thirty-two hours to save the life of the 23-year-old graduate student who had just suffered her final cardiac arrest.

The resident slid a large manila envelope across the desk top. "Take a look at this," he said. "Routine screening chest x-ray, taken 10 months ago. The tumor is right there, and it was curable—then. By the time the second film was taken 8 months later, because she was complaining of pain, it was too late. The tumor had spread everywhere, and the odds were hopelessly against her. Everything we've done since then has really just been wishful thinking. We missed our chance. She missed her chance." Exhausted, the resident put his head in his hands and cried.

Two months later, the Quality Assurance Committee completed its investigation. . . . "We find the inpatient care commendable in this tragic case," concluded the brief report, "although the failure to recognize the tumor in a potentially curable stage 10 months earlier was unfortunate. . . ." Nowhere in this report was it written explicitly why the results of the first chest x-ray had not been translated into action. No one knew.

One year later. . . . it was 2:00 AM, and the night custodian was cleaning the radiologist's office. As he moved a filing cabinet aside to sweep behind it, he glimpsed a dusty tan envelope that had been stuck between the cabinet and the wall. The envelope contained a yellow radiology report slip, and the date on the report—nearly two years earlier—convinced the custodian that this was, indeed, garbage . . . He tossed it in with the other trash, and 4 hours later it was incinerated along with other useless things. (Berwick et al, 1990)

This patient may have had perfect access to care for an illness whose treatment is scientifically proved; she may have seen a physician who knew how to make the diagnosis and deliver the appropriate treatment; and yet the quality of her care was disastrously deficient. Dozens of people and hundreds of processes influence the care of one person with one illness. In her case, one person—perhaps a file clerk with a near-perfect record in handling thousands of radiology reports—lost control of one report, and the physician's office had no system to monitor whether or not x-ray reports had been received. The result was the most tragic of quality failures—the unnecessary death of a young person.

How health care systems and institutions are organized has a major impact on health care outcomes. For example, large multispecialty group practices in 22 metropolitan areas have better-quality measures at lower cost than dispersed physician practices in those

areas (Weeks et al, 2009). Studies have shown that hospitals with more RN staffing have lower surgical complication rates (Kovner and Gergen, 1998) and lower mortality rates (Aiken et al, 2002).

Oliver Hart lived in a city with a population of 80,000. He was admitted to Neighborhood Hospital with congestive heart failure caused by a defective mitral valve. He was told he needed semiurgent heart surgery to replace the valve. The cardiologist said "You can go to University Hospital 30 miles away or have the surgery done here." The cardiologist did not say that Neighborhood Hospital performed only seven cardiac surgeries last year. Mr. Hart elected to remain for the procedure. During the surgery, a key piece of equipment failed, and he died on the operating table.

Quality of care must be viewed in the context of regional systems of care (see Chapter 6), not simply within each health care institution. In one study, 27% of deaths related to coronary artery bypass graft (CABG) surgery at low-volume hospitals might have been prevented by referral of those patients to hospitals performing a higher volume of those surgeries (Dudley et al, 2000). Quality improves with the experience of those providing the care (Kizer, 2003; Peterson et al, 2004). Had Mr. Hart been told the relative surgical mortality rates at University Hospital, which performed 500 cardiac surgeries each year, and at Neighborhood Hospital, he would have chosen to be transferred 30 miles down the road. Not only does the volume of surgeries in a hospital matter; equally important is the volume of surgeries performed by the specific surgeon (Birkmeyer et al, 2003).

In the late 1980s, Dr. Donald Berwick (1989) and others realized that quality of care is not simply a question of whether or not a physician or other caregiver is competent. If poorly organized, the complex systems within and among medical institutions can thwart the best efforts of professionals to deliver high-quality care.

There are two approaches to the problem of improving quality . . . [One is] the Theory of Bad Apples, because those who subscribe to it believe that quality is best achieved by discovering bad apples and removing them from the lot. . . . The Theory of Bad Apples gives rise readily to what can be called the my-apple-is-just-fine-thank-you response . . . and seeks not understanding, but escape. [The other is] the Theory of Continuous Improvement . . . . Even when people were at the root of defects,. . . the problem was generally not one of motivation or effort, but rather of poor job design, failure of leadership, or unclear purpose. Quality can be improved much more when people are assumed to be trying hard already, and are not accused of sloth. Fear of the kind engendered by the disciplinary approach poisons improvement in quality, since it inevitably leads to the loss of the chance to learn.

Real improvement in quality depends . . . on continuous improvement throughout the organization through constant effort to reduce waste, rework, and complexity. When one is clear and constant in one's purpose, when fear does not control the atmosphere (and thus the data), when learning is guided by accurate information . . . and when the hearts and talents of all workers are enlisted in the pursuit of better ways, the potential for improvement in quality is nearly boundless . . . . A test result lost, a specialist who cannot be reached, a missing requisition, a misinterpreted order, duplicate paperwork, a vanished record, a long wait for the CT scan, an unreliable on-call system—these are all-too-familiar examples of waste, rework, complexity, and error in the physician's daily life . . . . For the average physician, quality fails when systems fail. (Berwick et al, 1989)

▶ The Components of Quality: Summary

Good-quality care can be compromised at a number of steps along the way.

Angie Roth has coronary heart disease and may need CABG surgery. (1) If she is uninsured and cannot get to a physician, high-quality care is impossible to obtain. (2) If clear evidence-based guidelines do not exist regarding who benefits from CABG and who does not, Ms. Roth's physician may make the wrong choice. (3) Even if clear guidelines exist, if Angie Roth's physician fails to evaluate her illness correctly or sends her to a surgeon with poor operative skills, quality may suffer. (4) If indications for surgery are not clear in Ms. Roth's case but the surgeon will benefit economically from the procedure, the surgery may be inappropriately performed. (5) Even if the surgery is appropriate and

Table 10–2. Quality aims as defined by the Institute of Medicine

- *Safe*—avoiding injuries to patients from the care that is intended to help them
- *Effective*—providing services based on scientific knowledge to all who could benefit and refraining from providing services to those not likely to benefit (avoiding underuse and overuse, respectively)
- *Patient-centered*—providing care that is respectful of and responsive to individual patient preferences, needs, and values and ensuring that patient values guide all clinical decisions
- *Timely*—reducing waits and sometimes harmful delays for both those who receive and those who give care
- *Efficient*—avoiding waste, including waste of equipment, supplies, ideas, and energy
- *Equitable*—providing care that does not vary in quality because of personal characteristics such as gender, ethnicity, geographic location, and socioeconomic status

Source: Institute of Medicine. *Crossing the Quality Chasm: A New Health System for the 21st Century.* Washington, DC: National Academies Press; 2001.

performed by an excellent surgeon, faulty equipment in the operating room or poor teamwork among the operating room surgeons, anesthesiologists, and nurses may lead to a poor outcome.

The Institute of Medicine, in its influential 2001 report *Crossing the Quality Chasm*, conceptualized six core dimensions of quality: safe, effective, patient-centered, timely, efficient, and equitable. These dimensions, defined in greater detail in Table 10–2, are consistent with the components of quality discussed earlier.

PROPOSALS FOR IMPROVING QUALITY

Several infants at a hospital received epinephrine in error and suffered serious medical consequences. An analysis revealed that several pharmacists had made the same mistake; the problem was caused by the identical appearance of vitamin E and epinephrine bottles in the pharmacy. This was a system error.

An epidemic of unexpected deaths on the cardiac ward was investigated. The times of the deaths were correlated with personnel schedules, leading to the conclusion that one nurse was responsible. It turned out that she was administering lethal doses of digoxin to patients. This was not a system error.

Quality issues must be investigated to determine if they are system errors or problems with a particular caregiver. Traditionally, quality assurance has focused on individual caregivers and institutions in a "bad apple" approach that relies heavily on sanctions. More recently, quality has been viewed through the lens of the continuous quality improvement (CQI) model that seeks to enhance the clinical performance of all systems of care, not just the outliers with flagrantly poor quality of care. The move to a CQI model has required development of more formalized standards of care that can be used as benchmarks for measuring quality, and more systematic collection of data to measure overall performance and not just performance in isolated cases (Tables 10–2).

▶ Traditional Quality Assurance: Licensure, Accreditation, and Peer Review

Traditionally, the health care system has placed great reliance on educational institutions and licensing and accrediting agencies to ensure the competence of individuals and institutions in health care. Health care professionals undergo rigorous training and pass special licensing examinations intended to ensure that caregivers have at least a basic level of knowledge and competence. However, not all individuals who have successfully completed their education and passed licensing examinations are competent clinicians. In some cases, this reflects a failure of the educational and licensing systems. In other cases, clinicians may have been competent practitioners at the time they took their examinations, but their skills lapsed or they developed impairment from alcohol or drug use, depression, or other conditions (Leape and Fromson, 2006).

Licensing agencies in the United States do not require periodic reexaminations. In most cases, licensing boards only respond to patient or health care professional complaints about negligent or unprofessional behavior. Many organizations that confer specialty board certification require physicians to pass examinations on a periodic basis to maintain active specialty certification. Some specialties also require physicians to perform and document systematic quality reviews of their own clinical practices for maintenance of certification. However, while some hospitals may require active specialty certification for a physician to be granted privileges to practice in the hospital, certification is not required for medical licensure, diluting some of the consequences of not participating in specialty recertification.

The traditional approach to quality assurance has also relied heavily on peer pressure within hospitals, HMOs, and the medical community at large. Peer review is the evaluation by health care practitioners of the appropriateness and quality of services performed by other practitioners, usually in the same specialty. Peer review has been a part of medicine for decades (eg, tissue committees study surgical specimens to determine whether appendectomies and hysterectomies have actually removed diseased organs; credentials committees review the qualifications of physicians for hospital staff privileges). But peer review moved to center stage with the passage of the law enacting Medicare in 1965.

Medicare anointed the Joint Commission on Accreditation of Hospitals (now named simply the Joint Commission) with the authority to terminate hospitals from the Medicare program if quality of care was found to be deficient. The Joint Commission requires hospital medical staff to set up peer review committees for the purpose of maintaining quality of care.

The Joint Commission uses criteria of structure, process, and outcome to assess quality of care. Structural criteria include such factors as whether the emergency department defibrillator works properly. Criteria of process include whether medical records are dictated and signed in a timely manner, or if the credentials committee keeps minutes of its meetings. Outcomes include such measures as mortality rates for surgical procedures, proportions of deaths that are preventable, and rates of adverse drug reactions and wound infections. Medicare also contracts with quality improvement organizations (QIOs) in each state to promote better quality of care among physicians caring for Medicare beneficiaries.

Angela Lopez, age 57, suffered from metastatic ovarian cancer but was feeling well and prayed she would live 9 months more. Her son was the first family member ever to attend college, and she hoped to see him graduate. It was decided to infuse chemotherapy directly into her peritoneal cavity.

As the solution poured into her abdomen, she felt increasing pressure. She asked the nurse to stop the fluid. The nurse called the physician, who said not to worry. Two hours later, Ms. Lopez became short of breath and demanded that the fluid be stopped. The nurse again called the physician, but an hour later Ms. Lopez died. Her abdomen was tense with fluid, which pushed on her lungs and stopped circulation through her inferior vena cava. The quality assurance committee reviewed the case as a preventable death and criticized the physician for giving too much fluid and failing to respond adequately to the nurse's call. The physician replied that he was not at fault; the nurse had not told him how sick the patient was. The case was closed.

The traditional quality assurance strategies of licensing and peer review have not been particularly effective tools for improving quality. Peer review often adheres to the theory of bad apples, attempting to discipline physicians (to remove them from the apple barrel) for mistakes rather than to improve their practice through education. The physician who caused Ms. Lopez's preventable death responded to peer criticism by blaming the nurse rather than learning from the mistake. With the hundreds of decisions physicians make each day, often in time-constrained situations, serious errors are relatively common in medical practice. Yet 42% of physicians recently surveyed had never disclosed a serious error to a patient (Gallagher et al, 2006). Hiding mistakes rather than correcting them is the legacy of a punitive quality assurance apparatus (Leape, 1994).

Even if sanctions against the truly bad apples had more teeth, these measures would not solve the quality problem. Removing the incontrovertibly bad apples from the barrel does not address all the quality problems that emanate from competent caregivers who are not performing optimally. Health care systems do need to ensure basic clinical competence and to forcefully sanction caregivers who, despite efforts at remediation, cannot operate at a basic standard of acceptable practice. But measures are also needed to "shift the curve" of overall clinical practice to a higher level of quality, not just to trim off the poor-quality outliers.

Peer reviewers frequently disagree as to whether the quality of care in particular cases is adequate or not (Laffel and Berwick, 1993). Because of these limitations,

Table 10–3. Proposals for improving quality

Identifying and sanctioning "bad apples"
Clinical practice guidelines
Measuring practice patterns
Continuous quality improvement
Computerized information systems
Public reporting of quality
Pay for reporting
Pay for performance
Financially neutral clinical decision making

efforts are underway to formalize standards of care using clinical practice guidelines and to move from individual case review to more systematic monitoring of overall practice patterns (Table 10–3).

▶ Clinical Practice Guidelines

Dr. Benjamin Waters was frustrated by patients who came in with urinary incontinence. He never learned about the problem in medical school, so he simply referred these patients to a urologist. In his managed care plan, Dr. Waters was known to overrefer, so he felt stuck. He could not handle the problem, yet he did not want to refer patients elsewhere. He solved his dilemma by prescribing incontinence pads and diapers, but did not feel good about it.

Dr. Denise Drier learned about urinary incontinence in family medicine residency but did not feel secure about caring for the problem. On the web, she found "Urinary Incontinence in Adults: Clinical Practice Guideline Update." She studied the material and applied it to her incontinence patients. After a few successes, she and the patients were feeling better about themselves.

For many conditions, there is a better and a worse way to make a diagnosis and prescribe treatment. Physicians may not be aware of the better way because of gaps in training, limited experience, or insufficient time or motivation to learn new techniques. For these problems, clinical practice guidelines can be helpful in improving quality of care. In 1989, Congress established the Agency for Health Care Policy and Research, now called the Agency for Healthcare Research and

Quality (AHRQ), to develop practice guidelines, among other tasks. Produced by panels of experts, practice guidelines make specific recommendations to physicians on how to treat clinical conditions such as diabetes, osteoporosis, urinary incontinence, or cataracts. However, some powerful physician interests, displeased by AHRQ practice guidelines that recommended against surgical treatment for most cases of back pain, pressured Congress to reduce AHRQ's budget and bar AHRQ from issuing its own guidelines.

More than 2000 guidelines exist; written by dozens of organizations, they vary in scientific reliability. Most are developed by societies of medical specialists (Steinbrook, 2007). Ideally, practice guidelines are based on a rigorous and objective review of scientific evidence, with explicit ratings of the quality of the evidence. However, 87% of clinical practice guideline authors in one survey had ties to the pharmaceutical industry, a bias often not disclosed to readers of the guidelines (Shaneyfelt and Centor, 2009). For example, eight of nine authors of widely used guidelines recommending broad use of cholesterol-lowering statin drugs had financial ties to companies making or selling statins (Abramson and Starfield, 2005). Moreover, clinical practice guidelines developed based on research on a narrowly defined population, such as nonelderly patients with a single chronic condition, may not be applicable to different patient populations, such as elderly patients with multiple diseases (Boyd et al, 2005).

Practice guidelines are not appropriate for many clinical situations. Uncertainty pervades clinical medicine, and practice guidelines are applicable only for those cases in which we enjoy "islands of knowledge in our seas of ignorance." Practice guidelines can assist but not replace clinical judgment in the quest for high-quality care.

Pedro Urrutia, age 59, noticed mild nocturia and urinary frequency. His friend had prostate cancer, and he became concerned. The urologist said that his prostate was only slightly enlarged, his prostate-specific antigen (blood test) was normal, and surgery was not needed. Mr. Urrutia wanted surgery and found another urologist to do it.

At age 82, James Chin noted nocturia and urinary hesitancy. He had two glasses of wine on his wife's birthday and later that night was unable to urinate.

He went to the emergency department, was found to have a large prostate without nodules, and was catheterized. The urologist strongly recommended a transurethral resection of the prostate. Mr. Chin refused, thinking that the urinary retention was caused by the alcohol. Five years later, he was in good health with his prostate intact.

The difficulty with creating a set of indications for surgery, for example surgery for benign enlargement of the prostate gland, is that patient preferences vary markedly. Some, like Mr. Urrutia, want prostate surgery, even though it is not clearly needed; others, like Mr. Chin, have strong reasons for surgery but do not want it. Practice guidelines must take into account not only scientific data, but also patient preferences (O'Connor et al, 2007).

Do practice guidelines in themselves improve quality of care? Studies reveal that by themselves they are unsuccessful in influencing physicians' practices (Cabana et al, 1999). However, guidelines can be an important foundation for more comprehensive quality improvement strategies, such as computer systems to remind physicians when patients are in need of certain services according to a guideline (eg, a reminder system about women due for a mammogram) or having trusted colleagues ("opinion leaders") or visiting experts ("academic detailing") conduct small group sessions with clinicians to review and reinforce practice guidelines (Bodenheimer and Grumbach, 2007).

▶ Measuring Practice Patterns

One of the central tenets of the CQI approach is the need to systematically monitor how well individual caregivers, institutions, and organizations are performing. There are two basic types of indicators that are used to evaluate clinical performance: process measures and outcome measures. *Process* of care refers to the types of services delivered by caregivers. Examples are prescribing aspirin to patients with coronary heart disease, or turning immobile patients in hospital beds on a regular schedule to prevent bed sores. *Outcomes* are death, symptoms, mental health, physical functioning, and related aspects of health status, and are the gold standard for measuring quality. However, outcomes (particularly those dealing with quality of life) may be difficult to measure. More easily counted outcomes such as mortality may be rare events, and therefore uninformative for evaluating quality of care for many conditions that are not immediately life-threatening. Also, outcomes may be heavily influenced by the underlying severity of illness and related patient characteristics, and not just by the quality of health care that patients received (King and Wheeler, 2007) When measuring patient outcomes, it is necessary to "risk adjust" these outcome measurements for differences in the underlying characteristics of different groups of patients. Because of these challenges in using outcomes as measures to monitor quality of care, process measures tend to be more commonly used. For process measures to be valid indicators of quality, there must first be solid research demonstrating that the processes do in fact influence patient outcomes.

Dr. Susan Cutter felt horrible. It was supposed to have been a routine hysterectomy. Somehow she had inadvertently lacerated the large intestine of the patient, a 45-year-old woman with symptomatic fibroids of the uterus but otherwise in good health prior to surgery. Bacteria from the intestine had leaked into the abdomen, and after a protracted battle in the ICU the patient died of septic shock.

Dr. Cutter met with the Chief of Surgery at her hospital. The Chief reviewed the case with Dr. Cutter, but also pulled out a report showing the statistics on all of Dr. Cutter's surgical cases over the previous 5 years. The report showed that Dr. Cutter's mortality and complication rates were among the lowest of surgeons on the hospital's staff. However, the Chief did note that another surgeon, Dr. Dehisce, had a complication rate that was much higher than that of all the other staff surgeons. The Chief of Surgery asked Dr. Cutter to serve on a departmental committee to review Dr. Dehisce's cases and to meet with Dr. Dehisce to consider ways to address his poor performance.

The contemporary approach to quality monitoring moves beyond examining a few isolated cases toward measuring processes or outcomes for a large population of patients. For example, a traditional peer review approach is to review every case of a patient who dies during surgery. Reviewing an individual case may help a surgeon and the operating team understand where errors may have occurred—a process known as "root cause" analysis. However, it does not indicate whether the case represented an aberrant bad outcome for a surgeon or team that usually has good surgical outcomes, or whether the case is indicative of more widespread problems. To answer these questions requires examining data on all the patients operated on by the surgeon and the operating team to measure the overall rate of surgical complications, and having some benchmark data that indicate whether this rate is higher than expected for similar types of patients.

Mel Litus was the nurse in charge of diabetes education for a large medical group. After seeing yet another patient return to clinic after having had a foot amputation or suffering a heart attack, Mel wondered how the clinic team could do a better job in preventing diabetic complications. The medical group had recently implemented a new computerized clinical information system. Mel met with the administrator in charge of the computer system and arranged to have a printout made of all the laboratory findings, referrals, and medications for the diabetic patients in the medical group. When Mel reviewed the printout, he noticed that many of the patients didn't attend appointments very regularly and were not receiving important services like regular ophthalmology visits and medications that protect the kidneys from diabetic damage. Mel met with the medical director for quality improvement to discuss a plan for sharing this information with the clinical staff and creating a system for more closely monitoring the care of diabetic patients.

Many practice organizations, from small groups of office-based physicians to huge, vertically integrated HMOs are starting to monitor patterns of care and provide feedback on this care to physicians and other staff in these organizations. The goal of this feedback is to alert caregivers and health care organizations about patterns of care that are not achieving optimal standards, in order to stimulate efforts to improve processes of care. The response may range from individual clinicians systematically reviewing their care of certain types of patients and clinical conditions, to entire organizations redesigning the system of care. A typical example of this practice profiling is measuring the rate at which diabetic patients receive recommended services, such as annual eye examinations, periodic testing of HbA_{1c} levels, and evaluation of kidney function. Process of care profiles alert individual caregivers to specific diabetic patients who need to be called in for certain tests, and point out patterns of care that suggest that the organization should implement systematic reforms, such as developing case management programs for diabetic patients in poor control (Bodenheimer and Grumbach, 2007).

Continuous Quality Improvement

Maximizing excellence for individual health care professionals is only one ingredient in the recipe for high-quality health care. Improving institutions is the other, through CQI techniques. CQI involves the identification of concrete problems and the formation of interdisciplinary teams to gather data and propose and implement solutions to the problems.

In LDS Hospital in Salt Lake City, variation in wound infection rates by different physicians was related to the timing of the administration of prophylactic antibiotics. Patients who received antibiotics 2 hours before surgery had the lowest infection rates. The surgery department adopted a policy that all patients receive antibiotics precisely 2 hours before surgery; the rate of postoperative wound infections dropped from 1.8% to 0.9%. (Burke, 2001)

Such successes only dot, but do not yet dominate, the health care quality landscape (Solberg, 2007). The Institute for Healthcare Improvement (IHI) has led efforts to spread CQI efforts by sponsoring "collaboratives" to assist institutions and groups of institutions to improve health care outcomes and access while ideally reducing costs. Hundreds of health care organizations have participated in collaboratives concerned with such topics as improving the care of chronic illness, reducing waiting times, improving care at the end of life, and reducing adverse drug events. Collaboratives involve learning sessions during which teams from various institutions meet and discuss the application of a rapid change methodology within institutions. Some of IHI's successes have taken place in the area of chronic disease, with a variety of institutions—from large integrated delivery systems to tiny rural community health centers—implementing the chronic care model to improve outcomes for conditions such as diabetes, asthma, and congestive heart failure (Bodenheimer et al, 2002). Collaboratives that assist institutions to implement the chronic care model have shown modest

improvement in patient outcomes compared with controls (Vargas et al, 2007). In the area of patient safety, in 2004, IHI launched the 100,000 Lives Campaign (www.ihi.org) to reduce mortality rates in hospitals, followed by a 5 Million Lives Campaign between 2006 and 2008; more than 4000 hospitals in the United States participated in these campaigns. There is evidence that these campaigns have contributed to reductions in hospital mortality, although there is debate about the magnitude of the impact (Berwick et al, 2006; Wachter and Pronovost, 2006).

Computerized Information Systems

The advent of computerized information systems has created opportunities to improve care and to monitor the process and outcomes of care for entire populations. Electronic medical records can create lists of patients who are overdue for services needed for preventive care or the management of chronic illness and can generate reminder prompts for physicians and patients (Baron, 2007). In-hospital medical errors related to drug prescribing are reduced with computerized physician order entry (CPOE), systems requiring physicians to enter hospital orders directly into a computer rather than handwriting them. The computer can alert the physician about inappropriate medication doses or medications to which the patient is known to be allergic (Kaushal et al, 2003). However, hospital-based electronic health records have not yet been proven to significantly improve quality (Eslami et al, 2007; DesRoches et al, 2010). By themselves, computerized information systems are unlikely to improve quality; computerization must be accompanied by changes in the organization of informational processes (Bodenheimer and Grumbach, 2007).

Public Reporting of Quality

The CQI approach emphasizes systematic monitoring of care to provide internal feedback to clinicians and health organizations to spur improved processes of care. A different approach to monitoring quality of care is to direct this information to the public. This approach views public release of systematic measurements of quality of care—commonly referred to as health care "report cards"—as a tool to empower health care consumers to select higher-quality caregivers and institutions. Advocates of this approach argue that armed with this information, patients and health care purchasers will make more informed decisions and preferentially seek out health care organizations with better report card grades.

An important experiment in individual physician report cards was initiated by the New York State Department of Health in 1990. The department released data on risk-adjusted mortality rates for coronary bypass surgery performed at each hospital in the state, and in 1992, mortality rates were also published for each cardiac surgeon. Each year's list was big news and highly controversial. However, difficulties in measurement were highlighted by the fact that within 1 year, 46% of the surgeons had moved from one-half of the ranked list to the other half.

Several fascinating results came of this project: (1) Patients did not switch from hospitals with high mortality rates to those with lower mortality rates. (2) With the release of each report, one in five bottom quartile surgeons relocated or ceased practicing within two years. (3) In 4 years, overall risk-adjusted coronary artery bypass mortality dropped by 41% in New York State. Mortality for this operation also dropped in states without report cards, but not as much. (4) Some surgeons, worried about the report cards, may have elected not to operate on the most risky patients in order to improve their report card ranking. It is possible that the reduction in surgical mortality in part resulted from withholding surgery for the sickest patients. The New York State experiment had less effect on changing the market decisions of patients and purchasers than on motivating quality improvements in hospitals that had poor surgical outcomes (Marshall et al, 2000; Jha and Epstein, 2006).

In 2011, the federal Centers for Medicare and Medicaid Services (CMS) launched its Physician Compare website, which will report on quality-of-care measures for specific physicians by 2015 (www.medicare.gov/find-a-doctor/provider-search.aspx).

The most important report card program is the Healthcare Effectiveness Data and Information Set (HEDIS). Developed by the National Committee for Quality Assurance (NCQA), a private organization controlled by large HMOs and large employers, HEDIS for 2010 is a list of 71 performance indicators including the percentage of children immunized; the percentage of enrollees of certain ages who have received Pap smears, colorectal screening, mammograms, and glaucoma screening; the percentage of pregnant women who received prenatal care in the first trimester; the percentage of diabetic patients who received retinal examinations; and the percentage of smokers for whom physicians made efforts at smoking cessation; the appropriateness of treatment for asthma, bronchitis, osteoporosis, depression, and others. NCQA chiefly reports on the performance of health plans; some critics believe that reporting on physicians and hospitals would be more helpful. Another problem is that few employers use quality data when selecting health plans for their employees; cost is the driving factor in most employer decisions (Galvin and Delbanco, 2005).

Report cards are based on a philosophy that says "if you can't count it, you can't improve it." Albert Einstein expressed an alternative philosophy that might illuminate the report card enterprise: "Not everything that can be counted counts, and not everything that counts can be counted." Increasingly, the focus on quality is switching to a focus on value, with value referring to quality divided by cost. Thus an increase in a quality measure associated with a growth in cost may not improve value, where improved quality with a stable or reduced cost increases value (Owens et al, 2011).

▶ Pay for Reporting

In 2003, the Medicare program initiated public reporting for hospitals, focusing on risk-adjusted quality of care for heart attacks, heart failure, and pneumonia. More recently, surgical care and other measures have been added. Reports on individual hospitals and an explanation of the program are available at www.hospitalcompare.hhs.gov. The program, the Hospital Quality Initiative, is voluntary but nonparticipating hospitals receive a reduction in their Medicare payments. One might say that the program is in essence no-pay for no-reporting. Hospital quality has improved for some measures that are reported (Chassin et al, 2010), but hospitals focus their quality activities on the specific measures prescribed by the program, at times to the detriment of other quality activities (Pham et al, 2006).

In 2007, Medicare began the Physician Quality Reporting System, under which physicians who report certain quality measures may receive a 2% increase in their Medicare fees. This is not a full-fledged pay for reporting program because the reports for individual physicians or physician practices are not made public (www.cms.hhs.gov/pqri/).

▶ Pay for Performance

By 2003, a new concept—"pay for performance"—was gaining widespread acceptance in health care (Epstein et al, 2004). Pay for performance (P4P) goes one step beyond pay for reporting; physicians or hospitals receive more money if their quality measures exceed certain benchmarks or if the measures improve from year to year.

One of the largest P4P programs is the Integrated Healthcare Association (IHA) program in California. IHA, representing employers, health plans, health systems and physician groups, launched the program in 2002 with a set of uniform performance measures. In 2010, seven health plans and 221 physician organizations— involving 35,000 physicians and 10 million patients— participated in the IHA program (www.iha.org).

In 2010, the health plans paid physician organizations $49 million in performance-based bonuses. The physician organizations receive funds for demonstrating improved clinical care (eg, cancer screening, immunizations, and management of asthma, diabetes, and cardiovascular disease), patient satisfaction, and development of information technology. In 2009, IHI added cost containment measures including inpatient utilization, hospital readmissions, and generic drug prescribing. Physician organizations distribute a substantial amount of the money to individual physicians but keep a portion of the bonus for organizationwide quality-enhancing initiatives. Quality measures have improved modestly since the program began, between 5% and 12%, but patient satisfaction did not. A limitation of the program is that the bonuses are small (about 2% of physician group revenues) and practices must spend money to organize and report their data (Damberg et al, 2009). Moreover, health plans are becoming less enthusiastic about P4P as they are not seeing the return on investment hoped for (Integrated Healthcare Organization, 2009).

The IHA program is unique for two reasons: All major health plans collaborated in choosing the measures upon which performance bonuses are based, and most physicians in California belong to a large medical group or independent practice association (see Chapter 6). If only one health plan sets up a P4P program with physicians, there may not be enough patients from that health plan to accurately measure the physician's quality; with all health plans participating, a substantial portion of a physician's patient panel is included in the measures. If P4P targets individual physicians rather than larger physician organizations, the small numbers of patients may distort the results. The ability of the California experience to aggregate a large number of patients allows for more accurate performance evaluation.

A P4P program initiated by large employers rather than health plans is Bridges to Excellence. This program involves more than 80 employers, large national health plans, and 3000 physicians in about 15 states. Physicians receive bonus payments for implementing computerized office systems and for improving the care of patients with diabetes, asthma, chronic lung disease, heart disease, back pain, and high blood pressure. Physicians practicing high-quality medicine in these areas receive public recognition and may receive bonuses, with the employers financing the program counting on higher-quality translating into lower costs. Performance is measured only for patients who are employees of the employers participating in the program, a small number for many physicians (www. bridgesto-excellence.org).

In 2003, Medicare launched a P4P program for 268 hospitals, measuring certain quality indicators for heart attack, heart failure, pneumonia, coronary artery bypass surgery, and hip and knee replacements. High-performing hospitals receive bonuses and the lowest performers may be subject to penalties. Performance on ten measures for heart attack, heart failure, and pneumonia in the P4P hospitals improved more than in control hospitals (Lindenauer, 2007). Another study looked at more than 100,000 heart attack patients treated at P4P and control hospitals; between 2003 and 2006, quality measures for these patients improved equally at P4P and control hospitals (Glickman et al, 2007). From 2003 to 2008, quality scores for participating hospitals improved by 18% (CMS, 2010), which was a 2% to 4% greater improvement than in control hospitals (Mehrotra et al, 2009).

A P4P program described as "an initiative to improve the quality of primary care that is the boldest such proposal attempted anywhere in the world" was launched in the United Kingdom in 2004 (Roland, 2004). This program is described in Chapter 14.

Some authors urge caution, pointing out that P4P programs could encourage physicians and hospitals to avoid high-risk patients in order to keep their performance scores up (McMahon et al, 2007). Another difficulty is that many patients see a large number of physicians in a given year, making it impossible to determine which physician should receive a performance bonus (Pham et al, 2007). Moreover, P4P programs could increase disparities in quality by preferentially rewarding physicians and hospitals caring for higher-income patients and having greater resources available to invest in quality improvement, and penalizing those institutions and physicians attending to more vulnerable populations in resource-poor environments (Casalino et al, 2007).

▶ Financially Neutral Clinical Decision Making

The quest for quality care encompasses a search for a financial structure that does not reward over- or under-treatment and that separates physicians' personal incomes from their clinical decisions. Balanced incentives (see Chapter 4), combining elements of capitation or salary and fee-for-service, may have the best chance of minimizing the payment–treatment nexus (Robinson, 1999), encouraging physicians to do more of what is truly beneficial for patients while not inducing inappropriate and harmful services. Completely financially neutral decision making will always be an ideal and not a reality.

WHERE DOES MALPRACTICE REFORM FIT IN?

During a coronary angiogram, emboli traveled to the brain of Ivan Romanov, resulting in a serious stroke, with loss of use of his left arm and leg. The angiogram was appropriate and performed without any technical errors. Mr. Romanov had suffered a medical injury (an injury caused by his medical treatment), but the event was not because of negligence.

During a dilation and curettage (D&C), Judy Morrison's physician unknowingly perforated her uterus and lacerated her colon. Ms. Morrison reported severe pain but was sent home without further evaluation. She returned 1 hour later to the emergency department with persistent pain and

internal bleeding. She required a two-stage surgical repair over the following 4 months. This medical injury was found by the legal system to be because of negligence.

A peculiar set of institutions called the malpractice liability system forms an important part of US health care (Sage and Kersh, 2006). The goals of the malpractice system are twofold: To financially compensate people who in the course of seeking medical care have suffered medical injuries and to prevent physicians and other health care personnel from negligently causing harm to their patients.

The existing malpractice system scores miserably on both counts. According to the Harvard Medical Practice Study, only 2% of patients who suffer adverse events caused by medical negligence file malpractice claims that would allow them to receive compensation, meaning that the malpractice system fails in its first goal. Moreover, the system does not deal with 98% of negligent acts performed by physicians, making it difficult to attain its second goal. More recent research has confirmed the findings of the Harvard study (Sage and Kersh, 2006).

On the other hand, as many as 40% of malpractice claims do not involve true medical errors (Studdert et al, 2006), with an even smaller proportion representing actual negligence. Nonetheless, one-quarter of these inappropriate claims result in the patient receiving monetary compensation. Overall, for every dollar in compensation received by patients in malpractice awards, legal costs and fees come to 54 cents (Studdert et al, 2006).

The malpractice system has serious negative side effects on medical practice (Localio et al, 1991).

1. The system assumes that punishment, which usually involves physicians paying large amounts of money to a malpractice insurer plus enduring the overwhelming stress of a malpractice jury trial, is a reasonable method for improving the quality of medical care. Berwick's analysis of the Theory of Bad Apples suggests that fear of a lawsuit closes physicians' minds to improvement and generates an "I didn't do it" response. The entire atmosphere created by malpractice litigation clouds a clear analytic assessment of quality.

2. The system is wasteful, with a huge portion of malpractice insurance premiums spent on lawyers,

court costs, and insurance overhead almost as costly as payments to patients (Mello et al, 2010). Many claims have no merit but create enormous waste and wreak an unnecessary stress upon physicians. Patients granted malpractice award payments sometimes experienced no negligent care, and patients subjected to negligent care often receive no malpractice payments (Brennan et al, 1996). Total costs of the malpractice system came to $55.6 billion in 2008, 2.4% of total national health spending (Mello et al, 2010).

3. The system is based on the assumption that trial by jury is the best method of determining whether there has been negligence, a highly questionable assumption.

4. People with lower incomes generally receive smaller awards (because wages lost from a medical injury are lower) and are therefore less attractive to lawyers, who are generally paid as a percentage of the award. Accordingly, low-income patients, who suffer more medical injury, are less likely than wealthier people to file malpractice claims (Burstin et al, 1993b).

In summary, the malpractice system is burdened with expensive, unfounded litigation that harasses physicians who have done nothing wrong, while failing to discipline or educate most physicians committing actual medical negligence and to compensate most true victims of negligence.

Mei Tagaloa underwent neurosurgery for compression of his spinal cord by a cervical disk. On awakening from the surgery, Mr. Tagaloa was unable to move his legs or arms at all. After 3 months of rehabilitation, he ended up as a wheelchair-bound paraplegic. He sued the neurosurgeon and his family physician. The physicians' malpractice insurer paid for lawyers to defend them. Mr. Tagaloa's lawyer used the system of contingency fees, whereby he would receive one-third of the settlement if Mr. Tagaloa won the case, but would receive nothing if Mr. Tagaloa lost.

After 18 months, the case went to trial; the physicians left their practices and sat in the courtroom for 3 weeks. Each physician spent many hours going over records and discussing the case with the lawyers. The family physician, who had nothing to do with the surgery, was so upset with the proceedings that he developed an ulcer. The jury found the family physician innocent and the neurosurgeon guilty of negligence. The family physician lost $8000 in income because of absence from his practice. The neurosurgeon's malpractice insurer paid $900,000 to Mr. Tagaloa, who paid $300,000 to the lawyer.

A number of proposals have been made for malpractice reform (Mello and Gallagher, 2010).

▶ **Tort Reform**

Medical malpractice fits into the larger legal field of torts (wrongful acts or injuries done willfully or negligently). The California Medical Injury Compensation Reform Act and the Indiana Medical Malpractice Act are examples of tort reform, placing caps on damages awarded to injured parties and limits on lawyers' contingency fees. Tort reform can help physicians by slowing the growth of malpractice insurance premiums. However, caps on awards can be unfair to patients, limiting payments to those with the worst injuries (Mello et al, 2003; Localio, 2010) (Table 10–4).

▶ **Alternative Dispute Resolution**

These programs would substitute mediation, arbitration, or private negotiated settlements for jury trials in the case of medical injury. Alternatives to the jury

Table 10–4. Malpractice reform options

Tort reform	Placing limits on malpractice awards paid to patients
Alternative dispute resolution	Substituting mediation and arbitration for jury trials
Use of practice guidelines	Improving the ability to determine whether a physician was negligent
No-fault reform	Providing compensation to patients suffering medical injury regardless of whether the injury is due to negligence
Enterprise liability	Making institutions responsible for compensating medical injuries on a no-fault basis, thereby creating incentives for institutions to improve the quality of care provided

trial could bring more compensation to injured parties by reducing legal costs and might shift the dispute settlement to a more scientific, less emotional theater.

No-Fault Malpractice Reform

Proposals have been made to switch compensation for medical injury from the tort system to a no-fault plan (Studdert and Brennan, 2001; Localio, 2010). Under no-fault malpractice, patients suffering medical injury would receive compensation whether or not the injury was caused by negligence. Without costly lawyers' fees and jury trials, overhead costs would drop from more than 50% to approximately 20%. A no-fault system would compensate far more people and would cost approximately the same as the current tort system (Johnson et al, 1992). In addition, the no-fault approach might allow physicians to be more inclined to identify and openly discuss medical errors for the purpose of correcting them (Studdert et al, 2004).

Enterprise Liability

A relatively new idea for malpractice reform is to make health care institutions—primarily hospitals and HMOs—responsible for compensating medical injuries (Studdert et al, 2004; Sage and Kersh, 2006; Chan, 2010). As with no-fault proposals, patients suffering medical injury would be compensated whether or not the injury is negligent. Enterprise liability improves upon the no-fault concept by making institutions pay higher insurance premiums if they are the site of more medical injuries (whether caused by system failure or physician error). Hospitals and HMOs would have a financial incentive to improve the quality of care.

CONCLUSION

Each year people in the United States make more than 1 billion visits to physicians' offices and spend more than 100 million days in acute care hospitals. While quality of care provided during most of these encounters is excellent, the goal of the health care system should be to deliver high-quality care every day to every patient. This goal presents an unending challenge to each health caregiver and health care institution. Physicians make hundreds of decisions each day, including which questions to ask in the patient history, which parts of the body to examine in the physical examination, which laboratory tests and x-rays to order

and how urgently, which diagnoses to entertain, which treatments to offer, when to have the patient return for follow-up, and whether other physicians need to be consulted. Nurse practitioners, physician assistants, nurses, and other caregivers face similar numbers of decisions. It is humanly impossible to make all of these decisions correctly every day. For health care to be of high quality, mistakes should be minimized, mistakes with serious consequences should be avoided, and systems should be in place that reduce, detect, and correct errors to the greatest extent possible. Even when all decisions are technically accurate, if caregivers are insensitive or fail to provide the patient with a full range of informed choices, quality is impaired.

For the clinician, each decision that influences quality of care may be simple, but the sum total of all decisions of all caregivers impacting on a patient's illness makes the achievement of high-quality care elusive. To safeguard quality of care, our nation needs laws and regulations, including standards for health care professional education, rules for licensure, boards with the authority to discipline clear violators, and measurement to inform institutions, practitioners, and patients about the quality of their care. Improvement of health care quality cannot solely rely on regulators in Washington, DC, in state capitals, or across town; it must come from within each institution, whether a huge academic center, a community hospital, or a small medical office.

REFERENCES

Abramson J, Starfield B. The effect of conflict of interest on biomedical research and clinical practice guidelines. *J Am Board Fam Pract*. 2005;18:414.

Agency for Healthcare Research and Quality. National Healthcare Disparities Report, 2009. www.ahrq.gov. Accessed August 22, 2011.

Ash JS et al. The extent and importance of unintended consequences related to computerized provider order entry. *J Am Med Inform Assoc*. 2007;14:415.

Ayanian JZ. Race, class, and the quality of medical care. *JAMA*. 1994;271:1207.

Baker AM et al. A web-based diabetes care management support system. *Jt Comm J Qual Improv*. 2001;27:179.

Baron RJ. Quality improvement with an electronic health record: Achievable but not automatic. *Ann Intern Med*. 2007;147:549.

Berenson RA et al. Hospital—physician relations: Cooperation, competition, or separation? *Health Aff Web Exclusive*. December 5, 2006:w31.

Berwick DM. Continuous improvement as an ideal in health care. *N Engl J Med.* 1989;320:53.

Berwick DM et al. *Curing Health Care.* San Francisco, CA: Jossey-Bass; 1990.

Berwick DM et al. IHI replies to "The 100,000 Lives Campaign: A scientific and policy review." *Jt Comm J Qual Patient Saf.* 2006;32:628.

Birkmeyer JD et al. Surgeon volume and operative mortality in the United States. *N Engl J Med.* 2003;349:2117.

Bodenheimer T et al. The primary care—specialty income gap: why it matters. *Ann Intern Med.* 2007;146:301.

Bodenheimer T, Grumbach K. *Improving Primary Care: Strategies and Tools for a Better Practice.* New York: McGraw-Hill; 2007.

Bodenheimer T et al. Improving primary care for patients with chronic illness. *JAMA.* 2002;288:1775, 1909.

Boyd CM et al. Clinical practice guidelines and quality of care for older patients with multiple comorbid diseases. *JAMA.* 2005;294:716.

Brennan TA et al. Incidence of adverse events and negligence in hospitalized patients. *N Engl J Med.* 1991;324:370.

Brennan TA et al. Relation between negligent adverse events and the outcomes of medical-malpractice litigation. *N Engl J Med.* 1996;335:1963.

Buerhaus PI. Is hospital patient care becoming safer? A conversation with Lucian Leape. *Health Aff Web Exclusive.* October 9, 2007:w687.

Bunker J. Surgical manpower. *N Engl J Med.* 1970;282:135.

Burke JP. Maximizing appropriate antibiotic prophylaxis for surgical patients. *Clin Infect Dis.* 2001;33(suppl 2):S78.

Burstin HR et al. The effect of hospital financial characteristics on quality of care. *JAMA.* 1993a;270:845.

Burstin HR et al. Do the poor sue more? *JAMA.* 1993b;270:1697.

Cabana MD et al. Why don't physicians follow clinical practice guidelines? *JAMA.* 1999;282:1458.

Casalino LP et al. Will pay-for-performance and quality reporting affect health care disparities? *Health Aff (Millwood).* 2007;26:405.

Casalino LP et al. Frequency of failure to inform patients of clinically significant outpatient test results. *Arch Intern Med.* 2009;169:1123.

Centers for Medicare and Medicaid Services (CMS). Hospital Premier Quality Incentive Demonstration Fact Sheet, December 2010. (www.cms.gov/HospitalQualityInits/35_HospitalPremier.asp).

Chan TE. Organisational liability in a health care system. *Torts Law Jl.* 2010;18(3): 228.

Chassin MR et al. The urgent need to improve health care quality. *JAMA.* 1998;280:1000.

Chassin MR et al. Accountability measures—using measurement to promote quality improvement. *N Engl J Med.* 2010;363:683.

Choudhry NK et al. Relationships between authors of clinical practice guidelines and the pharmaceutical industry. *JAMA.* 2002;287:612.

Damberg CL et al. Taking stock of pay-for-performance: A candid assessment from the front lines. *Health Aff (Millwood).* 2009;28:517.

DesRoches CM et al. Electronic health records' limited successes suggest more targeted uses. *Health Aff (Millwood).* 2010;29:639.

Deyo RA et al. Spinal fusion surgery—the case for restraint. *N Engl J Med.* 2004;350:722.

Dudley RA et al. Selective referral to high-volume hospitals: Estimating potentially avoidable deaths. *JAMA.* 2000; 283:1159.

Eddy DM. Three battles to watch in the 1990s. *JAMA.* 1993;270:520.

Egan BM et al. US trends in prevalence, awareness, treatment, and control of hypertension, 1988–2008. *JAMA.* 2010; 303:2043.

Epstein AM et al. Paying physicians for high-quality care. *N Engl J Med.* 2004;350:406.

Eslami S et al. Evaluation of outpatient computerized physician medication order entry systems. *J Am Med Inform Assoc.* 2007;14:400.

Fiscella K et al. Inequality in quality. *JAMA.* 2000;283:2579.

Fisher ES et al. The implications of regional variations in Medicare spending. Part 1: The content, quality, and accessibility of care. *Ann Intern Med.* 2003;138:273.

Gallagher TH et al. US and Canadian physicians' attitudes and experiences regarding disclosing errors to patients. *Arch Intern Med.* 2006;166:1605.

Galvin RS, Delbanco S. Why employers need to rethink how they buy health care. *Health Aff (Millwood).* 2005;24:1549.

Gandhi TK et al. Outpatient prescribing errors and the impact of computerized prescribing. *J Gen Intern Med.* 2005;20:837.

Glickman SW et al. Pay for performance, quality of care, and outcomes in acute myocardial infarction. *JAMA.* 2007;297:2373.

Hillman BJ et al. Frequency and costs of diagnostic imaging in office patients: A comparison of self-referring and radiologist-referring physicians. *N Engl J Med.* 1990;323:1604.

Hollingsworth JM et al. Physician-ownership of ambulatory surgery centers linked to higher volume of surgeries. *Health Aff (Millwood).* 2010;29:683.

Institute of Medicine. *To Err Is Human: Building a Safer Health System.* Washington, DC: National Academies Press; 1999.

Institute of Medicine. *Crossing the Quality Chasm: A New Health System for the 21st Century*. Washington, DC: National Academies Press; 2001.

Integrated Healthcare Organization. The California Pay For Performance Program, June 2009. www.iha.org.

Jha AK, Epstein AM. The predictive accuracy of the New York State coronary artery bypass surgery report-card system. *Health Aff (Millwood)*. 2006;25:844.

Johnson WG et al. The economic consequences of medical injuries: Implications for a no-fault insurance plan. *N Engl J Med*. 1992;267:2487.

Kaiser Family Foundation. *Annual Employer Health Benefits Survey* Menlo Park, CA: Kaiser Family Foundation; 2003.

Kaushal R et al. Effects of computerized physician order entry and clinical decision support systems on medication safety. *Arch Intern Med*. 2003;163:1409.

King TE, Wheeler MB. *Medical Management of Vulnerable and Underserved Patients*. New York: McGraw-Hill; 2007.

Kizer K. The volume-outcome conundrum. *N Engl J Med*. 2003;349:2159.

Laffel GL, Berwick DM. Quality health care. *JAMA*. 1993;270:254.

Leape LL et al. The nature of adverse events in hospitalized patients. *N Engl J Med*. 1991;324:377.

Leape LL. Unnecessary surgery. *Annu Rev Public Health*. 1992;13:363.

Leape LL. Error in medicine. *JAMA*. 1994;272:1851.

Leape LL, Fromson JA. Problem doctors: Is there a system-level solution? *Ann Intern Med*. 2006;144:107.

Lindenauer PK et al. Public reporting and pay for performance in hospital quality improvement. *N Engl J Med*. 2007;356:486.

Localio AR et al. Relation between malpractice claims and adverse events due to negligence. *N Engl J Med*. 1991;325:245.

Localio AR. Patient compensation without litigation: A promising development. *Ann Intern Med*. 2010;153:266.

Marshall MN, et al. The public release of performance data. *JAMA*. 2000;283:1866.

McGlynn EA et al. The quality of health care delivered to adults in the United States. *N Engl J Med*. 2003;348:2635.

McMahon LF et al. Physician-level P4P—DOA? *Am J Manag Care*. 2007;13:233.

Mehrotra A et al. Pay for performance in the hospital setting: What is the state of the evidence? *Am J Med Qual*. 2009;24:19.

Mello MM et al. The new medical malpractice crisis. *N Engl J Med*. 2003;348:2281.

Mello MM et al. National costs of the medical liability system. *Health Aff (Millwood)*. 2010;29:1569.

Mello MM, Gallagher TH. Malpractive reform—opportunities for leadership by health care institutions and liability insurers. *N Engl J Med*. 2010;362:1353.

Meurer LN et al. Excess mortality caused by medical injury. *Ann Fam Med*. 2006;4:410.

Mitchell JM, Scott E. New evidence of the prevalence and scope of physician joint ventures. *JAMA*. 1992;268:80.

Morrison J, Wickersham P. Physicians disciplined by a state medical board. *JAMA*. 1998;279:1889.

National Committee for Quality Assurance. *The State of Health Care Quality, 2009*. NCQA, 2010. www.ncqa.org.

O'Connor AM et al. Toward the "tipping point": Decision aids and informed patient choice. *Health Aff (Millwood)*. 2007;26:716.

Owens DK et al. High-value, cost-conscious health care. *Ann Intern Med*. 2011;154:174.

Peterson ED et al. Procedural volume as a marker of quality for CABG surgery. *JAMA*. 2004;291:195.

Pham HH et al. The impact of quality-reporting programs on hospital operations. *Health Aff (Millwood)*. 2006;25:1412.

Pham HH et al. Care patterns in Medicare and their implications for pay for performance. *N Engl J Med*. 2007;356:1130.

Phillips DP et al. Increase in US medication-error deaths between 1983 and 1993. *Lancet*. 1998;351:643.

Relman AS. *A Second Opinion: Rescuing America's Health Care*. New York: Public Affairs; 2007.

Robinson JC. Blended payment methods in physician organizations under managed care. *JAMA*. 1999;282:1258.

Roland M. Linking physicians' pay to the quality of care—a major experiment in the United Kingdom. *N Engl J Med*. 2004;351: 1448.

Rouf E et al. Computers in the exam room. *J Gen Intern Med*. 2007;22:43.

Sage WM, Kersh R. *Medical Malpractice and the US Health Care System*. New York: Cambridge University Press; 2006.

Saydah SH et al. Poor control of risk factors for vascular disease among adults with previously diagnosed diabetes. *JAMA*. 2004;291:335.

Schoen C et al. US health system performance: A national scorecard. *Health Aff Web Exclusive*. September 20, 2006:w457.

Schuster MA et al. How good is the quality of health care in the United States? *Milbank Q*. 1998;76:517.

Shaneyfelt TM, Centor RM. Reassessment of clinical practice guidelines. *JAMA*. 2009;301:868.

Smith-Bindman R. Is computed tomography safe? *N Engl J Med*. 2010;363:1.

Solberg LI. Improving medical practice: A conceptual framework. *Ann Fam Med*. 2007;5:251.

Steinbrook R. Guidance for guidelines. *N Engl J Med*. 2007;356:331.

Studdert DM, Brennan TA. No-fault compensation for medical injuries. *JAMA*. 2001;286:217.

Studdert DM et al. Medical malpractice. *N Engl J Med*. 2004;350:283.

Studdert DM et al. Claims, errors, and compensation payments in medical malpractice litigation. *N Engl J Med*. 2006;354:2024.

US Senate. Hearings Before the Permanent Subcommittee on Investigations, Committee on Government Operations, March 13 and 14, 1975. Prepaid Health Plans. US Government Printing Office; 1975.

Vargas RB et al. Can a chronic care model collaborative reduce heart disease risk in patients with diabetes? *J Gen Intern Med*. 2007;22:215.

Wachter RM. Why diagnostic errors don't get any respect—and what can be done about them. *Health Aff (Millwood)*. 2010;29:1605.

Wachter RM, Pronovost PJ. The 100,000 Lives Campaign: A scientific and policy review. *Jt Comm J Qual Patient Saf*. 2006;32:621.

Weeks WB et al. Higher health care quality and bigger savings found at large multispecialty medical groups. *Health Aff (Millwood)*. 2009;29:991.

Zahn C, Miller MR. Excess length of stay, charges, and mortality attributable to medical injuries during hospitalization. *JAMA*. 2003;290:1868.

Zhang Y et al. Geographic variation in the quality of prescribing. *N Engl J Med*. 2010;363:1985.

Prevention of Illness

WHAT IS PREVENTION?

In 2009, the United States spent $2.5 trillion on health care. Only 3% of this total was dedicated to government public health activities designed to prevent illness.

The renowned medical historian Henry Sigerist, writing in 1941, listed the main items that must be included in a national health program. The first three items were free education, including health education, for all; the best possible working and living conditions; and the best possible means of rest and recreation. Medical care rated only fourth on his list (Terris, 1992a). For Sigerist (1941), medical care was

A system of health institutions and medical personnel, available to all, responsible for the people's health, ready and able to advise and help them in the maintenance of health and in its restoration when prevention has broken down. (Sigerist, 1941)

Many people working in the fields of medical care and public health believe that "prevention has broken down" too often; sometimes because modern science has insufficient knowledge to prevent disease, but more often because society has dedicated insufficient resources and commitment to prevention.

Primary prevention seeks to avert the occurrence of a disease or injury (eg, immunization against polio; taxes on the sale of cigarettes to reduce their affordability, and thereby their use). *Secondary prevention* refers to early detection of a disease process and intervention to reverse or retard the condition from progressing (eg,

Pap smears to screen for premalignant and malignant lesions of the cervix, and mammograms for early detection of breast cancer).

The promotion of good health and the prevention of illness encompass three distinct levels or strategies (Terris, 1986; Table 11–1):

1. The first and broadest level includes measures to address the fundamental social determinants of illness; as evidence presented in Chapter 3 shows, lower income is associated with higher morbidity and mortality rates. Improvement in the standard of living and social equity (eg, through job creation programs to reduce or eliminate unemployment) may have a greater impact on preventing disease than specific public health programs or medical care services.

2. The second level of prevention involves public health interventions to reduce the incidence of illness in the population as a whole. Examples are water purification systems, the banning of cigarette smoking in the workplace, and public health education on human immunodeficiency virus (HIV) prevention in the schools. These strategies generally consist of primary prevention. The 3% figure cited in the opening paragraph represents these public health activities.

3. The third level of prevention involves individual health care providers performing preventive interventions for individual patients; these activities can be either primary or secondary prevention. The US Preventive Services Task Force and other organizations have established regular schedules for preventive

Table 11–1. Strategies of prevention

Strategy	Examples
1. Improvement in the standard of living	Job creation Increase in minimum wage
2. Public health interventions to reduce the incidence of illness in the population	Water purification systems in underdeveloped nations Increased tobacco taxes to reduce the purchase of cigarettes Mass education on the dangers of high-fat diets
3. Preventive medical care, performed by health care providers	Screening and treatment of hypertension Periodic breast examinations and mammograms Prenatal care

medical care services (US Preventive Services Task Force, 2010).

THE FIRST EPIDEMIOLOGIC REVOLUTION

Until modern times, the conditions that produced the greatest amount of illness and death in the population were infectious diseases. The initial decline of infectious disease mortality rates took place even before the cause of these illnesses was understood. In the eighteenth and nineteenth centuries, food production increased markedly throughout the Western world. By the early nineteenth century, infectious disease mortality rates were dropping in England, Wales, and Scandinavia, probably as a result of improved nutrition that allowed individuals, particularly children, to resist infectious agents. Thus, the initial success of illness prevention took place through the improvement of overall living conditions rather than from specific public health or medical interventions (McKeown, 1990).

In the nineteenth century, scientists and public health practitioners discovered many of the agents causing infectious diseases. By comprehending the causes (such as bacteria and viruses) and the risk factors (eg, poverty, overcrowding, poor nutrition, and contaminated water) associated with these illnesses, public health measures (such as water purification, sewage disposal, and pasteurization of milk) were implemented that drastically reduced their incidence. This was the first epidemiologic revolution (Terris, 1985).

From 1870 to 1930, the death rate from infectious diseases fell rapidly. Medical interventions, whether immunizations or treatment with antibiotics, were introduced only after much of the decline in infectious disease mortality had taken place. The first effective treatment against tuberculosis, the antibiotic streptomycin, was developed in 1947, but its contribution to the decrease in the tuberculosis death rate since the early nineteenth century has been estimated to be a mere 3%. For whooping cough, measles, scarlet fever, bronchitis, and pneumonia, mortality rates had fallen to similarly low levels before immunization or antibiotic therapy became available. Pasteurization and water purification were probably the main reason for the decline in infant mortality rates (McKeown, 1990).

Some illnesses are exceptions to the rule that infectious disease mortality is influenced more by improved living standards and public health measures than by medical interventions. Immunization for smallpox, polio, and tetanus and antimicrobial therapy for syphilis had a substantial impact on mortality rates from those illnesses. Considering infectious diseases as a group, however, medical measures probably account for less than 5% of the decrease in mortality rates for these conditions over the past century (McKinlay et al, 1989; McKeown, 1990).

As infectious diseases waned in importance during the first half of the twentieth century and as life expectancy increased, rates of noninfectious chronic illness grew rapidly. Eleven major infectious diseases accounted for 40% of total deaths in the United States in 1900, but less than 10% in 1980. In contrast, heart disease, cancer, and stroke (cerebrovascular disease) caused 16% of total deaths in 1900 but 64% by 1980 (McKinlay et al, 1989).

THE SECOND EPIDEMIOLOGIC REVOLUTION

Fifty years ago, epidemiologists did not understand the causes of noninfectious chronic diseases.

Unable to prevent the occurrence of these diseases, we retreated to a second line of defense, namely, early detection and treatment—so-called secondary prevention. But secondary prevention has—with few exceptions—proved disappointing; it cannot compare in effectiveness with measures for primary prevention. The periodic physical examination, the cancer detection center, multiphasic screening, and a host of variations on these themes have incurred enormous expenditures for relatively modest benefits . . . Major exceptions are cancer of the cervix, for which early detection has proved dramatically effective, and, to a lesser extent, cancer of the breast.

Beginning in 1950, dramatic breakthroughs occurred in the epidemiology of the noninfectious diseases. During the next three decades, our epidemiologists forged powerful weapons to combat most of the major causes of death. In doing so, they initiated a second epidemiologic revolution, which, if we act appropriately, will result in an enormous reduction in premature death and disability. (Terris, 1992b)

During the second epidemiologic revolution, it was learned that the major illnesses in the United States have a few central causes and are in large part preventable. In 2007, 2.4 million people died in the United States (Table 11–2). A surprisingly small number of

Table 11–2. Causes of death in the United States, 2007[a]

Total	2,424,000
Top 10 causes	
Heart disease	616,000
Cancer	563,000
Cerebrovascular disease	136,000
Chronic obstructive pulmonary disease	128,000
Unintentional injuries (accidents)	124,000
Diabetes	71,000
Pneumonia and influenza	53,000
Kidney disease	46,000
Septicemia	35,000
Top 3 contributors to mortality (2006)	
Tobacco	435,000
Diet and inactivity	365,000
Alcohol	85,000

[a]Xu J et al. Deaths: final data for 2007. National Vital Statistics Reports, Vol 59, No. 19. US Centers for Disease Control and Prevention, May 2010. www.cdc.gov; Heron MP et al. Deaths: final data for 2006. National Vital Statistics Report, Vol 57, No. 14. *Center for Disease Control and Prevention, 2009.* www.cdc.gov

risk factors are implicated in 37% of these deaths. It has been estimated that use of tobacco causes 435,000 fatalities, a high-fat diet and inactivity contributes to 365,000 more, and alcohol is responsible for 85,000 deaths annually in the United States (Heron et al, 2009; Xu et al, 2010). By discovering and educating the population about the risk factors of smoking, rich diet, and lack of exercise, the second epidemiologic revolution has already been very successful. From 1980 to 2006, age-adjusted mortality rates for coronary heart disease (CHD) declined by an astonishing 61%. This decline was associated with reduced rates of tobacco use and lowered mean serum cholesterol levels in the population. As with infectious diseases a century earlier, this decline was in substantial part related to public health interventions regarding smoking and diet (US Department of Health and Human Services, 2009). The unfortunate side of this success story is that those in the poorest socioeconomic position and the least education have considerably higher mortality rates than those with higher socioeconomic status (Loucks, 2009).

INDIVIDUAL OR POPULATION?

Chronic disease prevention may be viewed from two distinct perspectives: that of the individual and that of the population (Rose, 1985). The medical model seeks to identify high-risk individuals and offer them individual protection, often by counseling on such topics as smoking cessation and low-fat diet. The public health approach seeks to reduce disease in the population as a whole, using such methods as mass education campaigns to counter drinking and driving, the taxation of tobacco to drive up its price, and the labeling of foods to indicate fat and cholesterol content. Both approaches have merits but the medical model suffers from some drawbacks.

The individual-centered approach of the medical model may produce tunnel vision regarding the causation, and thus the prevention, of disease. Let us take the example of cholesterol.

Ancel Keys (1970) performed a famous study comparing CHD in different nations. In east Finland, CHD was common, 20% of diet calories came from saturated fat, and 56% of men aged 40 to 59 years had cholesterol levels greater than 250 mg/dL. In Japan, CHD was rare, 3% of calories were provided by saturated fat, and only 7% of men aged 40 to 59 years had cholesterol levels above 250 mg/dL. If we compared two individuals in east Finland who eat the same diet, one with a cholesterol level of 200 mg/dL and the other with a level of 300 mg/dL, we might conclude that the variation in cholesterol levels among individuals is caused by genetic or other factors, but not diet. If, on the other hand, we remove our individual blinders and look at entire populations, studying the average cholesterol level and the percentage of fat in the diet in east Finland and in Japan, we will conclude that high-fat diets correlate with high levels of cholesterol and with high rates of CHD.

Individual variations within each country are often of less importance than variations between one nation and another. The clues to the causes of diseases "must be sought from differences between populations or from changes within populations over time" (Rose, 1985).

The medical model may also target its interventions to the wrong individuals. Let us continue with the cholesterol example. In the United States, most people with high cholesterol levels remain healthy for years, and some people with low levels have heart attacks at an early age. Why is this so? Because the risk of CHD for persons with high cholesterol levels or low cholesterol levels is not so different; even for the low-risk individual, CHD is the most likely cause of death. Everyone in the United States is at risk for this disease. A "low" cholesterol level of 180 mg/dL is low by US standards, but high when compared with levels in poor nations. A large number of people at small risk for a disease may give rise to more cases of the disease than the smaller number of people who are at high risk (Brown et al, 1992). This fact limits the utility of the medical model's "high-risk" approach to prevention. A public health approach (eg, mass educational campaigns on the health effects of rich diets and the labeling of foods) strives to reduce the mean population cholesterol level. A 10% reduction in the serum cholesterol distribution of the entire population would do far more to reduce the incidence of heart disease than a 30% reduction in the cholesterol levels of those relatively few individuals with counts greater than 300 mg/dL.

A coherent ideology underlies the medical model of chronic disease prevention—the concept that in the arena of noninfectious chronic disease, individuals play a major role in causing their own illnesses by such behaviors as smoking, drinking alcohol, and eating high-fat foods. The corollary to this view is that chronic disease mortality rates can be reduced by persuading individuals to change their lifestyles. These statements are true, but they do not tell the whole story.

An alternative ideology, which fits more closely with the public health approach to chronic disease prevention, argues that modern industrial society, rather than the individuals living in that society, creates the conditions leading to heart disease, cancer, stroke, and other major chronic diseases of the developed world. Tobacco advertising; processed high-fat, high-salt foods in "supersized" portions; easy availability of alcoholic beverages; societal stress; an urbanized and suburbanized existence that substitutes automobile travel for exercise; and a markedly unequal distribution of wealth are the substrates upon which the modern epidemic of chronic disease has flourished. Such a worldview leads to an emphasis on societal rather than individual strategies for chronic disease prevention (Fee and Krieger, 1993).

Both the medical and the public health models (seeing responsibility as both individual and societal) must be joined to further implement the second epidemiologic revolution; medical caregivers must attempt to change high-risk lifestyles of their individual patients, and society must search for ways to reduce the consumption of tobacco, alcohol, and rich foods. One model that bridges the medical and public health approaches is community-oriented primary care. In this model, primary care clinicians systematically define a target population, determine its health needs, and develop community-based interventions to address these needs (Nutting, 1990). The target population could be as simple as the patients enrolled in a primary care practice, or more ambitiously, an entire neighborhood. For example, a pediatrician might review data on her enrolled patients and find that many children are obese. In addition to counseling individual families in her practice, in the Community Oriented Primary Care model the pediatrician would also work with community members and agencies on broader public health interventions, such as advocating for improved school lunch programs and more time for physical education classes in the local schools, or encouraging the local health department to launch a media campaign promoting consumption of water instead of sweetened beverages.

MODELS OF PREVENTION

To provide examples of different approaches to preventing illness, we have chosen to discuss two serious health problems in the United States: coronary heart disease and breast cancer.

▶ Coronary Heart Disease

Coronary heart disease (CHD) is associated with four major risk factors: the eating of a rich diet (the principal cause of the CHD epidemic), elevated levels of serum cholesterol, cigarette smoking, and hypertension (Stamler, 1992a).

Primary prevention strategies are available for CHD because the causes of the disease are well understood. Primary CHD prevention involves risk factor reduction, including cessation of cigarette smoking, replacement of rich diets by low-fat diets, and control of hypertension. These strategies have been largely responsible for the large decrease in CHD death rates (Figure 11–1).

Cigarette Smoking

Tobacco has been called the smallpox virus of chronic disease—a harmful agent whose elimination from the planet would benefit humankind (Fee and Krieger, 1993). Since the 1964 release of the first Surgeon General's Report on the Health Consequences of Smoking, the smoking behavior of the US population has changed dramatically. Between 1965 and 2007, the age-adjusted percentage of adult men who were current smokers dropped from 51% to 22%; for adult women, the decline was from 34% to 18% (Figure 11–2). These reductions in smoking prevalence avoided an estimated 3 million deaths between 1964 and 2000—a major public health achievement (Warner, 1989). However, rates of smoking are far higher among people with lower educational levels and smoking continues to be the leading cause of death in the United States (US Department of Health and Human Services, 2009).

Antismoking campaigns have been relatively successful for well-educated people, but less so for people with less education, who also tend to be poorer.

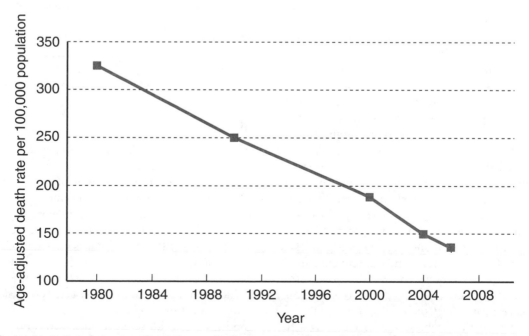

▲ **Figure 11–1.** Trends in age-adjusted mortality from coronary heart disease in the United States, 1980–2006.

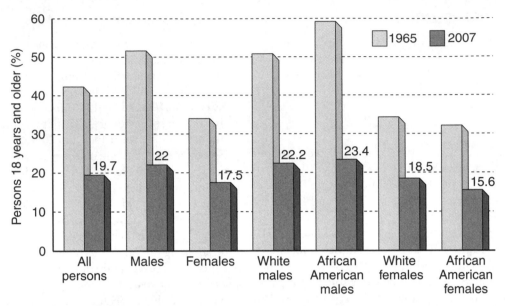

▲ **Figure 11–2.** Cigarette smoking by persons 18 years and older in the United States in 1965 (light blue bars) and 2007 (dark blue bars). Percentages are age adjusted. (US Department of Health and Human Services. *Health United States*. 2009.)

Between 1974 and 2007, cigarette smoking declined 38% among the least educated persons, while it dropped 67% among the most educated. In 2006, 30% of the least educated persons smoked cigarettes, compared with only 9% of the most educated (US Department of Health and Human Services, 2009).

Since the 1969 ban on radio and television cigarette advertising, the tobacco industry has increased its advertising expenditures dramatically in the print media and through sponsorship of community events. In 2005, tobacco advertising expenditures exceeded $13 billion, almost double the 1999 figure (Bayer et al, 2002; Cokkinides et al, 2009). Tobacco industry documents prove that the principal target group for cigarette advertising is young adults (Ling and Glantz, 2002). The antismoking campaign of the past 30 years has merged the medical and public health models of prevention. Physician counseling can influence smokers to quit. In 2006, however, only 34% of low-income smokers had smoking cessation discussions with their health care provider (Cokkinides et al, 2009) and relapse rates for those who quit after receiving active treatment are 77% at 12 months (Mannino, 2009).

Public health measures are more effective, including public education, cigarette taxes, and restriction of smoking in public places. A 10% increase in the price of cigarettes reduces cigarette consumption by 3% to 5%. Yet compared with other developed nations, the United States has relatively low taxes on tobacco (Cokkinides et al, 2009; Schroeder and Warner, 2010).

Rich Diet

A rich diet is a diet high in fat, saturated fat, cholesterol, salt, and often alcohol, and one with a high caloric intake in relation to the amount of energy expended (Stamler, 1992a). The rich diet produces CHD primarily by causing an increase in low-density-lipoprotein cholesterol. Lowering cholesterol levels has been shown to reduce the risk of heart attacks caused by CHD.

In the late 1980s, a major national campaign was launched by the National Institutes of Health (NIH) to reduce serum cholesterol levels. This National Cholesterol Education Program is based on the medical model, with health care providers screening individuals for elevated cholesterol and aggressively treating hyperlipidemic patients with diet, cholesterol-lowering medications, or both (Grundy et al, 2004).

Public health analysts have criticized the NIH strategy as relying too heavily on a medical model of prevention that is expensive and of potentially limited effectiveness. The NIH approach targets more than 100 million people who need dietary changes and recommends drug treatment for many of these individuals.

The use of statin drugs to treat hyperlipidemia in people with known CHD (secondary prevention) and without CHD (primary prevention) has been shown to reduce deaths from CHD and deaths from all causes (Steinberg and Gotto, 1999). However, the effectiveness of drug treatment is far greater if it is used in secondary rather than primary prevention (Hayward et al, 2010). For primary prevention, 53 patients would have to take a statin drug for 5 years to prevent one patient from experiencing a fatal or nonfatal coronary event. For secondary prevention (patients with known CHD), statin drugs can prevent approximately one nonfatal myocardial infarction or death for every 10 patients treated, at a far lower cost for every year of life saved (Pharoah and Hollingworth, 1996; Lloyd-Jones, 2001).

The NIH cholesterol reduction strategy highlights the paradox of primary prevention: Prevention within a population of healthy individuals may be better (and less expensively) served by broad public health efforts to reduce risk among the majority of people at moderate risk than by concentrating intensive medical interventions on the smaller number of high-risk persons (Rose, 1985). The traditional orientation of physicians toward individual patients (the medical model) has led the medical profession and the NIH to emphasize identification and treatment of high-risk individuals with elevated cholesterol levels. Pharmaceutical manufacturers also have an interest in promoting a medical model of prevention that relies on prescribing medications. Reducing the mean cholesterol level of the US population rather than reducing the individual cholesterol counts of hyperlipidemic patients may have better long-term results for primary prevention.

Currently, public health efforts to curb the consumption of rich foods are failing; 74% of adults in the United States were classified as overweight or obese in 2008, compared with 46% in the early 1960s (Ogden and Carroll, 2010). The food industry spends billions of dollars on advertising, a substantial portion of which promotes high-fat fast foods. Proposals have been made to copy the strategy used by tobacco prevention campaigns in reducing the availability of high-fat foods; for example, taxing unhealthy foods, changing school lunch programs to reduce their fat content, restricting food advertising directed at children, and eliminating school-based candy and soft-drink vending machines are primary preventive measures that are gaining public acceptance (Frieden et al, 2010). Growing attention is also being paid to the billions of dollars annually in federal government subsidies to agribusinesses for growing corn, which has contributed to the flooding of the nation with low-cost, high fructose corn sweeteners and other high calorie processed foods. Public health advocates have called for reforms to the federal farm bill to reduce subsidies for obesogenic foods and to provide more support for sustainable farming of healthful fruits and vegetables (Pollan, 2007; Wallinga, 2010).

Hypertension

Risk factors for hypertension include high salt intake, low potassium intake, high ratio of dietary sodium to potassium, obesity, and excess alcohol intake; other important risk factors likely exist. Prior to the advent of modern agriculture, intake of sodium was low and intake of potassium high, and high levels of physical exertion prevented persons from being overweight.

CHD risk is associated with increased blood pressure, even at relatively moderate levels of blood pressure elevation. Individuals with systolic blood pressures of 130 to 140 mm Hg have almost twice the cardiovascular risk of those with systolic blood pressures less than 110 mm Hg. One quarter of hypertension-related cardiovascular deaths take place among borderline hypertensives, and in the United States, 90% of men aged 35 to 57 years have blood pressure levels that create excess cardiovascular risk. Thus, it can be said that high blood pressure as a risk factor for CHD is a problem for the entire population and not simply a problem for the 20% to 25% of the population with frank hypertension. Similarly to the cholesterol situation, the greatest impact in reducing hypertension-related CHD mortality rates will come from a reduction in the blood pressure of the large number of borderline hypertensives rather than from focusing solely on people with very high blood pressure (Stamler, 1992b).

Primary prevention of high blood pressure can be accomplished by a reduction in the daily intake of salt by 3 g per person. Currently, the average man in the United States consumes 10.4 g of salt per day, with women eating 7.3 g. Such a change would reduce the number of new CHD cases by 60,000 per year. This public health approach would be as effective as the use of medical treatment to control the blood pressures of the 65 million people in the United States with hypertension (Bibbins-Domingo et al, 2010).

Prevention of hypertension has focused on screening and early treatment of elevated blood pressure. These measures are considered secondary prevention (early diagnosis and intervention) with respect to high blood pressure as a disease but are categorized as primary prevention (averting the occurrence) with respect to CHD. American medicine has a poor record in lowering elevated blood pressures; only 50% of hypertensives are adequately controlled (Egan et al, 2010)

▶ Breast Cancer

Whereas mortality rates for cardiovascular disease declined since the late 1960s, cancer mortality rates continued to increase through 1990. Between 1990 and 2006, cancer mortality rates dropped by 16%, probably as a result of reductions in cigarette smoking. Breast cancer mortality rates have also decreased during those years, but are considerably higher for African American women than for white women (US Department of Health and Human Services, 2009).

The designing of effective primary prevention for a disease generally depends on an understanding of the epidemiology of that disease. In the case of lung cancer, the discovery of the link with cigarette smoking allowed a widespread primary prevention program to be developed—the antismoking campaign. But the causes of many cancers are still unclear, meaning that preventive strategies must use secondary rather than primary prevention. Pap smears for early detection of cervical cancer, fecal occult blood testing and colonoscopy for early detection of colorectal cancer, and mammography for early detection of breast cancer are examples of secondary prevention.

Multiple risk factors for breast cancer have been uncovered, including age greater than 65 years, a family history of breast cancer, atypical hyperplasia on breast biopsy, birth in North America or northern Europe, and genetic susceptibility related to the BRCA genotype. Women with more years of ovulatory menstrual cycles have a greater risk, indicating a hormonal influence on the disease (American Cancer Society, 2011).

However, only one-fourth of breast cancer cases can be accounted for by these risk factors. The differences between high and low age-adjusted breast cancer risk in the United States are small compared with the differences between such high-incidence nations as the United States and low-incidence (generally underdeveloped) nations. Perhaps unknown agents related to modern industrialization are the primary causes of breast cancer, while such influences as female hormones are secondary promoters of the disease.

The age-adjusted incidence (new cases) of breast cancer fell sharply in 2003 compared with 2002 and continued to fall slightly through 2006, a phenomenon temporally related to the drop in the use of hormone replacement therapy by women in the United States, occasioned by the widely publicized report from the Women's Health Initiative providing new data on the risks of hormone replacement therapy (Ravdin et al, 2007). This association suggests that estrogen is an important cause or facilitator of breast cancer.

Evidence linking dietary fat to cancer of the breast is inconsistent and weak, and further research is needed on the role of environmental carcinogens (American Cancer Society, 2011). From the 1940s to the 1980s, industrial production of synthetic organic chemicals rose from 1 billion to 400 billion pounds annually, and the volume of hazardous wastes also increased 400-fold during that period (Epstein, 1990, 1994). One study estimated that toxic chemicals encountered at workplaces are responsible for 20% of all human cancers (Landrigan, 1992). Estrogens have been used as additives to poultry and cattle feed, and pesticide residues contain estrogen-like compounds that may contribute to breast cancer causation (Davis and Bradlow, 1995). Some studies have linked breast cancer risk to organochlorine insecticides, polycyclic aromatic hydrocarbons, and organic solvents, but research on these environmental causes of breast cancer has been inadequate and inconsistent (Brody and Rudel, 2003).

Lack of knowledge has forced modern medicine to retreat to secondary prevention (ie, early diagnosis through breast examinations and mammography) to reduce mortality rates in women with the disease.

Thankfully, breast cancer, like cervical cancer, lends itself to secondary prevention techniques. Periodic mammograms can reduce breast cancer mortality rates in women aged above 50 years. Yet many breast cancer activists decry the relatively paltry sums going for basic epidemiologic research to determine the causes of breast cancer.

▶ Summary

The examples of CHD and breast cancer illustrate different aspects of illness prevention. Primary prevention has been successful in reducing mortality rates for CHD. Both public health and medical approaches have been used, with far greater emphasis given to the latter strategy. Secondary prevention has had some success in reducing breast cancer mortality rates, but the incidence of the disease remains high and primary prevention is badly needed.

DOES PREVENTION REDUCE MEDICAL CARE COSTS?

The influence of prevention on medical care costs is a complex one. As a rule, primary prevention using public health measures is far more cost-effective than primary prevention through medical care; public health measures do not require many millions of expensive one-to-one interactions with medical care providers.

In the arena of individual medical care prevention, some measures save money and some do not. Every dollar invested in measles, mumps, and rubella immunizations saves many more dollars in averted medical care costs. Physician counseling on smoking cessation is a low-cost activity that can reduce the multibillion dollar cost of caring for people with tobacco-related illness. These preventive care activities do reduce health care spending in the long run. In contrast, medical care to reduce cholesterol and high blood pressure are unlikely to result in significant savings to the health care system (Cohen et al, 2008).

Primary prevention through public health action can be enormously effective in reducing the burden of human suffering and the cost of treating disease. From 1900 to 1940, the nation's public health efforts achieved a 97% reduction in the death rate for typhoid fever; 97% for diphtheria; 92% for infectious diarrhea; 91% for measles, scarlet fever, and whooping cough; and 77% for tuberculosis (Winslow, 1944). The imposition of a $2-per-pack increase in the tobacco tax could substantially reduce the $50-plus billion annual cost of tobacco-related disease, while at the same time yielding tens of billions of dollars per year in tax revenues—an ideal preventive measure that actually earns money. If the three primary preventive methods known to reduce the incidence of coronary heart disease, cancer, and stroke (ie, reduction in smoking, cholesterol levels, and blood pressure) were intensified, the medical care costs of these illnesses could be reduced by 50%. These three illnesses account for 20% of personal health care costs in the United States and reducing their incidence could yield a cost savings of billions of dollars per year. However, these savings are overstated because money saved by preventing disease X will ultimately be spent on the treatment of disease Y or Z, which will strike those people spared from disease X.

CONCLUSION

The goals of disease prevention are to delay disability and death and to maximize illness-free years of life. Improvements in living standards, public health measures, and preventive medical care have made enormous contributions toward the achievement of these goals. Producing further improvements in the overall health of society will likely depend on reducing the growing gap between the rich and the poor and shifting a greater proportion of the health dollar to disease prevention.

REFERENCES

American Cancer Society. What are the risk factors for breast cancer, 2011. www.cancer.org/cancer/breastcancer/detailedguide/breast-cancer-risk-factors. Accessed November 15, 2011.

Bayer R et al. Tobacco advertising in the United States. *JAMA*. 2002;287:2990.

Bibbins-Domingo K et al. Projected effect of dietary salt reductions on future cardiovascular disease. *N Engl J Med*. 2010;362:590.

Brody JG, Rudel RA. Environmental pollutants and breast cancer. *Environ Health Perspect*. 2003;111:1007.

Brown EY, Viscoli CM, Horwitz RI. Preventive health strategies and the policy makers? paradox. *Ann Intern Med*. 1992;116:593.

Cohen JT et al. Does preventive care save money? *N Engl J Med*. 2008;358:661.

Cokkinides V et al. Tobacco control in the United States: recent progress and opportunities. *CA Cancer J Clin*. 2009;59:352.

Davis DL, Bradlow HL. Can environmental estrogens cause breast cancer? *Sci Am.* 1995;273:167.

Egan BM et al. US trends in prevalence, awareness, treatment, and control of hypertension, 1988–2008. *JAMA.* 2010; 303:2043.

Epstein SS. Losing the war against cancer: Who's to blame and what to do about it. *Int J Health Serv.* 1990;20:53.

Epstein SS. Environmental and occupational pollutants are avoidable causes of breast cancer. *Int J Health Serv.* 1994;24:145.

Fee E, Krieger N. Thinking and rethinking AIDS: Implications for health policy. *Int J Health Serv.* 1993;23:323.

Frieden TR et al. Reducing childhood obesity through policy change. *Health Aff (Millwood).* 2010;29:357.

Grundy SM et al. Implications of recent clinical trials for the National Cholesterol Education Program Adult Treatment Panel III guidelines. *Circulation.* 2004;110:227.

Hayward RA et al. Optimizing statin treatment for primary prevention of coronary artery disease. *Ann Intern Med.* 2010;152:69.

Heron MP et al. Deaths: Final data for 2006. *Natl Vital Stat Rep.* 2009;57(14):1–134.

Keys A. Coronary heart disease in seven countries. *Circulation.* 1970;41(suppl 1):11.

Landrigan PJ. Commentary: Environmental disease: A preventable epidemic. *Am J Public Health.* 1992;82:941.

Ling PM, Glantz SA. Using tobacco industry marketing research to design more effective tobacco control campaigns. *JAMA.* 2002;287:2983.

Lloyd-Jones DM et al. Applicability of cholesterol-lowering primary prevention trials to a general population. *Arch Intern Med.* 2001;161:949.

Loucks EB et al. Life-course socioeconomic position and incidence of coronary heart disease. *Am J Epidemiol* 2009;169:829.

Mannino DM. Why won't our patients stop smoking? *Diabetes Care.* 2009;32(suppl 2):S426.

McKeown T. Determinants of health. In: Lee PR, Estes CL, eds. *The Nation's Health.* Boston, MA: Jones & Bartlett; 1990.

McKinlay JB et al. A review of the evidence concerning the impact of medical measures on recent mortality and morbidity in the United States. *Int J Health Serv.* 1989;19:181.

Nutting PA, ed. *Community Oriented Primary Care: From Principle to Practice.* Albuquerque, NM: University New Mexico Press; 1990.

Ogden CL, Carroll MD. Prevalence of overweight, obesity, and extreme obesity among adults: United States, trends 1976–1980 through 2007–2008. June 2010. www.cdc.gov.

Pharoah PD, Hollingworth W. Cost effectiveness of lowering cholesterol concentration with statins in patients with and without pre-existing coronary heart disease. *Br Med J.* 1996; 312:1443.

Pollan M. You are what you grow. *N Y Times Mag.* April 22, 2007.

Ravdin PM et al. The decrease in breast-cancer incidence in 2003 in the United States. *N Engl J Med.* 2007;356:1670.

Rose G. Sick individuals and sick populations. *Int J Epidemiol.* 1985;14:32.

Schroeder SA, Warner KE. Don't forget tobacco. *N Engl J Med.* 2010;363;201.

Sigerist HE. *Medicine and Human Welfare.* New Haven, CT: Yale University Press; 1941.

Stamler J. Established major coronary risk factors. In: Marmot M, Elliott P, eds. *Coronary Heart Disease Epidemiology.* New York: Oxford University Press; 1992a.

Stamler R. The primary prevention of hypertension and the population blood pressure problem. In: Marmot M, Elliott P, eds. *Coronary Heart Disease Epidemiology.* New York: Oxford University Press; 1992b.

Steinberg D, Gotto AM. Preventing coronary artery disease by lowering cholesterol levels. *JAMA.* 1999;282:2043.

Terris M. The changing relationships of epidemiology and society: The Robert Cruikshank Lecture. *J Public Health Policy.* 1985;6:15.

Terris M. What is health promotion? *J Public Health Policy.* 1986;7:147.

Terris M. Concepts of health promotion: Dualities in public health theory. *J Public Health Policy.* 1992a;13:267.

Terris M. Healthy lifestyles: The perspective of epidemiology. *J Public Health Policy.* 1992b;13:186.

US Department of Health and Human Services. Health United States. 2009. www.cdc.gov.

US Preventive Services Task Force. *Guide to Clinical Preventive Services.* 2010–2011. August 2010. www.ahrq.gov.

Wallinga D. Agricultural policy and childhood obesity. *Health Aff (Millwood).* 2010;29:405.

Warner KE. Smoking and health: A 25-year perspective. *Am J Public Health.* 1989;79:141.

Winslow CEA. Who killed Cock Robin? *Am J Public Health.* 1944;34:658.

Xu J et al. Deaths: final data for 2007. *Natl Vital Stat Rep.* 2010;59(19):1–135.

Long-Term Care

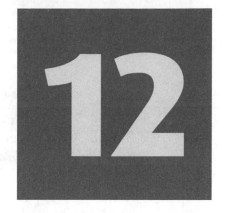

Eddie Taylor awoke one morning at his home in California unable to speak or to move the right side of his body, but able to understand other people around him. After 3 terrifying days in a hospital and 3 frustrating weeks in a stroke rehabilitation center, Mr. Taylor failed to improve. Because he no longer required hospital-level care, he became ineligible for Medicare hospital coverage. Since Mrs. Taylor was wheelchair-bound with crippling rheumatoid arthritis and unable to care for him, he was transferred to a nursing home. Medicare did not cover the $220 per day cost. After 2 years, Medicaid began to pick up the nursing home bills. Much of the family's life savings—earned during the 50 years Mr. Taylor worked in a men's clothing store—had been spent to allow Medicaid eligibility. Because Medicaid paid only $140 per day, few recreational activities were offered, and Mr. Taylor spent each day lying in bed next to a demented patient, who screamed for hours at a time. Unable to voice his complaints at the inhuman conditions of his life, he became severely depressed, stopped eating, and within 3 months was dead.

On high school graduation night, Lyle celebrated with a few drinks and drove to his girlfriend's house. He lost control of the car, hit a tree, and suffered a fractured cervical spine, unable to move his arms or legs. After 9 months in a rehabilitation unit, Lyle remained quadriplegic. He returned home, with a home care agency providing total 24-hour-a-day care at a cost of $300 per day, not covered by insurance. Lyle's father, a businessman, became increasingly angry at his wife, the principal

flutist in the city's professional orchestra, because she refused to leave the orchestra to care for Lyle. After 1 year and $110,000 in long-term care expenses, Lyle's parents were close to divorce. One night Lyle's father awoke in a cold sweat; in his dream, he had placed a plastic bag over Lyle's head and suffocated him.

Time and again physicians and other caregivers witness the tragedy of chronic illness compounded by the failure of the nation's health care system to meet the social needs created by the illness. The crisis of long-term care is twofold: Thousands of families each year lose their savings to pay for the chronic illness of a family member, and long-term care often takes place in dehumanizing institutions that rob their occupants of their last remaining vestiges of independence.

Long-term care includes those health, social, housing, transportation, and other supportive services needed by persons with physical, mental, or cognitive limitations sufficient to compromise independent living. The need for long-term care services is usually determined by evaluating a person's impairment of activities of daily living (ADLs; eg, eating, dressing, bathing, toileting, and getting in or out of bed or a chair) and in instrumental activities of daily living (IADLs; eg, laundry, housework, meal preparation, grocery shopping, transportation, financial management, taking medications, and telephoning) (Table 12–1). Twelve million people in the United States require assistance with one or more ADLs or IADLs, and can therefore be considered as needing long-term care services (Kaye et al, 2010).

Table 12–1. Activities requiring assistance in long-term care

Activities of daily living (ADLs) (basic human functions)
  Feeding
  Dressing
  Bathing or showering
  Getting to and from the toilet
  Getting in and out of a bed or chair
  Dealing with incontinence
Instrumental activities of daily living (IADLs) (activities necessary to remain independent)
  Doing housework and laundry
  Preparing meals
  Shopping for groceries
  Using transportation
  Managing finances
Making and keeping appointments
  Taking medications
  Telephoning

Projections of growth for the elderly population in the United States are startling. In 2000, the population 65 years of age and older numbered 35 million; this figure is expected to reach 72 million by the year 2030. The number of people 85 years and older will more than double from 4.2 million in 2000 to 8.7 million in 2030. Those 80 years and older are most likely to need long-term care because 56% have severe disability (Administration on Aging, 2010). As more and more people need long-term care, the answers to two questions become increasingly urgent: How shall the nation finance long-term care? Should most long-term care be delivered through institutions or in people's homes and communities?

WHO PAYS FOR LONG-TERM CARE?

Phoebe McKinnon was in good health until she fell, broke her hip, and suffered a postoperative joint infection. She was placed on complete bed rest with oral antibiotics for 3 months, after which time she would have another surgery. Widowed, Ms. McKinnon lived alone; her only daughter lived 1500 miles away. Because Ms. McKinnon required 24-hour-a-day help, the social worker, after carefully researching the financial options, reluctantly suggested that Ms. McKinnon spend the 3 months in a nursing home. Ms. McKinnon and her daughter agreed but were shocked when the social worker explained that the cost would be $220 a day, for a total bill of $19,800.

The United States spent $205 billion on long-term care in 2009, including $137 billion on nursing home care (Martin et al, 2011). In 2006, a 1-year nursing home stay cost an average of $76,000.

In 2009, direct out-of-pocket payments by patients and their families financed 22% of long-term care services in the United States. A common scenario is that of Eddie Taylor: After a portion of their life savings are spent for long-term care, families finally become eligible for Medicaid long-term care coverage. Medicaid pays for 34% of US long-term care expenditures (Table 12–2). Many people expect the Medicare program to pay for nursing home stays, and like Phoebe McKinnon and her daughter, are surprised and shocked when they find that Medicare will not assist them. Only 28% of long-term care costs are financed by Medicare (Martin et al, 2011).

Average out-of-pocket expenses for health care paid by the Medicare beneficiaries amounted to 20% of

Table 12–2. Long-term care financing, 2009[a]

	Out of Pocket	Private Insurance	Medicare	Medicaid	Other
Nursing home care	29%	8%	20%	34%	9%
Home care	9%	7%	44%	36%	4%
Total long-term care[b]	22%	8%	28%	34%	8%

[a]Martin A et al: Recession contributes to slowest annual rate of increase in health spending in five decades. *Health Affairs* 2011;30:11.
[b]These figures do not include long-term care items such as adult day care, other community-based services, durable medical equipment, or unpaid care provided by family members at home.

family income in 2005. One-fifth of these expenses went to nursing homes (Kaiser Family Foundation, 2009).

What are the precise roles of Medicare, Medicaid, and private insurance in the financing of long-term care services?

Medicare Long-Term Coverage

Glenn Whitehorse, who was a diabetic, developed gangrene of his right leg requiring above-the-knee amputation. He was transferred from the acute care hospital to the hospital's skilled nursing facility, where he received physical therapy services. Because he was generally frail, he was unable to move from bed to chair without assistance. Mr. Whitehorse's physical and occupational therapists felt he might do better at home, where he could receive home physical therapy and nursing care. All these services were covered by Medicare.

Mrs. Whitehorse had Parkinson's disease and was unable to assist her husband in bathing, getting out of bed, and going to the bathroom; she was forced to hire someone to assist with these custodial functions, which were not covered by Medicare. When Mr. Whitehorse no longer showed any potential for improvement, Medicare discontinued coverage of his home health services. The situation became too difficult, and he was placed in a nursing home for custodial care. Medicare did not cover the nursing home costs.

Which services provided in a nursing facility or at home are covered by Medicare? The key distinction is between "skilled care," for which Medicare pays, and "custodial care," which is usually not covered. A related issue is that of postacute versus chronic care. Medicare usually covers services needed for a few weeks or months after an acute hospitalization but often does not pay for care required by a stable chronic condition.

What are some examples of skilled care versus custodial services? Registered nurses in a hospital nursing facility, nursing home, or home care agency provide a wide variety of services, such as changing the dressing on a wound, taking blood pressures, listening to the heart and lungs to detect heart failure or pneumonia, reviewing patient compliance with medications, and providing patient education about diabetes, hypertension, heart failure, and other illnesses. Physical and occupational therapists work with stroke, hip fracture, and other patients to help them reach their maximum potential level of functioning. Speech therapists perform the difficult task of teaching stroke patients with speech deficits how to communicate. These are all skilled services, usually covered by Medicare.

Custodial services involve assistance with ADLs and IADLs rather than treatment or rehabilitative care related to a disease process; these are tasks such as cooking, cleaning house, shopping, or helping a patient to the toilet. These services, usually provided by nurses' aides, home health aides, homemakers, or family members, are considered unskilled and are often not covered by Medicare.

Medicaid Long-Term Coverage

Willie Robinson, who lived alone, suffered from deforming degenerative arthritis and was unable to do anything more active than sitting in a chair. Because Mr. Robinson had no skilled care medical needs, Medicare would not provide any assistance. Medicaid and the county welfare agency paid for a homemaker to provide 20 hours of help per week, but that was not sufficient. Mr. Robinson had no choice but to enter a nursing home, because that was the only way he could obtain 24-hour-a-day help paid for by Medicaid.

Medicaid differs from Medicare in paying the costs of nursing home care. For home health care, however, Medicaid generally does not cover 24-hour-a-day custodial services for people unable to care for themselves. The completeness of Medicaid's nursing home coverage, in contrast to the limited nature of Medicaid-financed home health care, forces many low-income disabled people like Willie Robinson to go into nursing homes unless they have families capable of providing 24-hour-a-day custodial care. In order to qualify for Medicaid nursing home coverage, families may be forced to spend their savings down to low levels, although in some states, Medicaid allows spouses of nursing home residents to keep some of their assets.

Medicaid's coverage of home health services has increased as a result of home- and community-based care 1915(c) waivers, initially authorized in 1981 (Ng et al, 2010). This program, which attempts to prevent nursing home admissions, allows Medicaid recipients to receive more home care services than previously. Whereas Oregon allocated 71% of its long-term care Medicaid dollars to this program in 2005, nationally Medicaid spent 35% of long-term care dollars for home and community-based care (Kaiser Family Foundation, 2006a).

▶ Private Long-Term Care Insurance

Sue and Lew MacPherson, both age 72, were worried about their future. They remembered their cousin, who was turned down for private long-term care insurance because of his high blood pressure and later spent his entire savings on nursing home bills. Hoping to protect their $32,000 in savings, they decided to apply for long-term care insurance before an illness would make them uninsurable. Their insurance agent calculated the cost of two policies at $6000 per year, or 30% of their $20,000 per year income. At that price, Sue and Lew would spend most of their savings on insurance premiums within a few years. They declined the insurance.

Private insurance plays a minor role in long-term care financing, with only 8% of long-term care costs covered by private policies (Table 12–2). Experience rating (see Chapter 2) has had a profound effect on the dynamics of private long-term care insurance. The largest market for this type of insurance is the elderly population. Under experience-rated insurance, the elderly are charged high premiums because they are at considerable risk of requiring long-term care services. The 2009 median income of people over 65 is $31,000 (US Census Bureau, 2010). Only 17% of households with the head of the household aged 70 to 74 years could afford the average long-term care insurance policy (Kaiser Family Foundation, 2006b). The major attractive market for long-term care insurers is the younger employed population, but only a tiny fraction of this group is interested in long-term care insurance because the prospects of needing such care are so remote.

People purchasing long-term care insurance may find it to be a poor investment. Some private policies specify that a policyholder must be dependent in three or more ADLs before receiving benefits for home health services. Yet many people with fewer than three ADL impairments need long-term care services; for these people, their insurance may pay nothing.

Long-term care policies usually have a large deductible (measured in nursing home days) for nursing home care, and most policies pay a fixed daily fee rather than reimbursing actual charges. A typical policy might provide $150 per day after a 90-day deductible. The 2006 average daily nursing home charge was $220, meaning that $70 would be the patient's responsibility. Thus a year's stay would require out-of-pocket expenditures totaling $39,050 (90 days × $220 = $19,800 plus 275 days × $70 = $19,250) over and above payment of the insurance premium. Most policies limit their coverage to a few years, which places a cap on how much the insurance will pay.

WHO PROVIDES LONG-TERM CARE?

▶ Informal Caregivers

Since her husband died, Mrs. Dora Whitney has lived alone. At age 71, she became forgetful and one day left the gas stove on, causing a fire in the kitchen. Two months later, she was unable to find her way home after going to the store and was found by the police wandering in the streets. Her daughter, Kimberly, brought her to the university hospital, where she was diagnosed with Alzheimer's dementia. After a team conference with her mother's physicians, nurses, occupational therapist, and social worker, Kimberly admitted that her only option was to abandon her career as a teacher to care for her mother. Kimberly refused to place her mother in a nursing home, and funds were not available to hire the needed 24-hour-a-day help.

Most people needing long-term care services receive them from their family and friends. In 2007, about 52 million people served as unpaid family caregivers, of whom the majority were women. For men, their wives often provide long-term care, and for women, their daughters are frequently caregivers. A growing number of the elderly do not have family living near enough to them to provide informal care; the absence of an informal caregiver is a common reason for nursing home placement. On average, informal caregivers provide 20 hours per week of care, and the estimated economic value of their unpaid contributions was approximately $375 billion in 2007. Thirty-seven percent of informal caregivers to persons age 50 and older reported quitting their job or reducing their work hours in order to assist their family members. Elderly people with caregivers have shorter hospital stays, fewer readmissions, and lower inpatient expenses, demonstrating that unpaid caregivers create a great deal of value for the health care system (Levine, 1999; AARP, 2008).

Community-Based and Home Health Services

Ana Dominguez insisted that her daughter Juana accept the Yale scholarship. Though at age 49 Ms. Dominguez was bed- and wheelchair-bound with multiple sclerosis, she would feel too guilty if Juana remained in San Antonio, TX, just to care for her. Before Juana left, she arranged with the home care agency to have her mother transported to an adult day health center 3 days a week; for nursing, physical, and occupational therapy 3 times a week; and for meals-on-wheels. Medicare paid for these services. But Ms. Dominguez needed someone at home 24 hours a day, a service not covered by Medicare. For $15 a day, Juana was able to hire Vilma, an undocumented teenager from El Salvador, to live at home. Adding Vilma's pay and the cost of her food, Juana figured they would spend $35,000 of their $42,000 in savings by the time she graduated from Yale.

Community-based long-term care is delivered through a variety of programs, such as home care, adult day care, assisted living settings, home-delivered meals, board and care homes, hospice care for the terminally ill, mental health programs, and others. During the 1970s, the independent living movement among disabled people created a strong push away from institutional (hospital and nursing home) care toward community-based and home care that fostered the greatest possible independence. During the 1980s, AIDS activists furthered the development of hospice programs that provide intensive home care services for people with terminal cancer and AIDS. The home is usually a more therapeutic, comforting environment than the hospital or nursing home.

As a product of the intersection of the popular movement toward home care and the DRG-created incentive to reduce Medicare hospital stays, home health services expanded rapidly from 1980 to 1997. This, in turn, prompted changes in Medicare payment policies to rein in home care expenditures. After concerns were voiced about excessive cuts in Medicare home care payments, in 2000 Medicare instituted a prospective payment system for home care based on the episode-of-illness model (see Chapter 4). Home care agencies are paid a lump sum (which, like DRG hospital payments varies with the severity of the illness) for 60 days of care.

Many categories of health caregivers function in teams to perform home care, including nurses, physical, occupational, speech, and respiratory therapists, social workers, home health aides, case managers, and drivers delivering meals-on-wheels. Yet home care, designed to help fill the once low-tech niche in the health care system that assists the disabled with ADLs and IADLs, has become increasingly specialized. Home care agencies now offer intravenous antibiotic infusions, morphine pumps, indwelling central venous lines, and home renal dialysis, administered by highly skilled intravenous and wound care nurses, respiratory therapists, and other health care professionals. These developments are a major advance in shifting medical care from hospital to home, but they have not been matched by growth in the paid personal custodial care needed to allow disabled people to remain safely in their homes. Similarly, hospice care, while providing excellent nursing services for patients with terminal illnesses, is limited in the ADL support it provides. Hospice programs may not accept terminal patients without an informal caregiver at home; thus, the people who may need home hospice services the most cannot receive them.

Assisted living, which provides housing with a graded intensity of services depending on the functional capabilities of its residents, has been growing rapidly. However, the average annual cost in 2009 was $34,000, most of which comes from out-of-pocket payments, thereby pricing assisting living out of the reach of low- and moderate-income families (Stevenson and Grabowski, 2010).

Nursing Homes

Each morning, more than one and a quarter million Americans awaken in nursing homes. Most of them are very old and very feeble. Most will stay in the nursing home for a long time. For most, it will be the last place they ever live. . . . [Nursing home] residents live out the last of their days in an enclosed society without privacy, dignity, or pleasure, subsisting on minimally palatable diets, multiple sedatives, and large doses of television—eventually dying, one suspects at least partially of boredom. (Vladeck, 1980)

Often, informal help and formal home health services are unable to provide the care required for severely disabled people. Such people may be placed in nursing homes with 24-hour-a-day care provided by health aides and orderlies under the supervision of nurses. In 2007, 1.8 million people resided in US nursing homes. Sixty-seven percent of nursing home residents are women, who more often outlive their spouses (Kaye et al, 2010). Frequently, after caring for a sick husband at home, women will themselves fall ill and be placed in a nursing home because no one is left to care for them at home. People who reach the age of 65 have a 40% chance of entering a nursing home at some time in their life (www.medicare.gov/longtermcare/static/home.asp).

Seventy-six percent of nursing home residents have cognitive impairment and 93% have restricted mobility (Kaye et al, 2010). There are two main differences between the chronically ill inside and outside nursing homes: Nursing home residents have no family able to care for them, and a far larger proportion of nursing home patients suffer from dementia, a condition whose care is extremely difficult to provide at home by family members.

Nursing homes vary widely in quality. The Omnibus Budget Reconciliation Act of 1987 set standards for nursing home quality and mandated surveys to enforce these standards. Serious quality problems persist; the average number of deficiencies per facility increased from 5.7 in 1999 to 7.1 in 2005. Only 9% of nursing homes had no deficiencies in 2005. The most frequently cited deficiencies in 2005 were inadequate food sanitation, quality of care, professional standards, accident prevention, housekeeping, comprehensive care plans, infection control, pressure sores, and dignity (Harrington et al, 2006; Werner and Konetzka, 2010). Compared with non-Hispanic whites, Hispanics requiring nursing home are more likely to be placed in low-quality facilities (Fennell et al, 2010).

Lower-income people are housed in close quarters with several other patients and become totally dependent on an underpaid, inadequately trained staff. Hour after hour may be spent lying in bed or sitting in a chair in front of a TV. While quality of life varies between one nursing home and another, placement in a nursing home almost always thwarts the human yearning for some degree of independence of action and for companionship. A sense of futility overwhelms many nursing home residents, and the desire to live often wanes (Vladeck, 1980).

To keep down costs, most care in nursing homes is provided by nurse's aides, who are paid very little, receive minimal training, are inadequately supervised, and are required to care for more residents than they can properly serve. The job of the nursing home aide is very difficult, involving bathing, feeding, walking residents, cleaning them when they are incontinent, lifting them, and hearing their complaints. In 2005, 66% of all nursing homes were under for-profit ownership, many operated by large corporate chains (Harrington et al, 2006). For-profit ownership has been associated with lower staffing levels and poorer quality of care compared with nonprofit ownership (Comondore, 2009).

Offering a humane existence to severely disabled people housed together in close quarters is a nearly impossible task. One view of nursing home reform holds that only the abolition of most nursing homes and the development of adequately financed home and community-based care can solve the nursing home problem.

IMPROVING LONG-TERM CARE

▶ Financing Long-Term Care

Boomer was mad. As a self-employed person, his family's health insurance coverage was costing $600 each month, in addition to his out-of-pocket dental bills. To make matters worse, a big chunk of his social security payments went to Medicare each year, not to mention federal and state income taxes and sales taxes going to finance Medicare and Medicaid, so that other people could get health care. While spending all this money, Boomer was healthy and had not seen a physician for 6 years.

One day Boomer's father, Abraham, suffered a devastating stroke. After weeks in the hospital, largely paid for by Medicare, Abraham was transferred to a nursing home. Because Medicare does not cover most long-term care, Boomer's mother paid the bills out of her savings until most of the money ran out. Abraham then became eligible for Medicaid, which took care of the nursing home bills. After Abraham's illness, Boomer stopped complaining about his social security and tax payments going to medical care. Even though Boomer was paying more than he was receiving, Abraham was receiving far more than he was paying. Boomer was grateful for the care his father received and figured that he might be in Abraham's shoes some day.

In the early 1960s, it was recognized that private insurance was unable to solve the problem of health care financing for people older than 65. The costs of health care for the elderly were too great, making experience-rated health insurance premiums unaffordable for most elderly people. Accordingly, Medicare, a social insurance program, was passed (see Chapter 2). An identical problem confronts long-term care financing: As shown earlier in this chapter, most people who might wish to purchase long-term care insurance are unable to afford an adequate policy. Table 12–3 lists some proposals for improving long-term care.

The Pepper Commission (1990) recommended that the nation institute a social insurance program to finance long-term care. This program, like Medicare Part A, could be financed by an increase in the rate of social security contributions by employers and employees. It would pay for caregivers to provide those services not currently covered by Medicare, especially in-home help in feeding, dressing, bathing, toileting, housework, grocery shopping, transportation, and other assistance with ADLs and IADLs. A similar proposal was offered by Physicians for a National Health Program (Harrington et al, 1991).

▶ Providing Long-Term Care

Mei Soon Wang was desperate to go home. Since a brain tumor had paralyzed her left side and left her

incontinent, she had been confined to a nursing home because she had no family in San Francisco to care for her. Her daughter, visiting from Portland, heard of On Lok Senior Health Services, which cared for the frail elderly in their homes. On Lok accepted Ms. Wang, placed her in adult day care, arranged for meals to be delivered to her home, and paid for part-time help on evenings and weekends.

Because a reasonable quality of life and personal independence, within the confines of a patient's illness, are so difficult to achieve in the nursing home environment, long-term care reformers often advocate that most long-term care be provided at home. The first step toward deinstitutionalizing long-term care is a financing mechanism that pays for more comprehensive community-based and home long-term care services.

The ideal long-term caregivers are the patient's family and friends; thus, it can be argued that long-term care reform should support, assist, and pay informal caregivers, not replace them. Teams of nurses, physical and occupational therapists, physicians (who often know the least about long-term care), social workers, and attendants can train and work with informal caregivers, and personnel can be available to provide respite care so informal caregivers can have some relief from the 24-hours-a-day, 7-days-a-week burden. If informal caregivers are not available, all possible efforts can still be made to deliver long-term care in people's homes rather than in nursing homes (Harrington et al, 1991).

An innovative long-term care program that has achieved great success is the On Lok program in San Francisco. Translated from Chinese, On Lok means peaceful, happy abode. Begun in 1971 in San Francisco's Chinatown, On Lok merges adult day services, in-home care, home-delivered meals, housing assistance, comprehensive medical care, respite care for caregivers, hospital care, and skilled nursing care into one program. Persons eligible for On Lok have chronic illness sufficiently severe to qualify them for nursing home placement, but only 15% ever spend time in a nursing home. Services for each participant are organized by a multidisciplinary team, including physicians, nurses, social workers, rehabilitation and recreation therapists, and nutritionists.

Table 12–3. Proposals for improving long-term care

Developing social insurance to finance long-term care

Shifting from nursing home care to community-based care by improved financing of community-based care

Training and supporting family members as caregivers

Expanding the number of comprehensive acute and long-term care organizations modeled on On Lok Senior Health Services, which reduce costs by keeping the elderly out of the hospital as much as possible

In 1983, On Lok became the first organization in the United States to assume full financial risk for the care of a frail elderly population, receiving monthly capitation payments from Medicare and Medicaid to cover all services. Whereas 45% of US personal health care expenditures go to hospital and nursing home services, On Lok spent a mere 17% on these items, making 83% of the health care dollar available for ambulatory home- and community-based services. While its services are far more comprehensive, On Lok's costs are no higher than those for a similar frail elderly population under traditional Medicare and Medicaid (Eng et al, 1997; Bodenheimer, 1999). Seventy-five On Lok "look alikes" now exist in 29 states under the Program of All-Inclusive Care for the Elderly (PACE). However, PACE sites care for fewer than 25,000 of the 3 million frail elderly and disabled people in the United States.

The United States has not implemented a social insurance program for long-term care. However, other nations have been more proactive in addressing the needs of their aging populations. In 1995, Germany enacted a system of near-universal social insurance for long-term care—a program that the public has accepted as both affordable and beneficial (Harrington et al, 2002). A major expansion of the PACE concept combined with comprehensive social insurance for long-term care could provide a badly needed solution to the problems of long-term care in the United States.

REFERENCES

AARP. *Valuing the invaluable: the economic value of family caregiving, 2008 update.* AARP Public Policy Institute. November 2008. www.aarp.org/ppi.

Administration on Aging. *A Profile of Older Americans, 2010.* US Department of Health and Human Services; 2010. www.aoa.gov/aoaroot/aging_statistics/Profile/2010/docs/2010profile.pdf. Accessed November 16, 2011.

Bodenheimer T. Long-term care for frail elderly people—the On Lok model. *N Engl J Med.* 1999;341:1324.

Comondore VR. Quality of care in for-profit and not-for-profit nursing homes: Systematic review and meta-analysis. *BMJ.* 2009;339:b2732.

Eng C et al. Program of All-inclusive Care for the Elderly (PACE). *J Am Geriatr Soc.* 1997;45:223.

Fennell ML et al. Elderly Hispanics more likely to reside in poor quality nursing homes. *Health Aff (Millwood).* 2010;29:65.

Harrington C et al. A national long-term care program for the United States: A caring vision. *JAMA.* 1991;266:3023.

Harrington C et al. Germany's long-term care insurance model: Lessons for the United States. *J Public Health Policy.* 2002;23:44.

Harrington C et al. Nursing Facilities, Staffing, Residents, and Facility Deficiencies, 1999 through 2005. University of California at San Francisco, September 2006. www.nccnhr.org.

Kaiser Family Foundation. Medicaid and long-term care services. July 2006a. www.kff.org/medicaid/upload/Medicaid-and-Long-Term-Care-Services-PDF.pdf. Accessed November 16, 2011.

Kaiser Family Foundation. Private long-term care insurance: A viable option for low and middle-income seniors? July 2006b. www.kff.org/uninsured/upload/7459.pdf. Accessed November 16, 2011.

Kaiser Family Foundation. Revisiting "skin in the game" among Medicare beneficiaries. February 2009. www.kff.org/medicare/upload/7860.pdf. Accessed November 16, 2011.

Kaye HS et al. Long-term care: who gets it, how provides it, who pays, and how much? *Health Aff (Millwood).* 2010;29:11.

Levine C. The loneliness of the long-term care giver. *N Engl J Med.* 1999;340:1587.

Martin A et al. Recession contributes to slowest annual rate of increase in health spending in five decades. *Health Aff (Millwood).* 2011;30:11.

Ng T et al. Medicare and Medicaid in long-term care. *Health Aff (Millwood).* 2010;29:22.

Pepper Commission. *A Call for Action.* Washington, DC: US Government Printing Office; 1990.

Stevenson DG, Grabowski DC. Sizing up the market for assisted living. *Health Aff (Millwood).* 2010;29:35.

US Census Bureau. *Income, Poverty, and Health Insurance Coverage in the United States, 2009.* P60–238, September, 2010.

Vladeck BC. *Unloving Care: The Nursing Home Tragedy.* New York: Basic Books; 1980.

Werner RM, Konetzka RT. Advancing nursing home quality through quality improvement itself. *Health Aff (Millwood).* 2010;29:81.

Medical Ethics and Rationing of Health Care

For those who work in the healing professions, ethical values play a special role. The specific content of medical ethics was first formulated centuries ago, based on the sayings of Hippocrates and others. The refinement of medical ethics has continued up to the present by practicing health caregivers, health professional and religious organizations, and individual ethicists. As medical technology, health care financing, and the organization of health care transform themselves, so must the content of medical ethics change in order to acknowledge and guide new circumstances.

FOUR PRINCIPLES OF MEDICAL ETHICS

Over the years, participants in and observers of medical care have distilled widely shared human beliefs about healing the sick into four major ethical principles: beneficence, nonmaleficence, autonomy, and justice (Beauchamp and Childress, 2008) (Table 13–1).

Beneficence is the obligation of health care providers to help people in need.

Dr. Rolando Bueno is a hard-working family physician practicing in a low-income neighborhood of a large city. He shows concern for his patients, and his knowledge and judgment are respected by his medical and nursing colleagues. On one occasion, he was called before the hospital quality assurance committee when one of his patients unexpectedly died; he agreed that he had made mistakes in his care and incorporated the lessons of the case into his future practice.

Dr. Bueno tries to live up to the ideal of beneficence. He does not always succeed; like all physicians, he sometimes makes clinical errors. Overall, he treats his patients to the best of his ability. The principle of beneficence in the healing professions is the obligation to care for patients to the best of one's ability.

Nonmaleficence is the duty of health care providers to do no harm.

Mrs. Lucy Knight suffers from insomnia and Parkinson's disease. The insomnia does not bother her, because she likes to read at night, but it irritates her husband. Mr. Knight requests his wife's physician to order strong sleeping pills for her, but the physician declines, saying that the combination of sleeping pills and Parkinson's disease places Mrs. Knight at high risk for a serious fall.

The modern array of medical interventions has the capacity to do good or harm or both, thereby enmeshing the principle of nonmaleficence with the principle of beneficence. In the case of Mrs. Knight, the prescribing of sedatives has far more potential for harm than for good, particularly because Mrs. Knight does not see her insomnia as a problem.

Autonomy is the right of a person to choose and follow his or her own plan of life and action.

Mr. Winter is a frail 88-year-old found by Dr. James Washington, his family physician, to have colon cancer, which has spread to the liver. The cancer is causing no symptoms. An oncologist gives Mr. Winter the option of transfusions, parenteral nutrition, and surgery, followed by chemotherapy; or watchful waiting with palliative and hospice

Table 13–1. The four principles of medical ethics

Beneficence	The obligation of health care providers to help people in need
Nonmaleficence	The duty of health care providers to do no harm
Autonomy	The right of patients to make choices regarding their health care
Justice	The concept of treating everyone in a fair manner

care when symptoms appear. Mr. Winter is terrified of hospitals and prefers to remain at home. He feels that he might live a comfortable couple of years before the cancer claims his life. After talking it over with Dr. Washington, he chooses the second option.

The principle of autonomy adds another consideration to the interrelated principles of beneficence and nonmaleficence. Would Mr. Winter enjoy a longer life by submitting himself to aggressive cancer therapy that does harm in order to do good? Or, does he sense that the harm may exceed the good? The balance of risks and benefits confronts each physician on a daily basis (Eddy, 1990). But the decision cannot be made solely by a risk–benefit analysis; the patient's preference is a critical addition to the equation.

Autonomy is founded in the overall desire of most human beings to control their own destiny, to have choices in life, and to live in a society that places value on individual freedom. In medical ethics, autonomy refers to the right of competent adult patients to consent to or refuse treatment. While the physician has an obligation to respect the patient's wishes, he or she also has a duty to fully inform the patient of the probable consequences of those wishes. For children and for adults unable to make medical decisions, a parent, guardian, other family member, or surrogate decision maker named in a legal document becomes the autonomous agent on behalf of the patient.

Justice refers to the ethical concept of treating everyone in a fair manner.

Joe, a white businessman in the suburbs, suffers crushing chest pain and within 5 minutes is taken to a nearby private emergency department, where he receives immediate coronary angioplasty and

state-of-the-art treatment for a heart attack. Five miles away, in a poor neighborhood, Josephine, an African American woman, experiences severe chest pain, calls 911, waits 25 minutes for help to arrive, and is brought to a public hospital whose emergency department staff is attending to five other acutely ill patients. Before receiving appropriate attention, she suffers an arrhythmia and dies.

The principle of justice as applied to medical ethics is newer, more controversial, and harder to define than the principles of beneficence, nonmaleficence, and autonomy. In a general sense, people are treated justly when they receive what they deserve. It is unjust not to grant a medical degree to someone who completes medical school and passes all the necessary examinations. It is unjust to punish a person who did not commit a crime. In another meaning, *justice* refers to universal rights: to receive enough to eat, to be afforded shelter, to have access to basic medical care and education, and to be able to speak freely. If these rights are denied, justice has been violated. In yet another version, justice connotes equal opportunity: All people should have an equal chance to realize their human potential. Justice might be linked to the golden rule: Treat others as you would want others to treat you. While there is no clear agreement on the precise meaning of justice, most people would agree that the differential treatment of Joe and Josephine is unjust.

▶ Distributive Justice

In exploring the concept of justice, one area of concern is the allocation of benefits and burdens in society. This realm of ethical thinking is called *distributive justice*, and it involves such questions as: Who receives what amount of wealth, of education, or of medical care? Who pays what amount of taxes?

The principle of justice is linked to the idea of fairness. In the arena of distributive justice, no agreement exists on what formula for allocating benefits and costs is fair. Should each person get an equal share? Should those who work harder receive more? Should the proper formula be "to each according to ability to pay," as determined by a free market? Or "to each according to need?" In allocating costs, should each person pay an equal share or should those with greater wealth pay more? Most societies construct a mixture of these allocation formulas. Unemployment benefits consider effort (having had a job) and need (having lost the job). Welfare benefits are primarily based on need. Job promotions may be based on merit. Many goods are distributed according to ability to pay. Primary education in theory (but not always in practice) is founded on the belief that everyone should receive an equal share (Beauchamp and Childress, 2008; Jonsen et al, 2010).

How is the principle of distributive justice formulated for medical care? Throughout the history of the developed world, the concept that health care is a privilege that should be allocated according to ability to pay has competed with the idea that health care is a right and should be distributed according to need. In most developed nations, the allocation of health care according to need has become the dominant political belief, as demonstrated by the passage of universal or near-universal health insurance laws. In the United States, the failure of the 100-year battle to enact national health insurance, and the widely divergent opinions on the 2010 Affordable Care Act, attest to the ongoing debate between health care as a privilege and health care as a right (see Chapter 15).

If the overwhelming opinion in the developed world holds that health care should be allocated according to need, then all people should have equal access to a reasonable level of medical care without financial barriers (ie, people should have a right to health care). In this chapter, therefore, we consider that the principle of distributive justice requires all people to equally receive a reasonable level of medical services based on medical need without regard to ability to pay.

ETHICAL DILEMMAS, OLD AND NEW

Ethical dilemmas (Lo, 2009) are situations in which a provider of medical care is forced to make a decision that violates one of the four principles of medical ethics in order to adhere to another of the principles. Ethical dilemmas always involve disputes in which both sides have an ethical underpinning to their position. Financial conflicts of interest on the part of physicians (see Chapters 4 and 10), in contrast, pit ethical behavior against individual gain and are not ethical dilemmas.

Anthony, a 22-year-old Jehovah's Witness, is admitted to the intensive care unit for gastrointestinal bleeding. His blood pressure is 80/60 mm Hg, and in the past 4 hours, his hematocrit has fallen from 38% to 21%. The medical resident implores

Anthony to accept life-saving transfusions, but he refuses, saying that his religion teaches him that death is preferable to receiving blood products. When the blood pressure reaches 60/20 mm Hg, the desperate resident decides to give the blood while Anthony is unconscious. The attending physician vetoes the plan, saying that the patient has the right to refuse treatment, even if an avoidable death is the outcome.

In Anthony's case, the ethical dilemma is a conflict between beneficence and autonomy. Which principle has priority depends on the particular situation, and in this case, autonomy supersedes beneficence. If the patient were a child without sufficient knowledge or reasoning capability to make an informed choice, the physician would not be obligated to withhold transfusions, even if the family so demanded (Jonsen et al, 2010).

Pedro Navarro has lung cancer that has metastasized to his brain. No effective treatment is available, and Mr. Navarro is confused and unable to understand his medical condition. Mrs. Navarro demands that her husband undergo craniotomy to remove the tumor. The neurosurgeon refuses, arguing that the operation will do Mr. Navarro no good whatsoever and will cause him additional suffering.

The case of Mr. Navarro pits the principle of autonomy against the principle of nonmaleficence. Mr. Navarro's rightful surrogate decision maker, his wife, wants a particular course of treatment, but the neurosurgeon knows that this treatment will cause Mr. Navarro considerable harm and do him no good. In this case, nonmaleficence triumphs. Whereas patient autonomy allows the right to refuse treatment, it does not include the right to demand a harmful or ineffectual treatment.

The traditional dilemmas described in many articles and books on medical ethics feature beneficence or nonmaleficence in conflict with autonomy. In two famous ethical dilemmas, the families of Karen Ann Quinlan and Nancy Cruzan, young women with severe brain damage (persistent vegetative state) asked that physicians discontinue a respirator (in the Quinlan case) and a feeding tube (in the Cruzan case). Both cases were adjudicated in the courts. The Quinlan decision promoted the right of patients or their surrogate decision makers to withdraw treatment, even if the treatment is necessary to sustain life. The outcome of the Cruzan case placed limits on autonomy by requiring that life-supporting treatment can be withdrawn only when a patient has stated his or her wishes clearly in advance (Annas, 2005).

In 2005, the case of Terri Schiavo, for 15 years in a persistent vegetative state similar to the situations of Karen Ann Quinlan and Nancy Cruzan, made national headlines. In spite of multiple decisions of state and federal courts—up to the Supreme Courts of Florida and the United States—supporting the right of Terri Schiavo's husband to discontinue Ms. Schiavo's feeding tube, the US Congress, encouraged by President George Bush, passed legislation reopening the option of reinserting the feeding tube. Eventually, based on the precedents of the Quinlan and Cruzan cases, the courts prevailed and Ms. Schiavo died (Annas, 2005).

Overall, medical ethics has moved in the direction of giving priority to the principle of autonomy over that of beneficence.

In the late twentieth century, a new generation of ethical dilemmas emerged, moving beyond the individual physician–patient relationship to involve the broader society. These social–ethical problems derive from the new reality that money may not be available to pay for a reasonable level of medical services for all people. When money and resources are bountiful, the issue of distributive justice refers to equality in medical care access and health outcomes (see Chapter 3). Is it fair that some people are unable to receive needed care because they lack money and insurance? When money and resources become scarce, the issue of justice takes on a new twist. Should limits be set on treatments given to people with high-cost medical needs, so that other people can receive basic services? If not, might health care consume so many resources that other social needs are sacrificed? If limits should be set, who decides these limits?

Angela and Amy Lakeberg [actual names] were Siamese twins sharing one heart. Without surgery, they would die shortly. With surgery, Amy would die and Angela's chance of survival would be less than 1%. On August 20, 1993, a team of 18 physicians and nurses at Children's Hospital of Philadelphia performed an all-day operation to separate the twins. Amy died. The cost of the treatment was $1 million. The Medicaid program covered $700 to $1000 per day, and the hospital underwrote the balance of the costs. On June 9, 1994, Angela died; she had spent her brief life on a respirator in the hospital.

The new fiscal reality has spawned two related dilemmas.

1. The first involves a conflict between the duty of the physician to follow the principles of beneficence and nonmaleficence and the growing sentiment that physicians should pay attention to issues of distributive justice. In the case of the Lakeberg twins, the hospital and the surgeons adhered strictly to the principle of beneficence: Even a remote chance of aiding one twin was seen as worthwhile. The hospital could have balked, arguing that its funding of the surgery would be unfairly shifted to other payers. The surgeons could have declined to operate on the grounds that the money spent on the Lakebergs could have been better used by patients with a greater chance of survival. But, the surgeons could argue, who can guarantee that the money saved would have gone to better use?

2. The second category of social–ethical dilemma is the conflict between the individual patient's right to autonomy and society's claim to distributive justice. In the Lakeberg case, individual autonomy won out. The Lakeberg parents could have decided that spending $1 million of society's money on a less than 1% chance of saving one of two infants was excessive and could indirectly harm other patients. On the other hand, would not most parents have done what the Lakebergs did?

Physicians take up the practice of medicine with a recognition that they have a duty to help and not harm their patients. Individuals claim a right to health care and do not want others to restrict that care. Yet the principle of distributive justice (recognizing that resources for health care are limited and should be fairly allocated among the entire population) might lead to physicians denying legitimate services or patients setting aside rightful claims to treatment.

The basis for the principle of justice is the desire shared by many human beings to live in a civilized society. To live in a state of harmony, each person must balance the concerns of the individual with the needs of the larger community. There is no right or wrong answer to the question of whether the Lakeberg surgery should have been done, but the surgery must be seen as a choice. The $1 million spent on the twins might have been spent on immunizing 10,000 children, with greater overall benefit. When health resources are scarce, the principle of justice creates ethical dilemmas that touch many people beyond those involved in an individual physician–patient relationship. The imperatives of cost control have thrust the principle of justice to the forefront of health policy in the debate over rationing.

WHAT IS RATIONING?

Dr. Everett Wall works in a health maintenance organization (HMO). Betty Ailes came to him with a headache and wanted a magnetic resonance imaging (MRI) scan. After a complete history and physical examination, Dr. Wall prescribed medication and denied the scan. Ms. Ailes wrote to the medical director, complaining that Dr. Wall was rationing services to her.

Perry Hiler arrives at Vacant Hospital with fever and severe cough. His chest x-ray shows an infiltrate near the hilum of the lung consistent with pneumonia or tumor. Since Mr. Hiler has no insurance, the emergency department physician sends him to the county hospital. At the time, Vacant Hospital has 35 empty beds and plenty of staff. When he recovers, Mr. Hiler calls the newspaper to complain. The next day, a headline appears: "Vacant Hospital Rations Care."

Jim Delacour is a 50-year-old man with terminal cardiomyopathy. His physician sends him to a transplant center, where an evaluation concludes that he is an ideal candidate for a heart transplant. Because the number of transplant candidates is larger than the supply of donor hearts available, Mr. Delacour is placed on the waiting list. After waiting 6 weeks, he dies.

When the emergency department called, Dr. Marco Intensivo's heart sank. The eight-bed intensive care unit is filled with extremely ill patients, all capable of full recovery if they survive their acute illnesses. He has worried all day about another patient needing intensive care: a 55-year-old with a heart attack complicated by unstable arrhythmias. Which one of the nine needy cases will not get

intensive care? Dr. Intensivo needs to make a decision, and fast.

The general public and the media often view rationing as a limitation of medical care such that "not all care expected to be beneficial is provided to all patients" (Aaron and Schwartz, 1984). Such a view only partially explains the concept of rationing. More precisely, rationing means a conscious policy of equitably distributing needed resources that are in limited supply (Reagan, 1988) (Table 13–2). Under this definition, only the last two cases presented above can be considered rationing. In the first case, Dr. Wall did not feel that the MRI was a resource needed by Betty Ailes. In the second, Vacant Hospital's refusal to care for Perry Hiler was simply a decision on the part of a private institution to place its financial well-being above a patient's health; there was no scarcity of health care resources. In the heart transplant and intensive care unit cases, in contrast, donor hearts and intensive care unit beds were in fact scarce. For Mr. Delacour, the scarcity was nationwide and prolonged; for Dr. Intensivo, the scarcity was within a particular hospital at a particular time. In both cases, decisions had to be made regarding the allocation of those resources.

During World War II, insufficient gasoline was available to both power the military machine and satisfy the demands of automobile owners in the United States. The government rationed gasoline, giving priority to the military, yet allowing each civilian to obtain a limited amount of fuel. In a rural area, there may be a shortage of health care providers; in an overcrowded urban public hospital, there may be an insufficient number of beds; in the transplant arena, donor organs are truly in short supply. These are cases of commodity scarcity, wherein specific items are in limited supply.

Table 13–2. Two definitions of rationing

Popular usage of the term "rationing":

A limitation of medical care such that not all care expected to be beneficial is provided to all patients.

Precise usage of the term "rationing":

The limitation of resources, including money, going to medical care such that not all care expected to be beneficial is provided to all patients; and the distribution of these limited resources in a fair manner.

The United States is a nation with an adequate supply of hospital beds and physicians in most communities; commodity scarcity in health care is the exception (eg, scarcity of primary care resources is becoming a reality). But a different kind of health resource is becoming scarce, and that is money. Those who pay the bills are insistent that the flow of money into the health sector be restricted. Most discussions of health care rationing presume fiscal scarcity, not commodity scarcity.

In summary, rationing in medical care means the limitation of resources, including money, going to medical care such that not all care expected to be beneficial is provided to all patients, and the fair distribution of these limited resources.

COMMODITY SCARCITY: THE CASE OF ORGAN TRANSPLANTS

While fiscal scarcity is the more common form of resource limitation, commodity scarcity provides an instructive example of the interaction of ethics and rationing.

Mr. George Olds is a 76-year-old nonsmoking retired business executive with end-stage heart failure. He has good pulmonary and renal function and is not diabetic; thus, he is medically a good candidate for a heart transplant. His life expectancy without a transplant is 1 month. He has a loving family, with the resources to pay the $300,000 cost of the procedure.

Mr. Matt Younger is a 46-year-old divorced man who is unemployed, having lost his job as an auto worker 3 years ago. He has a history of smoking and alcohol use. He suffers a heart attack, develops intractable heart failure, and will die within 1 month without a heart transplant. He has good pulmonary and renal function and is not diabetic, making him a good candidate for the procedure.

Mr. Olds and Mr. Younger are in the same hospital and cared for by the same cardiologist, who applied for donor hearts on behalf of both patients on the same day. The cardiologist receives a call that one donor heart—histocompatible with both patients—has become available. Who should receive it?

In 1951, the first kidney transplant was performed in Massachusetts. But it was in 1967, when Dr. Christiaan Barnard sewed a living heart into the chest of a person suffering end-stage cardiac disease, that modern medicine fully entered the age of transplantation. Since that time, thousands of people have been kept alive for many years by transplantation of the kidneys, hearts, lungs, and livers of their fellow human beings. In 2010, 17,000 kidney, 2300 heart, 6300 liver, and 1800 lung transplants were performed in the United States. Transplants are truly life saving in most cases. Seventy to eighty percent of patients receiving heart, liver, or kidney transplants survive at least 5 years after transplantation (http://optn.transplant.hrsa.gov).

Transplantation of organs is both a medical miracle and an ethical watershed. It has generated debate on such questions as these: When are people really dead (so that their organs can be harvested for use in transplantation)? What is the responsibility of the families of brain-dead people to allow their organs to be harvested? Who pays and who is paid for organ transplants? Who should receive organs that are in short supply? We will focus only on the last of these issues.

The number of persons on the national waiting list for organ transplants rose from 16,000 in 1988 to 111,000 in 2010, yet the pool of organ donors has been estimated at 14,500. Even if all potential donors became actual donors, the number of organs that could be harvested each year falls far short of the required number. Nineteen patients in the United States die each day awaiting organs (www.mayoclinic.org/transplant/organ-donation.html).

Transplantation presents a classic case of commodity scarcity: There is insufficient supply to meet demand. Explicit rationing, which is a system that determines who gets organs and who does not, is inevitable. For heart, lung, and liver transplants, rationing is all or nothing: Those who receive organs may live, while those who do not will die.

Given the supply and demand imbalance, which potential transplant patients actually receive new organs? In the early 1980s, the major heart transplant center at Stanford University excluded people with "a history of alcoholism, job instability, antisocial behavior, or psychiatric illness," and required transplant recipients to enjoy "a stable, rewarding family and/or vocational environment." Stanford's recipients had a better than 50% chance of surviving 5 years, signifying that acceptance or rejection from the program was a matter of life and death. The US Department of Health and Human Services was concerned about

Stanford's selection criteria, which favored those middle-class or wealthy people with satisfying jobs. Moreover, the $100,000 cost restricted heart transplants to those with insurance coverage or ability to pay out of pocket. Both the social and economic criteria for access to this life-saving surgery raised serious issues of distributive justice.

Following the passage of the National Organ Transplantation Act of 1984, the federal government designated the United Network for Organ Sharing (UNOS) as a national system for matching donated organs and potential recipients (www.unos.org). According to the Task Force on Organ Transplantation (1986), organ allocation should be governed by medical criteria, with the major factors being urgency of need and probability of success. The Task Force recommended that if two or more patients are equally good candidates for an organ according to the medical criteria, length of time on the waiting list is the fairest way to make the final selection. In 2006, the US Department of Health and Human Services issued updated guidelines and in 2007 the Medicare program promulgated conditions that hospitals with transplant programs needed to follow.

Overall, UNOS follows these recommendations, placing potential recipients of organ transplants on its computerized waiting list. Recipients are prioritized according to a point scale based on severity of illness, time on the waiting list, and probability of a successful outcome. A serious attempt has been made to allocate scarce organs on the basis of justice criteria. But haunting the ethics of the prioritization process is the issue of ability to pay. In 2008, the average kidney transplant cost $259,000 and liver transplant $534,400. Persons needing a transplant are often rejected if they lack health insurance coverage (Laurentine and Bramstedt, 2010).

FISCAL SCARCITY AND RESOURCE ALLOCATION

During the 1980s, technologic advances in medicine combined with the rapid rise in health care costs led to the belief that medical care rationing was upon us. The ethical issues raised by organ transplantation have thereby become generalized to all medical care. However, great differences separate the case of organ transplants from that of medical care as a whole.

1. Medical care in general is not a scarce resource; in many geographic areas, facilities and personnel are overabundant.

2. Whereas a nationwide structure is in place to decide who will receive a transplant, no such structure exists for medical care as a whole.

Dr. Ernest, who works in a for-profit HMO, wants to do her part to keep medical costs down. She prescribes low-cost amoxicillin at 20 cents per capsule rather than ciprofloxacin, which is priced at $1.50 for each dose. She teaches back pain patients home exercises at no cost rather than sending them to physical therapy visits at $75 per session. At the end of each year, she enjoys calculating how many thousands of dollars she has saved compared with one of her colleagues, who ignores costs in making medical decisions. Because of her efforts and those of other cost-conscious physicians, the HMO's pharmacy bill goes down, and HMO management is able to lay off one physical therapist, thereby raising its profit margin.

While Dr. Ernest can be praised for attempting to reduce costs without sacrificing quality, her cost savings had no impact on overall national health care expenditures. Nor were the savings used to provide more childhood immunizations or to hire a physician assistant for a nearby rural community without any health care provider. In the United States, there is no structure within which to effect a trade-off between savings in one area and benefits in another. According to analyst Joshua Wiener. (1992)

In countries that have a socially determined health budget, cuts in one area can be justified on the grounds that the money will be spent on other, higher-priority services. This closed system of funding provides a moral underpinning for resource allocation across a range of potentially unlimited demands. In the United States, it is difficult to refuse additional resources for patients, because there is no certainty that the funds will be put to better use elsewhere (Wiener, 1992).

In the United States, persuading physicians to save money on one patient in order to improve services for someone else is as illogical as telling a child to eat all the food on the plate because children in Africa are starving (Cassel, 1985).

In order for health care providers like Dr. Ernest to make their cost savings socially useful, two things are needed: a closed system of health care funding, whether governmental through a global budget or private through a network of HMOs; and a decision-making structure controlling such funding that has the responsibility to allocate budgets to health care interventions in a fair manner.

For the purposes of the following discussion, let us assume that the United States is in a position of fiscal scarcity and that a mechanism exists to fairly allocate medical care resources from one individual or population group to another. Which ethical conflicts arise between beneficence, nonmaleficence, and autonomy on the one hand and justice (equitable distribution of resources) on the other?

THE RELATIONSHIP OF RATIONING TO COST CONTROL

Assume that Limittown, USA, has a fixed budget of $250 million for medical care in 2011. Limittown has three imaging centers, each with an MRI scanner that is used only 4 hours each weekday. None of the medical facilities perform bone marrow transplantation, a procedure that can markedly prolong the lives of some leukemia patients. In 2010, Limittown spent $5 million to pay for bone marrow transplants at a university hospital 50 miles away.

Limittown's health commissioner projects that 2011 medical care expenditures will be $5 million over budget; she must implement cost savings. She considers two choices: (1) Two of the three MRI scanners could be closed, allowing the remaining scanner's cost per procedure to be drastically reduced or (2) Limittown could stop paying for bone marrow transplantation for leukemia patients.

Is rationing the same as cost containment? We have defined rationing in medical care as the limitation of resources, including money, going to medical care such that not all care expected to be beneficial is provided to all patients, and the fair distribution of these limited resources. While the limitation of money going to medical care is cost containment, not all cost containment reduces beneficial care to patients. In the case of Limittown, both options for saving $5 million can be considered cost containment, but only denial of coverage for bone marrow transplants requires rationing. Consolidating MRI scanning at a single facility would allow the same number of scans to be per-

Table 13–3. Rationing and cost control

Not all cost control is rationing.
Painless cost control is not rationing, because no limitation is placed on medical care expected to be beneficial.
Painful cost control may require rationing because limits are placed on medical care expected to be beneficial.

formed but at a substantially lower cost. Rationing is associated with painful cost control (reducing effective medical care), but cost containment (see Chapter 8) can be either painful or painless (not reducing effective medical care) (Table 13–3). The extent of unnecessary care and administrative waste has led many health experts over the past three decades to conclude that the United States may not need to ration effective medical services (Brook and Lohr, 1986; Relman, 1990). Other health policy experts feel that rationing is likely to take place, and the issue is whether rationing is rational, based on the most effective medical interventions, or irrational, based on income or health insurance (Dranove, 2003). Whether or not rationing is needed today, advances in medical technology guarantee that rationing of medically efficacious services will be necessary in the future. But to maximize beneficence and autonomy without violating distributive justice, no rationing of beneficial services should take place until all wasteful practices are curtailed; painless cost control should precede painful cost control.

▶ Care Provided to Profoundly Ill People

Lula Rogers is an 84-year-old diabetic woman with amputations of both legs; multiple strokes have rendered her unable to move, swallow, understand, or speak. She has been in a nursing home for three years during which time her medical condition has slowly deteriorated. Ms. Rogers' son wishes to remove her feeding tube, but her physician and the nursing staff feel it is cruel to cause her death by malnutrition and dehydration. Ms. Rogers continues to live for 3 more years, costing $300,000.

A hotly debated issue is the amount of health care that should be provided to the profoundly and incurably ill. Were Lula Rogers' caregivers right to prolong a life that had value to her? Or were they prolonging

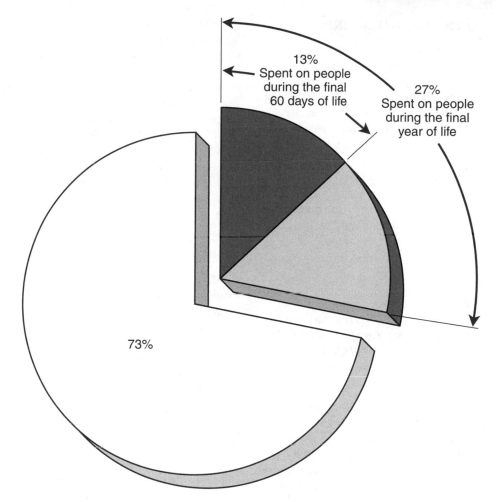

13%
Spent on people
during the final
60 days of life

27%
Spent on people
during the final
year of life

73%

▲ **Figure 13–1.** Medicare funds spent at the end of life.

Ms. Rogers' suffering and denying her a peaceful death? Should cost be a factor in such decisions, or should such matters of life and death be governed by autonomy, beneficence, and nonmaleficence alone (Luce, 1990)?

Twenty-seven percent of Medicare's budget is spent on people in their last year of life, with almost half of those funds ($68 billion in 2009) spent in the final 60 days (Lubitz and Riley, 1993; Hogan et al, 2001) (Figure 13–1). In 2000, an estimated 67% of people who died had their last place of care in the hospital or nursing home; 33% died at home, with half of patients dying at home cared for by hospice programs (Teno et al, 2004). Patients in hospice programs have lower end-of-life costs than those not in hospice programs (Emanuel et al, 2002), and family members of patients receiving hospice care at home are more satisfied with the care than families of patients dying in hospitals or nursing homes (Teno et al, 2004). Thus, a strong possibility exists that reduced expenditures can go hand in hand with better care. If these savings could be transferred to more efficacious therapies for other people, then improving the care of the incurably ill could promote all four of the ethical principles—beneficence, nonmaleficence, autonomy, and distributive justice.

RATIONING BY MEDICAL EFFECTIVENESS

We have seen that cost containment does not necessarily equal rationing and that eliminating administrative waste, medical waste, and unwanted interventions for the profoundly and incurably ill before rationing needed services best realizes the principles of beneficence and justice. However, if rationing of truly beneficial services is needed, the issues become even more difficult. If a health care system or program must compromise beneficence because of true fiscal scarcity, how can this compromise be made in a manner that yields the least harm and allocates the harm in the fairest possible way? In 2009 and 2010, federal legislation created a new structure for performing research on the comparative effectiveness of medical interventions (Benner et al, 2010)

> *Joy Fortune develops Hodgkin's disease, or cancer of the lymphatic system; she receives radiation therapy and is cured. Jessica Turner is moribund from advanced metastatic cancer of the pancreas. She undergoes chemotherapy and dies within 3 days.*

In the event of rationing, science is the best guide: The providing or withholding of care is ideally determined by the probability that the treatment will maximize benefits and minimize harm, that is by the criterion of medical effectiveness. Radiation therapy can often cure Hodgkin's disease, but chemotherapy is unlikely to provide much benefit to people with very advanced pancreatic cancer. If rationing is needed and only one of these therapies can be offered, a decision based on the criterion of medical effectiveness would allow for the treatment of Hodgkin's disease but not of terminal pancreatic cancer.

If intervention A increases person-years of reasonable-quality life more than intervention B, intervention A is more medically effective. The cost of the two interventions is not considered. Cost-effectiveness adds dollars to the equation: If intervention A increases person-years of reasonable-quality life per dollar spent more than intervention B, it is more cost-effective. Which is a better standard for rationing medical care: medical effectiveness or cost-effectiveness?

If money were not scarce, medical effectiveness (maximizing benefit and minimizing harm) would be the ideal standard upon which to ration care (ie, the less effective the therapy, the lower its priority on the list of treatments to be offered). But if money were not scarce, we would not need to ration. It is unrealistic to pretend that costs can be ignored (Garber and Sox, 2010). Suppose that bone marrow transplantation saves as many person-years of life by treating advanced cancers as does doxycycline by curing pneumonia. The former costs $150,000, while the latter can be obtained for $10. There is no reason to ration doxycycline, as its cost is negligible, whereas to make bone marrow transplantation similarly accessible is costly. Thus consideration of costs is essential as a means of deciding which services to ration.

▶ Rationing for Society as a Whole

> *Mrs. Smith's breast cancer has spread to her liver and bone. She has been told that her only slim hope lies in high-dose chemotherapy with autologous bone marrow transplantation (HDC-ABMT), costing $250,000. Even with the optimistic assumption that HDC-ABMT has a 5% cure rate, screening mammography is eight times as cost-effective as HDC-ABMT in person-years of life saved.*

In 1991, Dr. David Eddy (1991a) published a compelling article entitled "The individual vs society: Is there a conflict?" Dr. Eddy poses the preceding case of Mrs. Smith. If medical care must be rationed, it seems logical to spend funds on mammography rather than HDC-ABMT because the former intervention is more cost-effective. Dr. Eddy does not confine his analysis to cost-effectiveness, however, but moves on to the ethical issues.

> *Each of us can be in two positions when we make judgments about the value of different health care activities. We are in one position when we are healthy, contemplating diseases we might get, and writing out checks for taxes and insurance premiums. Call this the "first position." We are in a different position when we actually have a disease, are sitting in a physician's office, and have already paid our taxes and premiums (the "second position")…. Imagine that you are a 50-year-old woman employed by Mrs. Smith's corporation…. [The company] is considering two options: (1) cover screening for breast cancer…. or (2) cover HDC-ABMT…. Now imagine you are in the first*

position. . . . as long as you do not yet have the disease (the first position), option 1 will always deliver greater benefit at lower cost than option 2. . . . Now, let us switch you to the second position. Imagine that you already have breast cancer and have just been told that it has metastasized and is terminal. . . . The value to you of the screening option has plummeted because you already have breast cancer and can no longer benefit from screening. . . .

Maximizing care for individual patients attempts to maximize care for individuals when they are in the second position. Maximizing care for society expands the scope of concern to include individuals when they are in the first position. As this example illustrates, the program that delivers the most benefit for the least cost for society (option 1) is not necessarily best for the individual patient (option 2), and vice versa. But as this example also illustrates, individual patients and society are not distinct entities. Rather, they represent the different positions that each of us will be in at various times in our lives. When we serve ourselves in the second position, we can harm ourselves in the first. (Eddy, 1991a)

Physicians generally care for patients in Dr. Eddy's second position—when they are sick. But if the cost of treating those in the second position reduces resources available to prevent illness for the far larger number of people in the first position (who may not be seeing physicians because they feel fine), the individual principles of beneficence and autonomy are superseding the societal principle of justice. One could even say that choosing for individuals in the second position violates beneficence for those in the first position. On the other hand, if all resources go to those in the first position (eg, to cost-effective screening rather than highly technical treatment for those with life-threatening disease), injustice is committed in the other direction by ignoring the costly needs of the very ill.

Clearly, no ideal method of rationing medical care exists. The use of cost-effectiveness as a measuring stick raises ethical problems, and because of the difficulty in determining the cost-effectiveness of different interventions, has scientific limitations. All efforts should be made to control costs painlessly before resorting to the painful limitation of effective medical care. But if rationing is inevitable, a balance must be struck among many legitimate needs: The concerns of healthy people for illness prevention, the imperative for acutely sick people to obtain diagnosis and treatment, and the obligation to provide care and comfort to those with untreatable chronic illness.

▶ Rationing within One Health Program: The Oregon Health Plan

The previous discussion of rationing medical care nationwide presumes a mechanism that redirects savings from interventions not performed toward more cost-effective services. In fact, such a mechanism does not exist nationwide. Only in specific medical care programs do we find a decision-making apparatus for allocating expenditures. One example is the Oregon Health Plan (Bodenheimer, 1997).

In 1994, Oregon added 100,000 poor uninsured Oregonians to its Medicaid program. To control costs, a prioritized list of services was developed, and the state legislature decided how many services would be covered. The prioritized list was based on how much improvement in quantity and quality of life the treatment was likely to produce. The final list contained 745 condition–treatment pairs, and the State of Oregon paid for items above line 574 on the list; conditions below that line were not covered (Kilborn, 1999). What are some of the Oregon Health Plan's ethical implications?

1. The plan was more than a rationing proposal; its chief feature was to extend health care coverage to 100,000 more people. That aspect of the Oregon plan promotes the principle of justice.

2. Another positive feature of the plan was its attempt to prioritize medical care services on the basis of effectiveness, which, if rationing is needed, is a reasonable method for deciding which services to eliminate.

Other features of the Oregon plan must be viewed as negatively impacting distributive justice, or equal access to care without regard for ability to pay.

1. In 1996, 12% of beneficiaries reported being denied services because they were below the line on the priority list. Of those, 78% reported that the denial had worsened their health (Mitchell and Bentley, 2000). Medical services were rationed for Oregon's poor but not for anyone else.

2. The plan targeted beneficial medical services in a state with considerable medical waste. In 1988, many areas of Oregon had average hospital occupancy rates below 50%. The closing of unneeded hospital beds could have saved $50 million per year, enough to pay for some of the treatments eliminated in the plan (Fisher et al, 1992). Oregon did not exhaust its options for painless cost control before proceeding to potentially painful rationing.

By 2004, the Oregon Health Plan had unraveled (Oberlander, 2006). The state entered a period of budgetary woes, new premiums and copays were instituted, and Oregon Health Plan enrollees responded by dropping out of the program. The rate of uninsurance climbed from 11% to 17%. But the bold experiment in rational rationing remains alive in the minds of health care policymakers.

▶ Rationing within One Institution: Intensive Care

Ms. Wilson is a 71-year-old woman with a recently diagnosed lung cancer. Obstructing a bronchus, the tumor causes pneumonia, and Ms. Wilson is admitted to the hospital in her rural town. She deteriorates and becomes comatose, requiring a respirator. By the eighth hospital day, she is no better. On that day, Louis Ford, a previously healthy 27-year-old, is brought to the hospital with a crushed chest and pneumothorax suffered in an automobile accident. Mr. Ford is in immediate need of a respirator. None of the six patients in the intensive care unit can be removed from respirators without dying; of the six, Ms. Wilson has the poorest prognosis. She has no family. No other respirators exist within a 50-mile radius (Jonsen et al, 2010). Should Ms. Wilson be removed from the respirator in favor of Mr. Ford?

Resources may be scarce throughout an entire nation or within a small hospital. *Macroallocation* refers to the amount and distribution of resources within a society, whereas *microallocation* refers to resource constraints at the level of an individual physician or institution. Macroallocation decisions may be more significant, affecting thousands or millions of people. Microallocation choices can be more acute, bringing ethical dilemmas into stark, uncompromising focus and placing issues of resource allocation squarely in the lap of the practicing physician. The microallocation choice involving Ms. Wilson incorporates all four ethical principles, which must be weighed and acted on within minutes: (1) Beneficence: For whom? This ideal cannot be realized for both patients. (2) Nonmaleficence: If Ms. Wilson is removed from the respirator, harm is done to her, but the price of not harming her is great for Mr. Ford. (3) Autonomy: Withdrawal of therapy requires the consent of the patient or family, which is impossible in Ms. Wilson's case. (4) Justice: Should resources be distributed on a first-come first-served basis or according to need?

These are tragic decisions. Many physicians would remove Ms. Wilson from the respirator and make all efforts to save Mr. Ford. The main consideration would be medical effectiveness: Ms. Wilson's chance of living more than a few months is slim, while Mr. Ford could be cured and live for many decades.

Less stark but similar decisions face physicians on a daily basis. On a busy day, which patients get more of the physician's time? In a public hospital with an MRI waiting list, when should a physician call the radiologist and argue for an urgent scan, thereby pushing other people down on the waiting list? Situations involving microallocation demonstrate why, in real life, health care professionals are forced to balance the interests of one patient against those of another and the interests of individuals against the imperatives of society.

A BASIC LEVEL OF GUARANTEED MEDICAL BENEFITS

Don Rich is a bank executive who receives his care through a New York City HMO. He develops angina pectoris, which remains stable for over a year. An exercise treadmill test suggests mild coronary artery disease. Although this evaluation indicates that Mr. Rich's condition can be safely managed with medications, he asks his cardiologist to arrange a coronary angiogram with an angioplasty or coronary bypass if indicated. He is told that the HMO has finite resources for such procedures and limits their use to patients with unstable angina or highly abnormal treadmill tests, for whom the procedures are more efficacious. Mr. Rich flies to Texas, consults with a private cardiac surgeon, and receives a coronary angiogram at his own expense.

Most people in the United States believe that health care should be a right. But how much health care? If every person has a right to all beneficial health care, the nation may be unable to pay the bill or may be forced to limit other rights such as education or fire and police protection. One approach to this problem is to limit the health care right to a basic package of services. (In the case of Don Rich's HMO, angiography for stable angina pectoris is not within the basic package.) Any services beyond the basics can be purchased by individuals who choose to spend their own money. This solution creates an ethical problem. If a service that does produce medical benefit is not included in the basic package or is denied by an insurance company medical director, that service becomes available only to those who can afford it. Where should society draw the line between a basic level of care that should be equally available to all, and "more than basic" services that may be purchased according to individual ability and willingness to pay (Eddy, 1991b)? Unless the basic package covers all beneficial health services, the principle of distributive justice, that all people equally receive a reasonable level of medical services without regard to ability to pay, will be compromised.

THE ETHICS OF HEALTH CARE FINANCING

Yoshiko Takahashi's first heart attack came at age 59. It was minor, and she felt well the next day. Then came the real shock: because of her high blood pressure, her private insurance policy considers disease of the cardiovascular system a preexisting condition and will not cover costs for complications of hypertension. She demands to go home to limit her hospital bill. Twelve hours later comes the second heart attack, which is severe. She is readmitted to intensive care and remains in the hospital for 8 more days. Because of persistent pain, she is a candidate for coronary angiography, which she refuses on account of the cost. When she purchased the insurance, Ms. Takahashi had not understood its terms because her English skills were poor.

Decisions by physicians encompass only one aspect of resource allocation; the payers of health care have great power in the distribution of medical care. The policies of the private insurance industry, which covers the largest number of people in the United States, raise important ethical issues. In the case of Yoshiko Takahashi, the insurance company, rather than her physicians, largely determined what kind of medical care she received.

Private insurance may be experience rated (see Chapter 2), with premiums costing more for people or groups with a higher risk of illness. Under the practice of experience rating, people who need health care the most (because they have a chronic illness) are less likely to be able to purchase affordable health insurance. Many people feel that private insurers violate the justice principle because those most in need of services have the least chance of gaining coverage for those services.

Health insurance executives, however, have a different view, believing that private health insurance is fair. An advertisement sponsored by the insurance industry argued,

> *If insurance companies didn't put people into risk groups [experience rating], it would mean that low-risk people would be arbitrarily mixed in with high-risk people. . . . and [low-risk people] would have to pay higher rates. That would be unfair to everyone. (Light, 1992)*

According to this notion, it is unfair to force one person or group to pay for the needs or burdens of another. An alternative view, citing the principle of distributive justice, holds that young and healthy people should pay more in health costs than they use in health services so that older and less healthy people can receive health services at a reasonable cost. Even from the perspective of one's own long-term self-interest, it makes sense to pay more for health care while young and healthy, and to pay less when advanced age creates a greater risk of becoming sick.

A much-discussed issue involves individuals whose behavior, particularly smoking, eating unhealthy diets, and drinking alcohol in excess, is seen as contributing to their ill health.

> *Jim Butts, a heavy smoker, develops emphysema and has multiple hospitalizations for respiratory failure, including many days on the respirator. Randy Schipp, a former shipyard worker, develops work-related asbestosis and has multiple hospitalizations for respiratory failure, including many days on the respirator. Should Jim pay more for health insurance than Randy?*

Gene eats a low-fat diet, exercises regularly, but has a strong family history of heart disease; he suffers a heart attack at age 44. Mac eats fast food, does not exercise, and has a heart attack at age 44. Should Mac pay more for health care coverage than Gene?

One view holds that individuals who fall sick as a result of high-risk behavior such as smoking, substance abuse including use of alcohol, and consumption of high-fat foods are entirely responsible for their behavior and should pay higher health insurance premiums. Opponents of this idea see it as "blaming the victim" and argue that high-risk behaviors have a complex causation that may involve genetic and environmental factors including uncontrollable addiction. They cite a number of facts to support their position. The food industry spends billions of dollars each year on television advertising; the average child sees thousands of food commercials each year, most of them for products with poor nutritional value. The tobacco industry heavily advertises to teenagers. Illegal drug use is associated with poverty, hopelessness, and easy availability of drugs. Some evidence finds a genetic predisposition to alcoholism. To the extent that individuals are not entirely at fault for their high-risk behavior, it would be unfair to charge them more for health insurance. On the other hand, it seems sensible that users of tobacco and alcohol pay through taxes on those products.

WHO ALLOCATES HEALTH CARE RESOURCES?

The predicament of limited resources has been likened to a herd of cattle grazing on a common pasture. The total grazing area may be regarded as the entirety of economic resources in the United States. A smaller pasture, the *medical commons*, comprises that portion of the grazing area dedicated to health care. The herd represents the nation's physicians, using the resources of the commons in the process of providing care to patients. Physicians, guided by medicine's moral imperative to "do everything possible for the patient," continually attempt to extend the borders of the medical commons. But communities outside the medical commons have legitimate claims to societal resources and view the herd as encroaching on resources needed for other pursuits (Grumbach and Bodenheimer, 1990).

Who decides the magnitude of the medical commons, that is, the resources devoted to health care?

Physicians and other health care providers, whose interventions on behalf of their patients add up to the totality of medical resources used? The sum of individual consumer choices operating through a free market? Health insurance plans, watching over their particular piece of the commons? Or government, using the political process to set budgetary limits on the entire health care system?

Traditionally, physicians and patients have had a great deal to say about the size of the medical commons. In the United States, the medical commons traditionally has been an open range. The quantity and price of medical visits, hospital days, surgeries, diagnostic studies, pharmaceuticals, and other such interventions determine the total costs of medical care. This is not the case in other nations, where government health care budgets constitute a "fence" around the medical commons, setting a clear limit on the quantity of resources available. Some advocates of fence-building in the United States have considered parceling the medical commons into numerous subpastures, each representing an HMO or Accountable Care Organization (see Chapter 6) working within the constraints of fixed, prepaid budgets. Not all pastures would be equal in size, and the fences would have holes that allow patients to purchase additional services outside of the organized systems of care.

Ethical considerations play a role in both open and closed medical care systems. In the US open range, the principles of beneficence and autonomy have the upper hand, tending toward an expanding, though not equitable, system. Fenced-in systems, in contrast, balance the more expansive principles of beneficence and autonomy with the demands of distributive justice in order to allocate resources within the medical commons.

If the United States moves toward a more fenced-in medical commons, decisions will be needed about who gets what. Do all 90-year-old people with multiple organ failure receive kidney dialysis that may extend their lives only a few months? Are very low-birth-weight infants afforded neonatal intensive care even with a small chance of leading a normal life? Do individual physicians, interacting with their patients, have the final say in making these decisions? Should societal bodies such as government, commissions of interested parties, or professional associations set the rules?

Microallocation issues come down to daily clinical decisions about which individual patients will receive what types of care (Lo, 2009). Physicians and other caregivers may well recoil from the prospect of "bedside rationing," believing that allocative decision making unduly compromises their commitment to the principles of beneficence and autonomy. Levinsky (1984) has argued that physicians must maintain their single-mindedness in maximizing care for each patient:

There is increasing pressure on doctors to serve two masters. Physicians in practice are being enjoined to consider society's needs as well as each patient's needs in deciding what type and amount of medical care to deliver . . . . When practicing medicine, doctors cannot serve two masters. It is to the advantage both of our society and of the individuals it comprises that physicians retain their historic single-mindedness. The doctor's master must be the patient. (Levinsky, 1984)

Yet if physicians abstain from the arena of macroallocation decision making, who is to decide? Currently, these decisions are often made by medical directors of private insurance companies and the leaders of the Medicare and Medicaid programs. Studies have documented that such decisions vary from plan to plan, and even within a single insurance plan, a medical director may make different decisions on different days for similar patients (Light, 1994). If physicians refuse to accept two masters, then medicine will be granting allocation decisions to insurance company and governmental officials. The physician of the twenty-first century will continue to face individual patient responsibilities but will find it difficult to escape the obligation to balance the wishes of individual patients against the larger needs of society (Cassel, 1985; Morreim, 1989).

If physicians are to serve two masters (ie, to maintain their dedication to individual patients while at the same time responsibly managing resources), they need rules to assist them. These rules should operate at both a population and an individual level. At the population level, society should ideally decide which general treatments are to be collectively paid for through the process of universal health insurance. At the individual level, rules are needed to guide decisions about the prioritization of resources for specific patients. The workings of organ transplantation provide a model of how physicians can serve two masters: They do everything possible to procure organs for their transplant patients, but also accept the rules of the system that attempt to allocate organs in a fair manner (Benjamin et al, 1994). The modern health care professional is caught in a global ethical dilemma. On the one hand, patients and their families expect the best that modern technology can offer, paid for through private or public insurance. The imperatives of beneficence, nonmaleficence, and autonomy rule the bedside. On the other hand, grave injustices take place on a daily basis: An uninsured young person with a curable illness is unable to pay for care, while an insured, bedridden individual who had a stroke incurs vast medical bills during the last weeks of her ebbing life. Should not the physician at the stroke patient's bedside be concerned about both patients? However this dilemma is resolved, the principle of justice will relentlessly peek at the physician from under the bed.

REFERENCES

Aaron HJ, Schwartz WB. *The Painful Prescription.* Washington, DC: The Brookings Institution; 1984.

Annas GJ. "Culture of life" politics at the bedside—the case of Terri Schiavo. *N Engl J Med.* 2005;352:1710.

Beauchamp TL, Childress JF. *Principles of Biomedical Ethics.* 6th ed. New York: Oxford University Press; 2008.

Benjamin M et al. What transplantation can teach us about health care reform. *N Engl J Med.* 1994;330:858.

Benner JS et al. An evaluation of recent federal spending on comparative effectiveness research. *Health Affairs.* 2010;29:1768.

Bodenheimer T. The Oregon Health Plan: Lessons for the nation. *N Engl J Med.* 1997;337:651, 720.

Brook RH, Lohr KN. Will we need to ration effective health care? *Issues Sci Technol.* 1986;3:68.

Cassel CK. Doctors and allocation decisions: A new role in the new Medicare. *J Health Polit Policy Law.* 1985;10:549.

Dranove D. *What's Your Life Worth? Health Care Rationing... Who Lives? Who Dies? And Who Decides?* Upper Saddle River, NJ: Prentice Hall; 2003.

Eddy DM. Comparing benefits and harms: The balance sheet. *JAMA.* 1990;263:2493.

Eddy DM. The individual vs society: Is there a conflict? *JAMA.* 1991a;265:1446.

Eddy DM. What care is "essential?" What services are "basic?" *JAMA.* 1991b;265:782.

Emanuel EJ et al. Managed care, hospice use, site of death, and medical expenditures in the last year of life. *Arch Intern Med.* 2002;162:1722.

Fisher ES, Welch HG, Wennberg JE. Prioritizing Oregon's hospital resources. *JAMA*. 1992;267:1925.

Garber AM, Sox HC. The role of costs in comparative effectiveness research. *Health Aff*. 2010;29:1805.

Grumbach K, Bodenheimer T. Reins or fences: A physician's view of cost containment. *Health Aff*. 1990;9:120.

Hogan C et al. Medicare beneficiaries' costs of care in the last year of life. *Health Aff*. 2001;20:188.

Jonsen AR et al. *Clinical Ethics: A Practical Guide to Ethical Decisions in Clinical Medicine*. 7th ed. New York, NY: McGraw-Hill; 2010.

Kilborn PT. Oregon falters on a new path to health care. *New York Times*. January 3, 1999.

Laurentine KA, Bramstedt KA. Too poor for transplant: Finance and insurance issues in transplant ethics. *Prog Transplant*. 2010;20:178.

Levinsky NG. The doctor's master. *N Engl J Med*. 1984;311:1573.

Light DW. The practice and ethics of risk-rated health insurance. *JAMA*. 1992;267:2503.

Light DW. Life, death, and the insurance companies. *N Engl J Med*. 1994;330:498.

Lo B. *Resolving Ethical Dilemmas. A Guide for Clinicians*. 4th ed. Baltimore, MD: Lippincott Williams & Wilkins; 2009.

Lubitz JD, Riley GF. Trends in Medicare payments in the last year of life. *N Engl J Med*. 1993;328:1092.

Luce JM. Ethical principles in critical care. *JAMA*. 1990;263:696.

Mitchell JB, Bentley F. Impact of Oregon's priority list on Medicaid beneficiaries. *Med Care Res Rev*. 2000;57:216.

Morreim EH. Fiscal scarcity and the inevitability of bedside budget balancing. *Arch Intern Med*. 1989;149:1012.

Oberlander J. Health reform interrupted: The unraveling of the Oregon Health Plan. *Health Affairs*. 2006:w96–w105.

Reagan MD. Health care rationing: What does it mean? *N Engl J Med*. 1988;319:1149.

Relman AS. Is rationing inevitable? *N Engl J Med*. 1990;322:1809.

Task Force on Organ Transplantation. *Issues and Recommendations*. Washington, DC: US Department of Health and Human Services; 1986.

Teno JM et al. Family perspectives on end-of-life care at the last place of care. *JAMA*. 2004;291:88.

Wiener JM. Rationing in America: overt and covert. In: Strosberg MA et al, eds. *Rationing America's Medical Care: The Oregon Plan and Beyond*. Washington, DC: The Brookings Institution; 1992.

Health Care in Four Nations

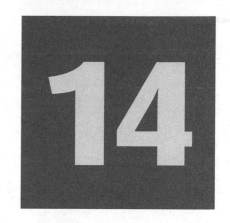

14

The financing and organization of medical care throughout the developed world spans a broad spectrum. In most countries, the preponderance of medical care is financed or delivered (or both) in the public sector; in others, like the United States, most people both pay for and receive their care through private institutions.

In this chapter, we describe the health care systems of four nations: Germany, Canada, the United Kingdom, and Japan. Each of these nations resides at a different point on the international health care continuum. Examining their diverse systems may aid us in our search for a suitable health care system for the United States.

Recall from Chapter 2 the four varieties of health care financing: out-of-pocket payments, individual private insurance, employment-based private insurance, and government financing. Germany, Canada, the United Kingdom, and Japan emphasize the last two modes of payment. Germany finances medical care through government-mandated, employment-based private insurance, though German private insurance is a world apart from that found in the United States. Canada and the United Kingdom feature government-financed systems. Japan's financing falls between the German method of financing and the government model of Canada and the United Kingdom. Regarding the delivery of medical care, the German, Japanese, and Canadian systems are predominantly private, while the United Kingdom's is largely public.

Although these four nations demonstrate great differences in their manner of financing and organizing medical care, in one respect they are identical: They all provide universal health care coverage, thereby guaranteeing to their populations financial access to medical services.

GERMANY

► Health Insurance

Hans Deutsch is a bank teller living in Germany. He and his family receive health insurance through a sickness fund that insures other employees and their families at his bank and at other workplaces in his city. When Hans went to work at the bank, he was required by law to join the sickness fund selected by his employer. The bank contributes 7.3% of Hans's salary to the sickness fund, and 8.2% is withheld from Hans's paycheck and sent to the fund. Hans's sickness fund collects the same 15.5% employer-employee contribution for all its members.

Germany was the first nation to enact compulsory health insurance legislation. Its pioneering law of 1883 required certain employers and employees to make payments to existing voluntary sickness funds, which would pay for the covered employees' medical care. Initially, only industrial wage earners with incomes less than $500 per year were included; the eligible population was extended in later years.

Almost 90% of Germans now receive their health insurance through the mandatory sickness funds, with 10% covered by voluntary insurance plans (Figure 14–1). Several categories of sickness funds exist. Thirty-seven percent of people (mostly blue-collar workers and their families) belong to funds organized by

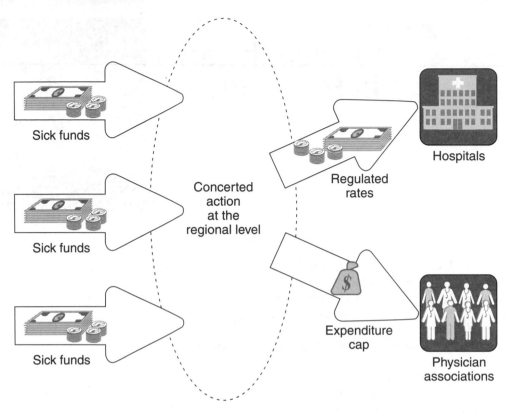

▲ **Figure 14–1.** The German national health insurance system.

geographic area; 33% (for the most part the families of white-collar workers) are in nationally based "substitute" funds; 21% are employees or dependents of employees who work in 700 companies that have their own sickness funds; and 6% are in funds covering all workers in a particular craft (Busse and Riesberg, 2004; Busse, 2008).

In 2010, the proportion of earnings going to a sickness fund was set at 15.5%, with employers paying 47% and employees 53% of that amount. These contributions formerly went directly to the sickness funds, which are nonprofit, closely regulated entities that lie somewhere between the private and public sectors. Since 2009, employee and employer contributions are collected by a government-run health fund, which then distributes the money to health funds based on a risk-adjusted (more for older and sicker people) amount per insured person (Ornyanova and Busse, 2009). The number of sickness funds is shrinking, down from 1000 to

less than 200 in 2011. The funds are not allowed to exclude people because of illness, or to raise contribution rates according to age or medical condition; that is, they may not use experience rating. The funds are required to cover a broad range of benefits, including hospital and physician services, prescription drugs, and dental, preventive, and maternity care. Because wages supporting health care financing are declining relative to health care costs, employers are proposing that their contribution be capped at 7% of earnings so that further increases are borne by employees (Zander et al, 2009).

Hans's father, Peter Deutsch, is retired from his job as a machinist in a steel plant. When he worked, his family received health insurance through a sickness fund set up for employees of the steel company. The fund was run by a board, half of whose members represented employees and the other half the employer. On retirement, Peter's family continued its coverage through the same sickness fund with no change in benefits. The sickness fund continues to pay approximately 60% of his family's health care costs (subsidized by the contributions of active workers and the employer), with 40% paid from Peter's retirement pension fund.

Hans has a cousin, Georg, who formerly worked for a gas station in Hans's city, but is now unemployed. Georg remained in his sickness fund after losing his job. His contribution to the fund is paid by the government. Hans's best friend at the bank was diagnosed with lymphoma and became permanently disabled and unable to work. He remained in the sickness fund, with his contribution paid by the government.

Upon retiring from or losing a job, people and their families retain membership in their sickness funds. Health insurance in Germany, as in the United States, is employment based, but German health insurance, unlike in the United States, must continue to cover its members whether or not they change jobs or stop working for any reason.

Hans's Uncle Karl is an assistant vice-president at the bank. Because he earns more than 49,500 Euros per year, he is not required to join a sickness fund, but can opt to purchase private health insurance. Many higher-paid employees choose a sickness fund; they are not required to join the fund selected by the employer for lower-paid workers but can join one of 15 national "substitute" funds.

Ten percent of Germans, with incomes more than 49,500 Euros per year (2011), choose voluntary private insurance. Private insurers pay higher fees to physicians than do sickness funds, often allowing their policyholders to receive preferential treatment. In summary, in Germany 88% of the populace belong to the mandatory sickness fund system, 10% opt for private insurance, 2% receive medical services as members of the armed forces or police, and less than 0.2% (all of whom are wealthy) have no coverage.

Germany finances health care through a merged social insurance and public assistance structure (see Chapters 2, 12, and 15 for discussion of these concepts), such that no distinctions are made between employed people who contribute to their health insurance, and unemployed people, whose contribution is made by the government.

▶ Medical Care

Hans Deutsch develops chest pain while walking, and it worries him. He does not have a physician, and a friend recommends a general practitioner (GP), Dr. Helmut Arzt. Because Hans is free to see any ambulatory care physician he chooses, he indeed visits Dr. Arzt, who diagnoses angina pectoris—coronary artery disease. Dr. Arzt prescribes some medications and a low-fat diet, but the pain persists. One morning, Hans awakens with severe, suffocating chest pain. He calls Dr. Arzt, who orders an ambulance to take Hans to a nearby hospital. Hans is admitted for a heart attack and is cared for by Dr. Edgar Hertz, a cardiologist. Dr. Arzt does not visit Hans in the hospital. Upon discharge, Dr. Hertz sends a report to Dr. Arzt, who then resumes Hans's medical care. Hans never receives a bill.

German medicine maintains a strict separation of ambulatory care physicians and hospital-based physicians. Most ambulatory care physicians are prohibited from treating patients in hospitals, and most hospital-based physicians do not have private offices for treating outpatients. People often have their own primary care physician (PCP) but are allowed to make appointments to see ambulatory care specialists without referral from the primary care physician. Fifty-one percent of Germany's physicians are generalists, compared with only 35% in the United States. The German system tends to use a dispersed model of medical care organization (see Chapter 5), with little coordination between ambulatory care physicians and hospitals (Busse and Riesberg, 2004).

▶ Paying Physicians and Hospitals

Dr. Arzt was used to billing his regional association of physicians and receiving a fee for each patient visit and for each procedure done during the visit. In 1986, he was shocked to find that spending caps had been placed on the total ambulatory physician budget. If in the first quarter of the year, the physicians in his regional association billed for more patient services than expected, each fee would be proportionally reduced during the next quarter. If the volume of services continued to increase, fees would drop again in the third and fourth quarters of the year. Dr. Arzt discussed the situation with his friend Dr. Hertz, but Dr. Hertz, as a hospital physician, received a salary and was not affected by the spending cap.

Ambulatory care physicians are required to join their regional physicians' association. Rather than paying physicians directly, sickness funds pay a global sum each year to the physicians' association in their region, which in turn pays physicians on the basis of a detailed fee schedule. These sums have been based on the number of patients cared for by the physicians in each regional association, but in 2007, a risk-adjustment factor is being introduced that increases payments for populations with greater health problems. Since 1986, physicians' associations, in an attempt to stay within their global budgets, have reduced fees on a quarterly basis if the volume of services delivered by their physicians was too high. Sickness funds pay hospitals on a basis similar to the diagnosis-related groups used in the US Medicare program. Included within this payment is the salary of hospital-based physicians (Busse and Riesberg, 2004).

▶ Cost Control

The 1977 German Cost Containment Act created a body called Concerted Action, made up of representatives of the nation's health providers, sickness funds, employers, unions, and different levels of government. Concerted Action is convened twice each year, and every spring, it sets guidelines for physician fees, hospital rates, and the prices of pharmaceuticals and other supplies. Based on these guidelines, negotiations are conducted at state, regional, and local levels between the sickness funds in a region, the regional physicians' association, and the hospitals to set physician fees and hospital rates that reflect Concerted Action guidelines. Since 1986, not only have physician fees been controlled, but as described in the above vignette about Dr. Arzt, the total amount of money flowing to physicians has been capped. As a result of these efforts, Germany's health expenditures as a percentage of the gross domestic product actually fell between 1985 and 1991 from 8.7% to 8.5%.

In 1991, however, German health care costs resumed an upward surge, paving the way for a 1993 cost control law restricting the growth of sickness fund budgets. In 2004, Germany raised copayments, ceased coverage of over-the-counter drugs, and enacted new controls on

pharmaceutical prices (Stock et al, 2006). While Germany's 2008 health care expenditures as a percent of GDP was the fifth highest among developed nations, this figure has remained stable since 2000, indicating that cost control measures limiting the size of sickness fund budgets are having success.

CANADA

▶ Health Insurance

The Maple family owns a small grocery store in Outer Snowshoe, a tiny Canadian town. Grandfather Maple has a heart condition for which he sees Dr. Rebecca North, his family physician, regularly. The rest of the family is healthy and goes to Dr. North for minor problems and preventive care, including children's immunizations. Neither as employers nor as health consumers do the Maples worry about health insurance. They receive a plastic card from their provincial government and show the card when they visit Dr. North.

The Maples do worry about taxes. The federal personal income tax, the goods and services tax, and the various provincial taxes take almost 40% of the family's income. But the Maples would never let anyone take away their health insurance system.

In 1947, the province of Saskatchewan initiated the first publicly financed universal hospital insurance program in North America. Other provinces followed suit, and in 1957, the Canadian government passed the Hospital Insurance Act, which was fully implemented by 1961. Hospital, but not physician, services were covered. In 1963, Saskatchewan again took the lead and enacted a medical insurance plan for physician services. The Canadian federal government passed universal medical insurance in 1966; the program was fully operational by 1971 (Taylor, 1990).

Canada has a tax-financed, public, single-payer health care system. In each Canadian province, the single payer is the provincial government (Figure 14–2). During the 1970s, federal taxes financed 50% of health services, but the federal share declined to 22% by 1996, generating acrimony between the federal and provincial governments. In response to this political debate, the federal contributions began to increase in 2001. Currently, the federal government funds approximately one-third of provincial health expenditures (Canadian

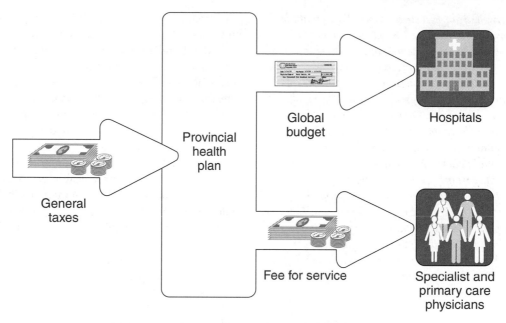

▲ **Figure 14–2.** The Canadian national health insurance system.

Institute for Health Information, 2010). Provincial taxes vary in type from province to province and include income taxes, payroll taxes, and sales taxes. Some provinces, for example British Columbia and Alberta, charge a compulsory health care premium—essentially an earmarked tax—to finance a portion of their health budgets.

Unlike Germany, Canada has severed the link between employment and health insurance. Wealthy or poor, employed or jobless, retired or younger than 18, every Canadian receives the same health insurance, financed in the same way. No Canadian would even imagine that leaving, changing, retiring from, or losing a job has anything to do with health insurance. In Canada, no distinction is made between the two public financing mechanisms of social insurance (in which only those who contribute receive benefits) and public assistance (in which people receive benefits based on need rather than on having contributed). Everyone contributes through the tax structure and everyone receives benefits.

The benefits provided by Canadian provinces are broad, including hospital, physician, and ancillary services. Provincial plans also pay for outpatient drugs, although the scope of drug coverage—and also long-term care benefits—varies across provinces.

The Canadian health care system is unique in its prohibition of private health insurance for coverage of services included in the provincial health plans. Hospitals and physicians that receive payments from the provincial health plans are not allowed to bill private insurers for such services, thereby avoiding the preferential treatment of privately insured patients that occurs in many health care systems. Canadians can purchase private health insurance policies for gaps in provincial health plan coverage or for such amenities as private hospital rooms.

▶ **Medical Care**

Grandfather Maple has had intermittent sensations of palpitations in his chest for a few weeks. He calls Dr. North, who tells him to come right over. An electrocardiogram reveals rapid atrial fibrillation, an abnormal heart rhythm. Because Mr. Maple is tolerating the rapid rhythm, Dr. North starts treatment with metoprolol in the office to gradually slow his heart rate, tells him to return the next day, and writes out a referral slip to see Dr. Jonathan Hartwell, a cardiologist in a nearby small city.

Dr. Hartwell arranges a stress echocardiogram at the local hospital to evaluate Mr. Maple's arrhythmia, finds severe coronary ischemia, and explains to Mr. Maple that his coronary arteries are narrowed. He recommends a coronary angiogram and possible coronary artery bypass surgery. Because Mr. Maple's condition is not urgent, Dr. Hartwell arranges for his patient to be placed on the waiting list at the University Hospital in the provincial capital 50 miles away. One month later, Mr. Maple awakens at 2 AM in a cold sweat, gasping for breath. His daughter calls Dr. North, who urgently sends for an ambulance to transport Mr. Maple to the University Hospital. There Mr. Maple is admitted to the coronary care unit, his condition is stabilized, and he undergoes emergency coronary artery bypass surgery the next day. Ten days later, Mr. Maple returns home, complaining of pain in his incision but otherwise feeling well.

Approximately half of Canadian physicians are family physicians (contrasted with the United States, where only 35% of physicians are generalists). Canadians have free choice of physician. As a rule, Canadians see their family physician for routine medical problems and visit specialists only through referral by the family physician. Specialists are allowed to see patients without referrals, but only receive the higher specialist fee if they specify the referring primary care physician in their billing; for that reason, most specialists will not see patients without a referral. Unlike the European model of separation between ambulatory and hospital physicians, Canadian family physicians are allowed to care for their patients in hospitals. Because of the close scientific interchange between Canada and the United States, the practice of Canadian medicine is similar to that in the United States; the differences lie in the financing system and the far greater use of primary care physicians. The treatment of Mr. Maple's heart condition is not significantly different from what would occur in the United States, with the exception that high-tech procedures such as cardiac surgery and magnetic resonance imaging (MRI) scans are regionalized in a limited number of facilities and performed far less frequently than in the United States. In 2007, Canada had 6.7 MRI scanners per million inhabitants compared with 25.9 in the United States (OECD, 2010).

Canadians on average wait longer for elective operations than do insured people in the United States and also have slightly more difficulty accessing primary care physicians (Schoen et al, 2010). Over the past ten years the federal and provincial governments have implemented successful policies to reduce elective surgery delays (Ross and Detsky, 2009). The median 2005 wait time for nonemergency surgery in Canada was 4 weeks (Willcox et al, 2007). Despite queues for elective procedures, only a tiny number of Canadians cross the border to seek care in the United States (Katz et al, 2002).

Canada's universal insurance program has created a fairer system for distributing health services. Canadians are much less likely than their counterparts in the United States to report experiencing financial barriers to medical care (Schoen et al, 2010). Low-income Canadians receive almost the same amount of medical services as Canadians from higher-income groups, whereas in the United States higher-income groups receive more health services than lower-income groups (Sanmartin et al, 2006). Nonetheless, inequities in care according to socioeconomic status remain in Canada despite universal insurance coverage (Guilfoyle, 2008).

▶ Paying Physicians and Hospitals

For Dr. Rebecca North, collecting fees is a simple matter. Each week she electronically bills the provincial government, listing the patients she saw and the services she provided. Within a month, she is paid in full according to a fee schedule. Dr. North wishes the fees were higher, but loves the simplicity of the billing process. Her staff spends 2 hours per week on billing, compared with the 30 hours of staff time her friend Dr. South in Michigan needs for billing purposes.

Dr. North is less happy about the global budget approach used to pay hospitals. She often begs the hospital administrator to hire more physical therapists, to speed up the reporting of laboratory results, and to institute a program of diabetic teaching. The administrator responds that he receives a fixed payment from the provincial government each year, and there is no extra money.

Most physicians in Canada—primary care physicians and specialists—are paid on a fee-for-service basis, with fee levels negotiated between provincial governments and provincial medical associations (Figure 14–2). Physicians participating in the provincial programs must accept the government rate as payment in full and cannot bill patients directly for additional payment. Because fee-for-service payment emphasizes volume over quality of care and makes cost control difficult (see Chapter 9), Canadian provinces are experimenting with alternative forms of payment such as salary or capitation for physicians in group practice and clinic settings. By 2009, many primary care physicians in the province of Ontario were being paid capitation with bonuses for high quality (Collier, 2009).

Canadian hospitals, most of which are private nonprofit institutions, negotiate a global budget with the provincial government each year. Hospitals have no need to prepare the itemized patient bills that are so administratively costly in the United States. Hospitals must receive approval from their provincial health plan for new capital projects such as the purchase of expensive new technology or the construction of new facilities. Canada also regulates pharmaceutical prices and provincial plans maintain formularies of drugs approved for coverage.

▶ Cost Control

The Canadian system has attracted the interest of many people in the United States because in contrast to the United States, the Canadians have found a way to deliver comprehensive care to their entire population at far less cost. In 1970, the year before Canada's single-payer system was fully in place, Canada and the United States spent approximately the same proportion of their gross domestic products on health care—7.2% and 7.4%, respectively. By 1990, Canada's health expenditures had risen to 9% of the gross domestic product, compared with 12% for the United States. In 2008, Canada dedicated 10.4% of its gross domestic product to health care while the United States reached 16% (OECD, 2010). The differences in cost between the United States and Canada are primarily accounted for by four items: (1) administrative costs, which are more than 300% greater per capita in the United States; (2) more widespread use of expensive high-tech services in the United States; (3) cost per patient day in hospitals, which reflects a greater intensity of service in the United States; and (4) physician fees and pharmaceutical prices, which are much higher in the United States (Anderson et al, 2003; Woolhandler et al, 2003; Reinhardt, 2008).

While 2008 Canadian per capita health care costs ($4079) were far lower than those in the United States ($7538), Canada was the fifth highest on that measure among developed nations (OECD, 2010). Canadian concern with cost increases began in the 1990s, when Canadian provinces put into effect caps on physician payments similar to those used in Germany (Barer et al, 1996).

However, the Canadian federal government's fiscal austerity policies of the 1990s appear to have shaken the public's traditionally high level of confidence in the Canadian health care system. In 2010, about one-quarter of Canadians were not confident that they would receive the care they needed (Schoen et al, 2010). This unrest in public opinion has prompted vigorous debate in Canada about whether to allow greater private financing of health care, raise taxes to increase public financing, or restructure services to improve efficiency (Steinbrook, 2006). By 2010, Canada had opted for the latter two options: a commitment of substantial increases in federal funds for provincial health plans coupled with reform of the organization of primary care and other services (Hutchison et al, 2011).

THE UNITED KINGDOM

▶ Health Insurance

Roderick Pound owns a small bicycle repair shop in the north of England; he lives with his wife and two children. His sister Jennifer is a lawyer in Scotland. Roderick's younger brother is a student at Oxford, and their widowed mother, a retired saleswoman, lives in London. Their cousin Anne is totally and permanently disabled from a tragic automobile accident. A distant relative, who became a US citizen 15 years before, recently arrived to help care for Anne.

Simply by virtue of existing on the soil of the United Kingdom—whether employed, retired, disabled, or a foreign visitor—each of the Pound family members is entitled to receive tax-supported medical care through the National Health Service (NHS).

In 1911, Great Britain established a system of health insurance similar to that of Germany. Approximately half the population was covered, and the insurance arrangements were highly complex, with contributions flowing to "friendly societies," trade union and

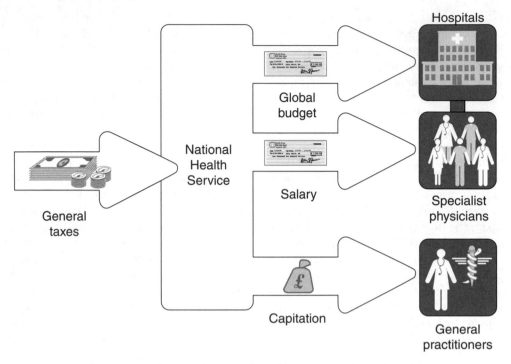

Figure 14–3. The British National Health Service: traditional model.

employer funds, commercial insurers, and county insurance committees. In 1942, the world's most renowned treatise on social insurance was published by Sir William Beveridge. The Beveridge Report proposed that Britain's diverse and complex social insurance and public assistance programs, including retirement, disability and unemployment benefits, welfare payments, and medical care, be financed and administered in a simple and uniform system. One part of Beveridge's vision was the creation of a national health service for the entire population. In 1948, the NHS began.

The great majority of NHS funding comes from taxes. As in Canada, the United Kingdom completely separates health insurance from employment, and no distinction exists between social insurance and public assistance financing. Unlike Canada, the United Kingdom allows private insurance companies to sell health insurance for services also covered by the NHS. A number of affluent people—12.5% of the population in 2007—purchase private insurance in order to receive preferential treatment, "hopping over" the queues for services present in parts of the NHS. Some employers

offer such supplemental insurance as a perk. People with private insurance are also paying taxes to support the NHS (Figure 14–3).

▶ Medical Care

Dr. Timothy Broadman is an English GP, whose list of patients numbers 1750. Included on his list is Roderick Pound and his family. One day, Roderick's son broke his leg playing soccer. He was brought to the NHS district hospital by ambulance and treated by Dr. Pettibone, the hospital orthopedist, without ever seeing Dr. Broadman.

Roderick's mother has severe degenerative arthritis of the hip, which Dr. Broadman cares for. A year ago, Dr. Broadman sent her to Dr. Pettibone to be evaluated for a hip replacement. Because this was not an emergency, Mrs. Pound required a referral from Dr. Broadman to see Dr. Pettibone. The orthopedist examined and x-rayed her hip and agreed that she needed a hip replacement, but not on an urgent basis. Mrs. Pound has been on the waiting list for her surgery for more than 6 months. Mrs. Pound has a wealthy friend with private health insurance who got her hip replacement within three weeks from Dr. Pettibone, who has a private practice in addition to his employment with the NHS.

Prior to the NHS, most primary medical care was delivered through GPs. The NHS maintained this tradition and formalized a gatekeeper system by which specialty and hospital services (except in emergencies) are available only by referral from a GP. Every person in the United Kingdom who wants to use the NHS must be enrolled on the list of a GP. There is free choice of GP (unless the GP's list of patients is full), and people can switch from one GP's list to another.

Whereas the creation of the NHS in 1948 left primary care essentially unchanged, it revolutionized Britain's hospital sector. As in the United States, hospitals had mainly been private nonprofit institutions or were run by local government; most of these hospitals were nationalized and arranged into administrative regions. Because the NHS unified the United Kingdom's hospitals under the national government, it was possible to institute a true regionalized plan (see Chapter 5).

Patient flow in a regionalized system tends to go from GP (primary care for common illnesses) to local hospital (secondary care for more serious illnesses) to regional or national teaching hospital (tertiary care for complex illnesses). Traditionally, most specialists have had their offices in hospitals. As in Germany, GPs do not provide care in hospitals. GPs have a tradition of working closely with social service agencies in the community, and home care is highly developed in the United Kingdom.

▶ Paying Physicians and Hospitals

Dr. Timothy Broadman does not think much about money when he goes to his surgery (office) each morning. He receives a payment from the NHS to cover part of the cost of running his office, and every month he receives a capitation payment for each of the 1750 patients on his list. Ten percent of his income has been coming from extra fees he receives when he gives vaccinations to the kids; does Pap smears, family planning, and other preventive care; and makes home visits after

hours. Recently, he also received a substantial bonus from the new pay-for-performance system.

Since early in the twentieth century, the major method of payment for British GPs has been capitation (see Chapter 4). This mode of payment did not change when the NHS took over in 1948. The NHS did add some fee-for-service payments as an encouragement to provide certain preventive services and home visits during nights and weekends. Consultants (specialists) are salaried employees of the NHS, although some consultants are allowed to see privately insured patients on the side, whom they bill fee-for-service.

In 2004, a major new payment mode began for GPs: pay for performance (P4P) (see Chapter 10), known in the United Kingdom as the Quality and Outcomes Framework. NHS management negotiated the program with the British Medical Association (BMA), and the success of the negotiations was in large part because of the government's policy of increasing payment to GP, whose average income rose by 60% from 2002 to 2007, with GP incomes approaching those of hospital specialists (Doran and Roland, 2010). The NHS and BMA agreed on dozens of clinical indicators measuring quality for preventive services and common chronic illnesses such as coronary heart disease, hypertension, diabetes, and asthma. In addition, physician practices are measured on practice organization—involving such measures as documentation in medical records, ability of patients to access the practice by phone, computerization, and safe management of medications—and on the patient experience as measured by patient surveys. Physician practices were awarded a maximum of 1050 points for GPs who performed well on all these measures. In 2005, each point was worth approximately £120 annually (more than $200). GP practices achieving maximum quality could potentially increase earnings by approximately $77,000 per physician (Roland, 2004).

In preparation for P4P, UK GP practices employed more nurses, established chronic disease clinics, and increased use of electronic medical records. In the first year of the program, practices in England scored a median of 1003 points, suggesting that a high level of quality was achieved. Moreover, performance improved faster among lower-quality practices, which narrowed inequalities in care. As a result, GP income increased markedly and the cost to the NHS was far greater than expected.

The extent to which actual quality was improved is unclear; successes may have been related in part to improved documentation rather than improved quality. Practices were allowed to exclude certain patients in the performance calculations on the basis of repeated no-shows, serious comorbidities, and other factors, introducing the possibility of "gaming" the system. An analysis of performance improvement prior to and following the introduction of P4P suggests that performance had been increasing before P4P, but that quality increased slightly faster after P4P for some chronic conditions. Nurses in GP practices were responsible for much of the quality improvement, as GPs delegated many preventive and chronic care tasks to them.

By 2009, an evaluation of the Quality and Outcomes Framework revealed that the rate of improvement in the quality of care increased for asthma and diabetes from 2003 to 2005, but not for heart disease. By 2007 the rate of improvement had slowed for all three conditions. Many practices had reached the quality benchmarks, which meant that the financial incentive to continue improving was blunted. Moreover, performance for quality measures removed from the Framework fell in some cases, suggesting that practices might neglect quality of care unassociated with financial rewards. No significant changes were found in patient reports of access to care and interpersonal aspect of care, but continuity of care decreased after the introduction of the Framework (Campbell et al, 2009; Doran and Roland, 2010).

▶ Cost Control

Health expenditures in the United Kingdom accounted for 7.0% of the gross domestic product (GDP) in 2000, far below the US figure of 13.4%. Believing that the NHS needed more resources, the government of Prime Minister Tony Blair infused the NHS with a major increase in funds. Between 1999 and 2004, the number of NHS physicians increased by 25%. In addition, the pay-for-performance system channeled the equivalent of several billion new dollars into physician practices (Roland, 2004; Klein, 2006). By 2008, health expenditures as a proportion of the GDP had risen to 8.7% and per capita spending had increased from $1837 (2000) to $3129 (2008), a 37% increase (OECD, 2010). In 2005, as a result of this large growth in health expenditures, the NHS found itself in a serious deficit and scaled back some of the increase in NHS staffing (Klein, 2006).

In spite of these developments, the United Kingdom continues to have a relatively low level of per capita health expenditures. Two major factors allow the United Kingdom to keep its health care costs low: the power of the governmental single payer to limit budgets and the mode of reimbursement of physicians. While Canada also has a single payer of health services, it pays most physicians fee-for-service and had to create physician expenditure caps (like Germany) in an attempt to control the inflationary tendencies of fee-for-service reimbursement. In contrast, the United Kingdom relies chiefly on capitation and salary to pay physicians; payment can more easily be controlled by limiting increases in capitation payments and salaries. Moreover, because consultants (specialists) in the United Kingdom are NHS employees, the NHS can and does tightly restrict the number of consultant slots, including those for surgeons. As a result, queues have developed for nonemergency consultant visits and elective surgeries (Hurst and Siciliani, 2003). From 2005 to 2007, 30% of patients with cerebrovascular events and an indication for carotid artery surgery experienced a delay of over 12 weeks in spite of national guidelines recommending surgery within 2 weeks of the onset of symptoms (Halliday et al, 2009). In 2006, the United Kingdom had 5.6 MRI scanners per million population compared with the US rate of 25.9 (OECD, 2010). Overall, the United Kingdom controls costs by controlling the supply of personnel and facilities and the budget for medical resources, and by investing heavily in a primary care system that has achieved some of the best quality measures in the developed world (Doran and Roland, 2010).

The United Kingdom is often viewed as a nation that rations certain kinds of health care. In fact, primary and preventive care are not rationed, and average waiting times to see a GP in the United Kingdom are significantly shorter than those for people in the US seeking medical appointments (Schoen et al, 2010). Overall, a striking characteristic of British medicine is its economy. British physicians simply do less of nearly everything—perform fewer surgeries, prescribe fewer medications, order fewer x-rays, and are more skeptical of new technologies than US physicians (Payer, 1988).

► Reforms of the National Health Service

A series of dramatic structural changes have been introduced into the NHS over the past 2 decades. In 1991, the Conservative government of Margaret Thatcher implemented market-style reforms requiring hospitals to compete for business by reducing delays for specialty and surgical care, and introducing general practitioner fundholding, by which GP practices could choose to receive a global budget to purchase all care for their panel of patients. In 1997, Tony Blair's Labor government abolished GP fundholding and replaced it with primary care trusts—a network of GPs working in the same district. All GP practices were required to join a primary care trust, which was given the responsibility for planning primary care and community health services in its area, contracting with hospitals and hospital consultants for specialty care, scrutinizing GP practice patterns, and implementing quality improvement activities. The average primary care trust had approximately 50 GP members, as well as additional primary care representatives from other professions, and covered a population of approximately 100,000 enrolled patients (Figure 14–4). Eighty-five percent of NHS funding flowed through the trusts, which were responsible for contracting for specialty and hospital services (Klein, 2004). As a result of the package of reforms (primary care trusts, the Quality and Outcomes Framework, and increased NHS funding), waiting times dropped, primary care access increased, chronic disease outcomes improved, and patient satisfaction grew.

In 2010, the new coalition government proposed yet another major structural reform, abolishing the primary care trusts but strengthening the policy of giving

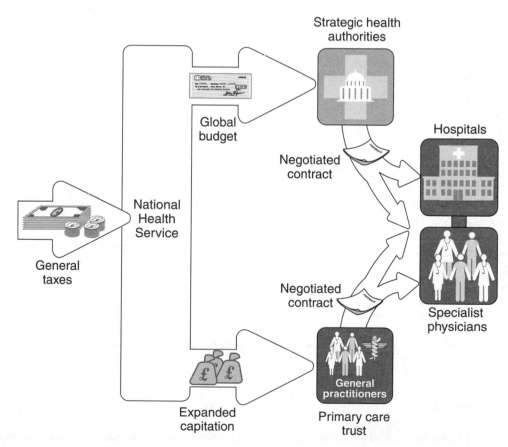

▲ **Figure 14–4.** The British National Health Service: Recent reforms.

groups of GPs large budgets from which they will fund primary care and buy specialty care for their patients. These GP commissioning groups will receive up to 70% of the NHS budget. GPs will either organize consortia to receive their budgets or be assigned to a consortium. This reform is touted as a shift in control from managers to physicians even though it is not clear that GPs want to manage budgets. As of early 2011, 170 consortia have been formed and 100 more are emerging. As the third major upheaval in 20 years, with each turnaround requiring several years to implement, it is unclear how health care providers and patients will fare in this constantly changing environment (Roland and Rosen, 2011), with critics complaining about a pattern of repeated "redisorganization" of the NHS from one governing party to the next.

JAPAN

▶ Health Insurance

Akiko Tanino works in the accounting department of the Mazda car company in Tokyo. Like all Mazda employees, she is enrolled in the health insurance plan directly operated by Mazda. Each month, 4% of Akiko's salary is deducted from her paycheck and paid to the Mazda health plan. Mazda makes an additional payment to its health plan equivalent to 4% of Akiko's salary.

Akiko's father Takeshi recently retired after working for many years as an engineer at Mazda. When he retired, his health insurance changed from the Mazda company plan to the community-based health insurance plan administered by the municipal government where he lives. Mazda makes payments to this health insurance plan to help pay for the health care costs of the company's retirees. In addition, the health insurance plan requires that Takeshi pay the plan a premium indexed to his income.

Akiko's brother Kazuo is a mechanic at a small auto repair shop in Tokyo. He is automatically enrolled in the government-managed health insurance plan operated by the Japanese national government. Kazuo and his employer each contribute payments equal to 4.1% of Kazuo's salary to the government plan.

Although Japanese society has a cultural history distinct from the other nations discussed in this chapter, its health care system draws heavily from European and North American traditions. Similar to Germany, Japan's modern health insurance system is rooted in an employment-linked social insurance program. Japan first legislated mandatory employment-based social insurance for many workers in 1922, building on preexisting voluntary mutual aid societies. The system was gradually expanded until universal coverage was achieved in 1961 with passage of the National Health Insurance Act. The Japanese insurance system differs from the German model by having different categories of health plans with even more numerous individual plans and less flexibility in choice of plan (Figure 14–5).

Employers with 700 or more employees are required to operate self-insured plans for their employees and dependents, known as "society-managed insurance" plans. Although these plans resemble the German industry-specific sickness funds, each company must operate its own individual health plan. Approximately 1800 different employer-based plans exist. Eighty-five percent of these society plans are operated by individual companies, with the balance operated as joint plans between two or more employers, although none involve as many companies as the typical German sickness fund. The boards of directors of society plans comprise 50% employee and 50% employer representatives. Employees and their dependents are required to enroll in their company's society plan, and the employee and the employer must contribute a premium to fund the society. Because each plan is self-insured, the premium rate varies (from 3% to 9.5% in 2006) depending on the average income and health risk of the company's employees, creating considerable inequities (Imai, 2002; Kemporen, 2007). Society-managed insurance plans cover 24% of the Japanese population.

Employees and dependents in companies with fewer than 700 employees are compulsorily enrolled in a single national health insurance plan for small businesses that is operated by the national government. This government-managed insurance plan, primarily financed by a premium (8.2% in 2006) on employers and employees, covers 28% of the population. The federal government also uses general tax revenues to subsidize the government-managed insurance plan.

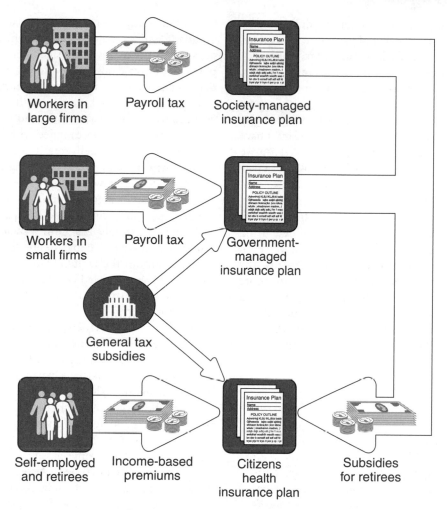

▲ **Figure 14–5.** The Japanese health system.

Yet a third type of health insurance, community-based health insurance (also called citizens' health insurance), covers self-employed workers and retirees (41% of the population). Each municipal government in Japan administers a local citizen's insurance plan and levies a compulsory premium on the self-employed workers and retirees in its jurisdiction. In addition, each employer-operated society-managed insurance plan and the single government-managed insurance plan must contribute payments to subsidize the costs for retirees. Approximately 40% of the financing for the citizens health insurance program comes from contributions from the society-managed and government-managed insurance plans, making employers liable for a large portion of the costs of their retirees' health care. Additional funds for the community-based health insurance plan come from general tax revenues.

A smattering of smaller insurance programs exist for government employees and other special categories of workers, and resemble the society-managed insurance plans. Persons who become unemployed remain enrolled in their health plan with the payroll tax waived. All plans are required to provide standard comprehensive benefits, including payment for hospital and physician services, prescription drugs, maternity care, and dental care. In addition, in 2000 Japan implemented a new long-term insurance plan, financed by general tax revenues and a new earmarked income tax, which provides comprehensive benefits to disabled adults, including payment for home care, case management, and institutional services.

Because Japan's society is aging more rapidly than any other developed nation, inequities and imbalances have developed in the financing of care for the most expensive patients—those at the highest age levels. In 2006, a new law was passed creating a more rational financing plan for retirees older than 75 (Kemporen, 2007).

In summary, Japan—like Germany—builds on an employment-based social insurance model, using additional general tax subsidies to create a universal insurance program. Compared with Germany, the national and local governments in Japan are more involved in directly administering health plans and a majority of Japanese are covered by government-run or government-managed plans rather than by employer-managed private plans (Kemporen, 2007).

▶ Medical Care

Takeshi Tanino's knee has been aching for several weeks. He makes an appointment at a clinic operated by an orthopedic surgeon. At the clinic Takeshi has a medical examination, an x-ray of the knee, and is scheduled for regular physical therapy. During the examination the orthopedist notes that Takeshi's blood pressure is high and recommends that Takeshi see an internist at a different clinic about this problem.

Six months later, Takeshi develops a cough and fever. He makes an appointment at the medical clinic of a nearby hospital run by Dr. Suzuki, is diagnosed with pneumonia, and is admitted to the medical ward. He is treated with intravenous antibiotics for 2 weeks and remains in the hospital for an additional 2 weeks after completing antibiotics for further intravenous hydration and nursing care.

Health plans place no restrictions on choice of hospital and physician and do not require preauthorization before using medical services. Most medical care is based on three types of settings: (1) independent clinics, each owned by a physician and staffed by the physician and other employees, with many clinics also

having small inpatient wards; (2) small hospitals with inpatient and outpatient departments, owned by a physician with employed physician staff; and (3) larger public and private hospitals with outpatient and inpatient departments and salaried physician staff. Facilities are organized by specialty, with larger hospitals having a wide range of specialties and smaller hospitals and clinics offering a more limited selection of specialty departments. Care is delivered in a specialty-specific manner, with a few organizations using a primary care–oriented gatekeeper model (Reid, 2009).

Physician entrepreneurship is a strong element in the organization of health care in Japan. Most clinics and small hospitals are family-owned businesses founded and operated by independent physicians. Unlike clinics in the United States such as the Mayo Clinic and Palo Alto Medical Foundation that began as family-owned institutions but evolved into nonprofit organizations with ownership shared among a larger group of physician partners, most clinics in Japan have remained under the ownership of a single physician, often passed down within a family from one generation to another. Many physicians expanded their clinics to become small hospitals, but the government builds and operates the larger medical centers. The distinction between clinics and hospitals in Japan is not as great as in most nations. Clinics are permitted to operate inpatient beds and only become classified as hospitals when they have more than 20 beds. Approximately 30% of clinics in Japan have inpatient beds. Virtually all physicians either own clinics and hospitals or work as employees of a clinic or hospital, and practice only within their single institution. Although many physician-owned clinics and hospitals are modest facilities, others are larger institutions offering a wide array of outpatient and inpatient services featuring the latest biomedical technology, electronic medical records, and automated dispensing of medications.

Rates of hospital admission are relatively low in Japan and rates of surgery are approximately one-third the rate in the United States. A cultural norm that makes patients reluctant to undergo invasive procedures in part explains the low surgical rate in Japan. When hospitalized, patients remain unusually long compared with most developed nations; average lengths of stay vary by hospital from 16 to 29 days. Patients are allowed long periods to convalesce while still in the hospital (Ikegami and Campbell, 2004).

Paying Physicians and Hospitals

One month after returning home from the hospital, Takeshi Tanino develops stomach pain that awakens him several nights. He makes an appointment at a general medical clinic run by Dr. Sansei. Dr. Sansei performs an endoscopy, which reveals gastritis. Dr. Sansei prescribes an H_2 blocker and arranges for Takeshi to return to the clinic every 4 weeks for the next 6 months. Takeshi's stomach ache improves after a few days of using the medication. At each follow-up visit, Dr. Sansei questions Takeshi about his symptoms and dispenses a new 4-week supply of medications.

Until recently, insurance plans paid both physicians and hospitals on a fee-for-service basis. In 2003, a per diem hospital payment based on diagnosis was introduced (Nawata et al, 2009) while physicians continue to be paid fee-for-service. The government strictly regulates physician fees, hospital payments, and medication prices, which are very low by US standards. The fee schedule is in many ways the opposite of US fees: In Japan, primary care services tend to command higher fees than do more specialized services such as surgical procedures and imaging studies. Services such as MRI scans that have shown large increases in volumes have had substantial cuts in fees (Ikegami and Campbell, 2004). Based on fee schedules in place in 2007, a family physician office visit might be reimbursed $5 or $10, one night's stay in a hospital $11, and a brain MRI $105 (Reid, 2009). Physicians make up for low fees with high volume, at times seeing 60 patients per day. In 2007 the number of physician visits per capita was 13.4, compared with 4.0 for the United States (OECD, 2010). Physicians are permitted to directly dispense medications, not just to prescribe them, and make a profit from the sale of pharmaceuticals. The government recently restricted how much physicians could charge patients for medications (Kemporen, 2007), but many physician visits are solely for the purpose of refilling medications. Quality of care in Japan is not systematically measured and is believed to vary greatly among physicians and hospitals (Henke et al, 2009).

Cost Control

Health care costs in Japan were only 8.1% of GDP in 2007. However this is a considerable rise from 1990's 6.0%, and concerns are mounting due to Japan's demographics. The health care system relies heavily on payroll taxes and thus requires a large employed population. But with, a plummeting birth rate and the longest life expectancy in the world, Japan's population is aging faster than that of other developed nations. The proportion of Japanese older than 65 years is projected to increase from 12% in 1990 to 40% in 2050 (Kemporen, 2007). In comparison, the proportion of the US population older than 65 years will increase much more modestly, from 12% to 21%, during this same period.

Through its fee schedule, the government has kept medical prices low, which is the main cost containment strategy. But physicians are unhappy and see too many patients for short visits, while many hospitals are old and underfunded. The stresses resulting from Japan's demographic reality and its overstretched health care providers make for an uncertain future (Reid, 2009).

CONCLUSION

Key issues in evaluating and comparing health care systems are access to care, level of health expenditures, public satisfaction with health care, and the overall quality of care as expressed by the health of the population. Germany, Canada, the United Kingdom, and Japan provide universal financial access to health care through government-run or government-mandated programs. These four nations have controlled health care costs more successfully than has the United States (Tables 14–1 and 14–2), though all four face challenges in containing their spending.

Sixteen percent of US adults surveyed in 2007 felt that the health system works well with only minor changes needed; 48% felt that fundamental change is needed, and 34% wanted the system rebuilt completely. Adults in Germany, Canada, and the United Kingdom had somewhat more favorable views of their health systems, though the majority in those countries also felt that major changes were needed (Schoen et al, 2007). Adults in the United States were much more likely than adults in Germany, the United Kingdom, and Canada to report problems with access to medical services due to costs (Figure 14–6).

Crossnational comparisons of health care quality are treacherous since it is difficult to disentangle the impacts of socioeconomic factors and medical care on the health status of the population. But such comparisons can convey rough impressions of whether a

Table 14-1. Total health expenditures as a percentage of gross domestic product (GDP), 1970–2008

	1970	1980	1990	2000	2008
Germany	5.5	7.9	8.3	10.3	10.5
United Kingdom	4.5	5.8	6.0	7.0	8.7
Canada	7.2	7.4	8.9	8.8	10.4
Japan	4.1	6.5	6.0	7.7	8.1 (2007)
United States	7.4	9.2	11.9	13.4	16.0

Source: Data from the Organisation for Economic Co-operation and Development, 2010. www.oecd.org.

Table 14-2. Per capita health spending in US dollars, 2008

Germany	$3737
United Kingdom	$3129
Canada	$4079
Japan	$2729 (2007)
United States	$7538

Source: Data from the Organisation for Economic Co-operation and Development, 2010. www.oecd.org.

health care system is functioning at a reasonable level of quality. From Table 14–3, it is clear that the United States has an infant mortality rate higher than Germany, Canada, the United Kingdom, and Japan, with the Japanese rate being the lowest. Japan also has the highest male and female life expectancy rates at birth. The life expectancy rate at age 65 is believed by some observers to measure the impact of medical care, especially its more high-tech component, more than it measures underlying socioeconomic influences. Even by this standard, the United States ranks

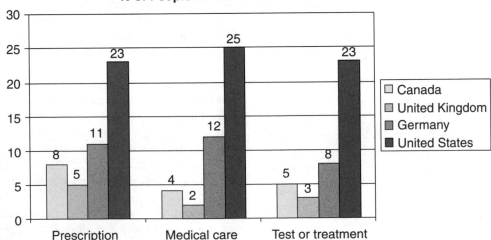

▲ **Figure 14-6.** Problems accessing medical services due to costs.

Table 14–3. Health outcome measures

	Infant Mortality, per 1000 Live Births[a]	Life Expectancy at Birth (years)[a]		Life Expectancy at Age 65 (years)[a]		Mortality Amenable to Health Care, 2002–3, Deaths per 100,000 Population[b]
		Men	Women	Men	Women	
Germany	3.5	77.6	82.7	17.6	20.7	90
United Kingdom	4.7	77.6	81.8	17.6	20.2	103
Canada	5.1	78.3	83.0	18.1	21.3	77
Japan	2.6	79.3	86.1	18.6	23.6	71
United States	6.7 (2006)	75.3	80.4	17.1	19.8	110

Infant mortality data and life expectancy data are for 2007 or 2008.
[a]Data from the Organisation for Economic Co-operation and Development, 2010. www.oecd.org.
[b]Data from Nolte and McKee, 2008.

below the other four nations (OECD, 2010). Researchers have developed another metric intended to assess the functioning of national health care systems, known as "mortality amenable to health care" (Nolte and McKee, 2008); the United States performs poorly on this metric as well relative to other nations (Table 14–3).

Just as epidemiologic studies often derive their most profound insights from comparisons of different populations (see Chapter 11), research into health services can glean insights from the experience of other nations. As the United States confronts the challenge of achieving universal access to high-quality health care at an affordable cost, lessons may be learned from examining how other nations have addressed this challenge.

REFERENCES

Anderson GF et al. It's the prices, stupid: Why the United States is so different from other countries. *Health Aff.* 2003;22(3):89.

Barer ML, Lomas J, Sanmartin C. Re-minding our Ps and Qs: Medical cost controls in Canada. *Health Aff.* 1996;15(2):216.

Busse R. The health system in Germany. *Eurohealth.* 2008;14(1):5.

Busse R, Riesberg A. *Health Care Systems in Transition: Germany.* Copenhagen: WHO Regional Office for Europe; 2004.

Campbell SM et al. Effects of pay for performance on the quality of primary care in England. *N Engl J Med.* 2009;261:368.

Canadian Institute for Health Information. Health Care in Canada, 2010, December 2010. www.cihi.ca.

Collier R. Shift toward capitation in Ontario. *Canadian Med Assoc J.* 2009;181:668.

Doran T, Roland M. Lessons from major initiatives to improve primary care in the United Kingdom. *Health Aff.* 2010;29:1023. https://www.mckinseyquarterly.com/Improving_Japans_health_care_system_2311. Accessed November 17, 2011.

Guilfoyle J. Prejudice in medicine. Our role in creating health care disparities. *Can Fam Physician.* 2008;54:1511.

Halliday AW et al. Waiting times for carotid endarterectomy in UK. *BMJ.* 2009;338:b1847.

Henke N et al. Improving Japan's health care system. *McKinsey Q.* 2009.

Hurst J, Siciliani L. *Tackling Excessive Waiting Times for Elective Surgery: A Comparison of Policies in Twelve OECD Countries.* Paris: Organisation for Economic Co-operation and Development; 2003.

Hutchison B et al. Primary health care in Canada: Systems in motion. *Milbank* Q. 2011:89(2):256.

Ikegami N, Campbell JC. Japan's health care system: Containing costs and attempting reform. *Health Aff.* 2004;23(3):26.

Imai Y. Health Care Reform in Japan. Organisation for Economic Co-operation and Development, February 2002. www.oecd.org.

Katz SJ et al. Phantoms in the snow: Canadians' use of health care services in the United States. *Health Aff.* 2002;21(3):19.

Kemporen (National Federation of Health Insurance Societies). Health Insurance, Long-Term Care Insurance and Health Insurance Societies in Japan, 2007. Kemporen, 2007.

Klein R. Britain's National Health Service revisited. *N Engl J Med.* 2004;350:937.

Klein R. The troubled transformation of Britain's National Health Service. *N Engl J Med.* 2006;355:409.

Nawata K, et al. Analysis of the new medical payment system in Japan, July 2009. www.mssanz.org.au/modsim09/A2/nawata.pdf.

Nolte E, McKee CM. Measuring the health of nations: Updating an earlier analysis. *Health Aff.* 2008;27:58. Erratum in: *Health Aff.* 2008;27:593.

Ornyanova D, Busse R. Health Fund now operational Health Policy Monitor, May 2009. www.hpm.org.

Organisation for Economic Co-operation and Development. OECD Health Data, 2010. www.oecd.org.

Payer L. *Medicine and Culture.* New York: Henry Holt; 1988.

Reid TR. *The Healing of America.* New York: The Penguin Press; 2009.

Reinhardt U. Why does US health care cost so much? *Economix.* November 14, 2008. http://economix.blogs.nytimes.com.

Roland M. Linking physicians' pay to the quality of care—a major experiment in the United Kingdom. *N Engl J Med.* 2004;351:1448.

Roland M, Rosen R. British NHS embarks on controversial and risky market-style reforms in health care. *N Engl J Med.* 2011;364:1360.

Ross JS, Detsky AS. Choice? Making health care decisions in the United States and Canada. *JAMA.* 2009;302:1803.

Sanmartin C et al. Comparing health and health care use in Canada and the United States. *Health Aff.* 2006;25:1133.

Schoen C et al. Toward higher-performance health systems: Adults' health care experiences in seven countries, 2007. *Health Aff.* 2007;26:w717.

Schoen C et al. How health insurance design affects access to care and costs: by income, in eleven countries. *Health Aff.* 2010;29:2323.

Steinbrook R. Private health care in Canada. *N Engl J Med.* 2006;354:1661.

Stock S et al. The influence of the labor market on German health care reforms. *Health Aff.* 2006;25:1143.

Taylor MG. *Insuring National Health Care. The Canadian Experience.* Chapel Hill, NC: University of North Carolina Press; 1990.

Willcox S et al. Measuring and reducing waiting times: A cross-national comparison of strategies. *Health Aff.* 2007;26:1078.

Woolhandler S et al. Costs of health care administration in the United States and Canada. *N Engl J Med.* 2003;349:768.

Zander B et al. Health policy in Germany after the election. *Health Policy Monitor.* November 2009. www.hpm.org.

Health Care Reform and National Health Insurance

For 100 years, reformers in the United States have argued for the passage of a national health insurance program, a government guarantee that every person is insured for basic health care. Finally in 2010, the United States took a major step forward toward universal health insurance.

The subject of national health insurance has seen six periods of intense legislative activity, alternating with times of political inattention. From 1912 to 1916, 1946 to 1949, 1963 to 1965, 1970 to 1974, 1991 to 1994, and 2009 to 2010, it was the topic of major national debate. In 1916, 1949, 1974, and 1994, national health insurance was defeated and temporarily consigned to the nation's back burner. Guaranteed health coverage for two groups—the elderly and some of the poor—was enacted in 1965 through Medicare and Medicaid. Expansion of coverage to over 30 million uninsured people was legislated with the Patient Protection and Affordable Care Act of 2010. National health insurance means the guarantee of health insurance for all the nation's residents—what is commonly referred to as "universal coverage." Most of the focus, as well as the political contentiousness, of national health insurance proposals tends to concern how to finance universal coverage. Because health care financing is so interwoven with provider reimbursement and cost containment, national health insurance proposals usually also address those topics.

The controversies that erupt over universal health care coverage become simpler to understand if one returns to the four basic modes of health care financing outlined in Chapter 2: out-of-pocket payment, individual private insurance, employment-based private insurance, and government financing. There is general agreement that out-of-pocket payment does not work as a sole financing method for costly contemporary health care. National health insurance involves the replacement of out-of-pocket payments by one, or a mixture, of the other three financing modes.

Under government-financed national health insurance plans, funds are collected by a government or quasigovernmental fund, which in turn pays hospitals, physicians, health maintenance organizations (HMOs), and other health care providers. Under private individual or employment-based national health insurance, funds are collected by private insurance companies, which then pay providers of care.

Historically, health care financing in the United States began with out-of-pocket payment and progressed through individual private insurance, then employment-based insurance, and finally government financing for Medicare and Medicaid (see Chapter 2). In the history of US national health insurance, the chronologic sequence is reversed. Early attempts at national health insurance legislation proposed government programs; private employment-based national health insurance was not seriously entertained until 1971, and individually purchased universal coverage was not suggested until the 1980s (Table 15–1). Following this historical progression, we shall first discuss government-financed national health insurance, followed by private employment-based and then individually purchased universal coverage. The most recent chapter of this history is the enactment under the administration of President Obama of the

Table 15-1. Attempts to legislate national health insurance

1912-1919	American Association for Labor Legislation
1946-1949	Wagner-Murray-Dingell bill supported by President Truman
1963-1965	Medicare and Medicaid passed as a first step toward national health insurance
1970-1974	Kennedy and Nixon proposals
1991-1994	A variety of proposals introduced, including President Clinton's Plan
2009-2010	Patient Protection and Affordable Care Act signed into law by President Obama

Patient Protection and Affordable Care Act of 2010, a pluralistic approach to national health insurance that draws on all three of these financing models: government financing, employment-based private insurance, and individually purchased private insurance.

GOVERNMENT-FINANCED NATIONAL HEALTH INSURANCE

▶ The American Association for Labor Legislation Plan

In the early 1900s, 25% to 40% of people who became sick did not receive any medical care. In 1915, the American Association for Labor Legislation (AALL) published a national health insurance proposal to provide medical care, sick pay, and funeral expenses to lower-paid workers—those earning less than $1200 a year—and to their dependents. The program would be run by states rather than the federal government and would be financed by a payroll tax–like contribution from employers and employees, perhaps with an additional contribution from state governments. Payments would go to regional funds (not private insurance companies) under extensive government control. The funds would pay physicians and hospitals. Thus, the first national health insurance proposal in the United States—because the money was collected by quasi-public funds through a mandatory tax—can be considered a government-financed program (Starr, 1982).

In 1910, Edgar Peoples worked as a clerk for Standard Oil, earning $800 a year. He lived with his wife and three sons. Under the AALL proposal, Standard

Oil and Mr. Peoples would each pay $13 per year into the regional health insurance fund, with the state government contributing $6. The total of $32 (4% of wages) would cover the Peoples family.

The AALL's road to national health insurance followed the example of European nations, which often began their programs with lower-paid workers and gradually extended coverage to other groups in the population. Key to the financing of national health insurance was its compulsory nature; mandatory payments were to be made on behalf of every eligible person, ensuring sufficient funds to pay for people who fell sick.

The AALL proposal initially had the support of the American Medical Association (AMA) leadership. However, the AMA reversed its position and the conservative branch of labor, the American Federation of Labor, along with business interests, opposed the plan (Starr, 1982). The first attempt at national health insurance failed.

▶ The Wagner–Murray–Dingell Bill

In 1943, Democratic Senators Robert Wagner of New York and James Murray of Montana, and Representative John Dingell of Michigan introduced a health insurance plan based on the social security system enacted in 1935. Employer and employee contributions to cover physician and hospital care would be paid to the federal social insurance trust fund, which would in turn pay health providers. The Wagner–Murray–Dingell bill had its lineage in the New Deal reforms enacted during the administration of President Franklin Delano Roosevelt. President Roosevelt had initially considered including a national health plan as part of the Social Security Act, but facing resistance from the AMA decided to omit health reform from the New Deal legislative package.

In the 1940s, Edgar Peoples' daughter Elena worked in a General Motors plant manufacturing trucks to be used in World War II. Elena earned $3500 per year. Under the 1943 Wagner–Murray–Dingell bill, General Motors would pay 6% of her wages up to $3000 into the social insurance trust fund for retirement, disability, unemployment, and health insurance. An identical 6% would be taken out of Elena's check for the same purpose. One-fourth of this total amount ($90) would be dedicated to the health *insurance portion of social security. If Elena or her children became sick, the social insurance trust fund would reimburse their physician and hospital.*

Edgar Peoples, in his seventies, would also receive health insurance under the Wagner–Murray–Dingell bill, because he was a social security beneficiary.

Elena's younger brother Marvin was permanently disabled and unable to work. Under the Wagner–Murray–Dingell bill he would not have received government health insurance unless his state added unemployed people to the program.

As discussed in Chapter 2, government-financed health insurance can be divided into two categories. Under the social insurance model, only those who pay into the program, usually through social security contributions, are eligible for the program's benefits. Under the public assistance (welfare) model, eligibility is based on a means test; those below a certain income may receive assistance. In the welfare model, those who benefit may not necessarily contribute, and those who contribute (usually through taxes) may not benefit (Bodenheimer and Grumbach, 1992). The Wagner–Murray–Dingell bill, like the AALL proposal, was a social insurance proposal. Working people and their dependents were eligible because they made social security contributions, and retired people receiving social security benefits were eligible because they paid into social security prior to their retirement. The permanently unemployed were not eligible.

In 1945, President Truman, embracing the general principles of the Wagner–Murray–Dingell legislation, became the first US president to strongly champion national health insurance. After Truman's surprise election in 1948, the AMA succeeded in a massive campaign to defeat the Wagner–Murray–Dingell bill. In 1950, national health insurance returned to obscurity (Starr, 1982).

▶ Medicare and Medicaid

In the late 1950s, less than 15% of the elderly had health insurance (see Chapter 2) and a strong social movement clamored for the federal government to come up with a solution. The Medicare law of 1965 took the Wagner–Murray–Dingell approach to national health insurance, narrowing it to people 65 years and older. Medicare was financed through social security contributions, federal income taxes, and individual premiums. Congress also enacted the Medicaid program in 1965, a public assistance or "welfare" model of government insurance that covered a portion of the low-income population. Medicaid was paid for by federal and state taxes.

In 1966, at age 66, Elena Peoples was automatically enrolled in the federal government's Medicare Part A hospital insurance plan, and she chose to sign up for the Medicare Part B physician insurance plan by paying a $3 monthly premium to the Social Security Administration. Elena's son, Tom, and Tom's employer helped to finance Medicare Part A; each paid 0.5% of wages (up to a wage level of $6600 per year) into a Medicare trust fund within the social security system. Elena's Part B coverage was financed in part by federal income taxes and in part by Elena's monthly premiums. In case of illness, Medicare would pay for most of Elena's hospital and physician bills.

Elena's disabled younger brother, Marvin, age 60, was too young to qualify for Medicare in 1966. Marvin instead became a recipient of Medicaid, the federal–state program for certain groups of low-income people. When Marvin required medical care, the state Medicaid program paid the hospital, physician, and pharmacy, and a substantial portion of the state's costs were picked up by the federal government.

Medicare is a social insurance program, requiring individuals or families to have made social security contributions to gain eligibility to the plan. Medicaid, in contrast, is a public assistance program that does not require recipients to make contributions but instead is financed from general tax revenues. Because of the rapid increase in Medicare costs, the social security contribution has risen substantially. In 1966, Medicare took 1% of wages, up to a $6600 wage level (0.5% each from employer and employee); in 2004, the payments had risen to 2.9% of all wages. The Part B premium has jumped from $3 per month in 1966 to $115.40 per month in 2011.

▶ The 1970 Kennedy Bill and the Single-Payer Plan of the 1990s

Many people believed that Medicare and Medicaid were a first step toward universal health insurance. European nations started their national health insurance programs by covering a portion of the population and later extending coverage to more people. Medicare and Medicaid seemed to fit that tradition. Shortly after Medicare and Medicaid became law, the labor movement, Senator Edward Kennedy of Massachusetts, and Representative Martha Griffiths of Michigan drafted legislation to cover the entire population through a national health insurance program. The 1970 Kennedy–Griffiths Health Security Act followed in the footsteps of the Wagner–Murray–Dingell bill, calling for a single federally operated health insurance system that would replace all public and private health insurance plans.

Under the Kennedy–Griffiths 1970 Health Security Program, Tom Peoples, who worked for Great Books, a small book publisher, would continue to see his family physician as before. Rather than receiving payment from Tom's private insurance company, his physician would be paid by the federal government, perhaps through a regional intermediary. Tom's employer would no longer make a social security contribution to Medicare (which would be folded into the Health Security Program) and would instead make a larger contribution of 3% of wages up to a wage level of $15,000 for each employee. Tom's employee contribution was set at 1% up to a wage level of $15,000. These social insurance contributions would pay for approximately 60% of the program; federal income taxes would pay for the other 40%.

Tom's Uncle Marvin, on Medicaid since 1966, would be included in the Health Security Program,

as would all residents of the United States. Medicaid would be phased out as a separate public assistance program.

The Health Security Act went one step further than the AALL and Wagner–Murray–Dingell proposals: It combined the social insurance and public assistance approaches into one unified program. In part because of the staunch opposition of the AMA and the private insurance industry, the legislation went the way of its predecessors: political defeat.

In 1989, Physicians for a National Health Program offered a new government-financed national health insurance proposal. The plan came to be known as the "single-payer" program, because it would establish a single government fund within each state to pay hospitals, physicians, and other health care providers, replacing the multipayer system of private insurance companies (Himmelstein and Woolhandler, 1989). Several versions of the single-payer plan were introduced into Congress in the 1990s, each bringing the entire population together into one health care financing system, merging the social insurance and public assistance approaches (Table 15–2). The California Legislature, with the backing of the California Nurses Association, passed a single-payer plan in 2006 and 2008, but the proposals were vetoed by the Governor.

THE EMPLOYER-MANDATE MODEL OF NATIONAL HEALTH INSURANCE

In response to Democratic Senator Kennedy's introduction of the 1970 Health Security Act, President Nixon, a Republican, countered with a plan of his own,

Table 15–2. Categories of national health insurance plans

1. Government-financed health insurance plans	Money is collected through taxes or premiums by a public or quasipublic fund that reimburses health care providers
2. Employer-mandated private health insurance plans	The government requires employers to pay for all or part of private health insurance policies for their employees
3. Individual-mandated private health insurance plans	The government requires individuals to purchase private health insurance, with subsidies for low-income people
4. Hybrid plans	Government-financed insurance for the elderly and the poor, employer-mandated private insurance for the employed and their dependents, individual-mandated private insurance for people without employment

the nation's first employment-based, privately administered national health insurance proposal. For 3 years, the Nixon and Kennedy approaches competed in the congressional battleground; however, because most of the population was covered under private insurance, Medicare, or Medicaid, there was relatively little public pressure on Congress. In 1974, the momentum for national health insurance collapsed, not to be seriously revived until the 1990s. The essence of the Nixon proposal was the employer mandate, under which the federal government requires (or mandates) employers to purchase private health insurance for their employees.

Tom Peoples' cousin Blanche was a receptionist in a physician's office in 1971. The physician did not provide health insurance to his employees. Under Nixon's 1971 plan, Blanche's employer would be required to pay 75% of the private health insurance premium for his employees; the employees would pay the other 25%.

Blanche's boyfriend, Al, had been laid off from his job in 1970 and was receiving unemployment benefits. He had no health insurance. Under Nixon's proposal, the federal government would pay a portion of Al's health insurance premium.

No longer was national health insurance equated with government financing. Employer mandate plans preserve and enlarge the role of the private health insurance industry rather than replacing it with tax-financed government-administered plans. While the Nixon plan preserved existing government programs such as Medicare and Medicaid, it proposed to expand coverage for the uninsured through a widening role for private, employment-based insurance. Government's new role under the Nixon plan would be to enforce private health insurance as a required benefit for employed people. The Nixon proposal changed the entire political landscape of national health insurance, moving it toward the private sector. In later years, Senator Kennedy embraced the employer mandate approach himself, fearing that the opposition of the insurance industry and organized medicine would kill any attempt to legislate government-financed national health insurance.

During the 1980s and 1990s, the number of people in the United States without any health insurance rose from 25 million to more than 40 million (see Chapter 3). Approximately three-quarters of the uninsured were

employed or were dependents of employed persons. The rapidly rising cost of health insurance premiums made insurance unaffordable for many businesses. In response to this crisis in health care access, President Clinton submitted legislation to Congress in 1993 calling for universal health insurance through an employer mandate, as well as broadened eligibility for Medicaid. Like the Nixon proposal, the essence of the Clinton plan was the requirement that employers pay for most of their employees' private insurance premiums.

A variation on the employer mandate type of national health insurance is the voluntary approach. Rather than requiring employers to purchase health insurance for employees, employers are given incentives such as tax credits to cover employees voluntarily. The attempt of some states to implement this type of voluntary approach has failed to significantly reduce the numbers of uninsured workers.

THE INDIVIDUAL-MANDATE MODEL OF NATIONAL HEALTH INSURANCE

In 1989, a new species of national health insurance appeared, sponsored by the conservative Heritage Foundation: the individual mandate. Just as many states require motor vehicle drivers to purchase automobile insurance, the Heritage plan called for the federal government to require all US residents to purchase individual health insurance policies. Tax credits would be made available on a sliding scale to individuals and families too poor to afford health insurance premiums (Butler, 1991). Under the most ambitious versions of universal individual insurance proposals, neither employer-sponsored group insurance nor government-administered insurance would continue to play a role in financing health care. These existing financing models would be dismantled and replaced by a universal, individual mandate program. Ironically, the individual insurance mandate shares at least one feature with the single-payer, government-financed approach to universal coverage: Both would severe the connection between employment and health insurance, allowing portability and continuity of coverage as workers moved from one employer to another or became self-employed.

Tom Peoples received health insurance through his employer, Great Books. Under an individual mandate plan, Tom would be legally required to purchase health insurance for his family. Great Books *could offer a health plan to Tom and his coworkers but would not be required to contribute anything to the premium. If Tom purchased private health insurance for his family at a cost of $8000 per year, he would receive a tax credit of $4000 (ie, he would pay $4000 less in income taxes). Tom's Uncle Marvin, formerly on Medicaid, would be given a voucher to purchase a private health insurance policy.*

With individual mandate health insurance, the tax credits may vary widely in their amount depending on characteristics such as household income and how much of a subsidy the architects of individual mandate proposals build into the plan. In a generous case, a family might receive a $10,000 tax credit, subsidizing much of its health insurance premium. If the family's tax liability is less than the value of the tax credit, the government would pay the family the difference between the family's tax liability and $10,000.

A related version of the individual mandate is a voucher system. Instead of issuing tax credits, the federal government would issue a voucher for a fixed dollar amount that could be used toward the purchase of health insurance, just as some local government jurisdictions issue vouchers that may be used to enroll children in private schools. In the most sweeping proposals, a tax-financed voucher system would completely replace existing insurance programs directly administered by government as well as employer-sponsorship of private insurance (Emanuel and Fuchs, 2005). Another version of individual health insurance expansion is the voluntary concept, which was proposed by President George W. Bush. Uninsured individuals would not be required to purchase individual insurance but would receive a tax credit if they chose to purchase insurance. The level of the tax credits in the Bush plan and similar proposals have been small compared to the cost of most health insurance policies, with the result that these voluntary approaches if enacted would have induced very few uninsured people to purchase coverage.

▶ The Massachusetts Individual Mandate Plan of 2006

Nearly 20 years after the Heritage Foundation drafted a proposal for a national individual mandate, Massachusetts enacted a state-level universal health coverage bill implementing the nation's first legislated individual mandate. The Massachusetts plan, enacted under the

leadership of Republican Governor Mitt Romney, mandates that every state resident must have health insurance coverage meeting a minimum standard set by the state. Individuals are required to provide proof of coverage at the time of filing their annual tax return, and face a financial penalty for failing to provide evidence of coverage. The state provides subsidies for purchase of private health insurance coverage to individuals with incomes below 300% of the federal poverty level if they are not covered by the state's Medicaid program or through employment-based insurance.

Brian Mayflower earns $16,000 a year as a waiter to support himself as an aspiring actor in Boston. He has chronic asthma, with his inhaler medications alone costing more than $1,000 annually. He is not eligible for Medicaid and is required under the Massachusetts Plan to purchase a private health plan. As a low-income person, Brian receives a state subsidy for most of the premium cost of the plan. The plan has a $500 per year deductible but pays for most of Brian's medications once he meets the annual deductible.

Brian's sister Dorothy Mayflower is a self-employed accountant living in Springfield and earning $58,000 a year. At her income level, the Massachusetts state subsidy for insurance coverage would leave her having to pay $3000 per year toward the premium for a plan that has a $2000 per year deductible. Dorothy is in good health and is having trouble paying the mortgage on her house, which recently ballooned. She decides she will not enroll in a health insurance plan and instead pays the $900 fine to the state for not complying with the individual mandate.

Like the Nixon employer mandate proposal, the Massachusetts individual mandate does not eliminate existing government insurance programs; it extends the reach of private insurance through a government mandate, in this case for individually purchased private insurance. State government provides an income-adjusted subsidy for individual coverage for people not eligible for employer-sponsored insurance and limits the degree to which private plans can experience-rate their premiums. The Massachusetts plan allows insurers to offer policies with large amounts of cost-sharing in the form of high deductibles and coinsurance. The plan also includes a weak employer mandate, requiring employers with more than 10 employees to either contribute toward insurance coverage for their employees or pay into the state fund that underwrites public subsidies for the individual mandate and related programs.

The Massachusetts Health Plan of 2006 is credited with reducing the uninsurance rate among nonelderly adults in Massachusetts from 13% in 2006 to 5% in 2009 (Long and Stockley, 2010). Some residents of the state, such as Dorothy Mayflower, continue to have trouble affording private insurance even with some degree of state subsidy, and the high levels of cost-sharing allowed under the minimum benefit standards leave many insured individuals with substantial out-of-pocket payments. In 2008, 18% of low-income people in Massachusetts reported unmet health care needs due to costs (copayments, deductibles, uncovered services) and about 20% of the entire population experienced difficulty accessing primary care due to the primary care shortage (Clark et al, 2011).

THE PLURALISTIC REFORM MODEL: THE PATIENT PROTECTION AND AFFORDABLE CARE ACT OF 2010

Following a year-long bitter debate, the Democrat-controlled House of Representatives and Senate passed the Affordable Care Act (ACA) without a single Republican vote. President Obama, on March 23, 2010, signed the most significant health legislation since Medicare and Medicaid in 1965 (Morone, 2010). Although the ACA was attacked as "socialized medicine" and a "government takeover of health care," its policy pedigree derives much more from the proposals of a Republican President (Nixon) and Republican Governor (Romney) than from the single-payer national health insurance tradition of Democratic Presidents Roosevelt and Truman. The pluralistic financing model of the ACA includes individual and employer mandates for private insurance and an expansion of the publicly financed Medicaid program. Ironically, despite the ACA's close resemblance to the Massachusetts Health Plan of 2006, Mitt Romney, the former Governor of Massachusetts who supported and signed that state's reform bill, upon turning his sights to his candidacy for the Republican nomination for the 2012 presidential election, called for repeal of the ACA.

In 2013, Mandy Must is uninsured and works for a small shipping company in Texas that does not offer health insurance benefits. In 2014, if the ACA survives legal and political challenges, she would be required to obtain private insurance coverage. Mandy earns about $35,000 per year, and in 2014 would receive a federal subsidy of about $2000 toward her purchase of an individual insurance policy with a premium cost of $5000.

In 2013, Walter Groop works full-time as a salesperson for a large department store in Miami which does not offer health insurance benefits to its workers. In 2014, he begins to apply for an individual policy to meet the requirements of the ACA, but his employer informs him that the department store would start contributing toward group health insurance coverage for its employees to avoid paying penalties under the ACA.

In 2013, Job Knaught has been an unemployed construction worker in St. Louis for over 18 months and, aside from an occasional odd job, has no regular source of income. Because he is not disabled, he does not qualify for Medicaid despite being poor. In 2014, Job becomes eligible for Missouri's Medicaid program.

The ACA has four main components to its reform of health care financing:

1. *Individual mandate:* Beginning in 2014, the ACA requires virtually all US citizens and legal residents to have insurance coverage meeting a federally determined "essential benefits" standard. This standard would allow high-deductible plans to qualify, with out-of-pocket cost-sharing capped at $5950 per individual and $11,900 per family, in 2010 dollars. Those who fail to purchase insurance and do not qualify for public programs such as Medicaid, Medicare, or veteran's health care benefits must pay a tax penalty which would be gradually phased in by 2016, when it would equal the greater of $695 per year for an individual (up to $2085 for a family) or 2.5% of household income. Individuals and families below 400% of the Federal Policy Level are eligible for income-based sliding-scale federal subsidies to help them purchase the required health insurance.

2. *Employer mandate:* Also beginning in 2014, employers with 50 or more full-time employees face a financial penalty if their employees are not enrolled in an employer-sponsored health plan meeting the essential

benefit standard and any of their employees apply for federal subsidies for individually purchased insurance. While this measure does not technically mandate large employers to provide health benefits to their full-time workers, it functionally has this effect by penalizing employers who do not provide insurance benefits and leave their employees to fend for themselves to comply with the individual mandate.

3. *Medicaid eligibility expansion*: As discussed in Chapter 2, Medicaid eligibility has traditionally required both a low income and a "categorical" eligibility requirement, such as being a child or an adult with a permanent disability. Effective in 2014, the ACA eliminates the categorical eligibility requirement and requires that states make all US citizens and legal residents below 133% of the Federal Poverty Level eligible for their Medicaid programs. In 2011, 133% of the Federal Poverty Level was $14,484 for a single person and $29,726 for a family of 4. The federal government pays states 100% of the Medicaid costs for beneficiaries qualifying under the expanded eligibility criteria for 2014 through 2016, with states contributing 10% after 2016. The benefit package is similar to current Medicaid benefits.

4. *Insurance market regulation*: The ACA also imposes some new rules on private insurance. One of the first measures of the ACA to be implemented in 2010 was a requirement that private health plans allow young adults up to age 26 to remain covered as dependents under their parents' health insurance policies. The ACA also eliminates caps on total insurance benefits payouts, prohibits denial of coverage based on preexisting conditions, and limits the extent of experience rating to a maximum ratio of 3-to-1 between a plan's highest and lowest premium charge for the same benefit package. The ACA also establishes state-based insurance exchanges to function as a clearing house to assist people seeking coverage under the individual mandate to shop for insurance plans meeting the federal standards (Kingsdale and Bertko, 2010). The benefit packages offered by plans in the exchanges would vary depending on whether individuals purchase a low-premium bronze plan with high out-of-pocket costs, a high-premium platinum plan with low out-of-pocket costs, or the intermediate silver or gold plans. These regulatory measures were deemed by many to be essential to the feasibility and fairness of an individual mandate. For example, mandates cannot work if insurers may deny coverage to individuals with preexisting conditions or steeply experience rate premiums. The insurance industry, for its part, balks at these types of market reforms in the absence of a mandate, fearing adverse disproportionate enrollment of high-risk individuals when coverage is voluntary.

The major coverage provisions of the ACA and their timeline for implementation are summarized in Table 15–3.

Table 15–3. Key coverage measures and implementation timeline for the Affordable Care Act of 2010

- High-risk health insurance pools for individuals with no insurance due to preexisting conditions (2010)
- Expansion of dependent coverage for young adults up to age 26 (2010)
- Elimination of provisions that allow health insurers to cap lifetime benefits or deny coverage to children based on preexisting conditions (2010)
- Reductions of the coverage gap for prescription medications under Medicare Part D (2011, phased in through 2020)
- Expansion of Medicaid to all individuals below 133% of the federal poverty level (2014)
- Individual health insurance mandate (2014)
- Subsidized health insurance exchanges for the uninsured to purchase insurance (2014)
- Elimination of provisions that allow health insurers to deny coverage based on preexisting conditions (2014)
- Requirement for employers with 50 or more employees to provide health care coverage or pay a penalty (2014)

Source: Kaiser Family Foundation. Summary of the New Health Reform Law, available at http://www.kff.org/ healthreform/upload/8061.pdf.

If the ACA is implemented in its entirety, 32 million of the 51 million uninsured Americans are expected to receive insurance coverage, an estimated 16 million through Medicaid expansion and 16 million through the individual mandate (Kaiser Family Foundation, 2010). None of the coverage expansion measures would benefit undocumented immigrants; they would not be eligible for federal premium subsidies under the individual mandate nor for Medicaid except for emergency care.

The ACA is expected to cost $938 billion over 10 years, with most of the costs associated with Medicaid expansion and individual mandate subsidies. The law is financed by a combination of new taxes and fees and by cost savings in the Medicare and Medicaid programs. Individuals with earnings over $200,000 and married couples with earnings over $250,000 would pay more for Medicare Part A. Health insurance companies, pharmaceutical firms, and medical device manufacturers would pay yearly fees. Medicare Advantage insurance plans and hospitals would receive less payment from the Medicare program. The Congressional Budget Office estimated that the new law would reduce the federal deficit by $124 billion over 10 years, though the CBO projection is not universally accepted.

In developing a proposal to expand coverage by building on the existing pluralistic funding model rather than turning to a single-payer model, President Obama and his congressional allies successfully calculated that they would be able to garner the political support of some powerful interest groups, such as the American Medical Association and pharmaceutical industry, that had been stalwart opponents of health reform proposals in prior eras (Morone, 2010). However, some conservative groups that opposed the ACA did not relent after the Act's passage, and the ACA has come under political and judicial threats since its enactment. One of the first acts passed by the House of Representatives in its 2011 session after Republicans regained a majority of seats in the House was repeal of the ACA. The ACA remained law because the Senate, with a Democratic majority, did not vote to repeal. Republican Governors and Attorney Generals in many states filed suits against the ACA, challenging the constitutionality of the federal government's mandating of individuals to purchase a private product. Federal judges in district courts have issued different rulings on the constitutionality of the ACA, and the case will ultimately be heard by the US Supreme Court.

SECONDARY FEATURES OF NATIONAL HEALTH INSURANCE PLANS

The primary distinction among national health insurance approaches is the mode of financing: government versus employment-based versus individual-based health insurance, or a mixture of all three. But while the overall financing approach may be considered the headline news of reform proposals, some of the details in the fine print are extremely important in determining whether a universal coverage plan will be able to deliver true health security to the public (Table 15–4). What are some of these secondary features?

▶ Benefit Package

An important feature of any health plan is its benefit package. Most national health insurance proposals cover hospital care, physician visits, laboratory, x-rays, physical and occupational therapy, inpatient pharmacy, and other services usually emphasizing acute care. One important benefit not included in the original Medicare program was coverage of outpatient medications. This coverage was later added in 2003 under Medicare Part D. Mental health services have often not been fully integrated into the benefit package of universal coverage proposals, a situation that has in part been addressed by the Mental Health Parity Act of 1996 and Mental Health Parity and Addiction Equity Act of 2008 which apply to group private health insurance plans. Neither the ACA nor most of its reform proposal precursors have included comprehensive benefits for dental care, long-term care, or complementary medicine services such as acupuncture.

▶ Patient Cost Sharing

Patient cost sharing involves payments made by patients at the time of receiving medical care services. It is sometimes broadened to include the amount of health insurance premium paid directly by an individual. Naturally, the breadth of the benefit package influences the amount of patient cost sharing: The more the services are not covered, the more the patients must

Table 15–4. Features of national health insurance plans

Primary Feature	
How the plan is financed	Government, employer mandate, and/or individual mandate?
Secondary Features	
Benefit package	Which services are covered?
Patient cost sharing	Will there still be considerable amounts of out-of-pocket payments in the form of patient share of premiums, deductibles, and copayments at the point of service?
Effect on existing programs	Do Medicare, Medicaid, and private insurance arrangements continue in their current form or are they largely dismantled?
Cost containment	Are cost controls introduced, and, if so, what type of controls?
Delivery system reform	Is only health care financing addressed, or does the plan call for changes in the organization and structure for delivering care?

pay out of pocket. Many plans impose patient cost sharing requirements on covered services, usually in the form of deductibles (a lump sum each year), coinsurance payments (a percentage of the cost of the service), or copayments (a fixed fee, eg, $10 per visit or per prescription). In general, single payer proposals restrict cost sharing to minimal levels, financing most benefits from taxes. In comparison, the individual mandate provisions of the Massachusetts Health Act and the ACA include considerable amounts of cost sharing. The ACA, for example, would require an individual such as Mandy Must with an income between 300% and 400% of the federal poverty level to pay up to 9.5% of her income toward a health insurance premium, in addition to having to potentially pay thousands of dollars per year in deductibles and copayments at the time of service. Critics have argued that this degree of out-of-pocket payment raises questions about whether the Affordable Care Act is a bit of a misnomer and that people of modest incomes will continue to be underinsured and subject to large amounts of out-of-pocket expenses. The arguments for and against cost sharing as a cost containment tool are discussed in Chapter 9.

▶ Effects on Medicare, Medicaid, and Private Insurance

Any national health insurance program must interact with existing health care programs, whether Medicare, Medicaid, or private insurance plans. Single-payer proposals make among the most far-reaching changes:

Medicaid and private insurance are eliminated in their current form and are melded into a single insurance program that resembles a Medicare-type program for all Americans. The most sweeping versions of individual mandate plans, such as that proposed by the Heritage Foundation, would dismantle both employment-based private insurance and government-administered insurance programs. Employer mandates, which extend rather than supplant employment-based coverage, tend to have the least effect on existing dollar flow in the health care system, as do pluralistic models such as the ACA that preserve and extend existing financing models through mandates for private insurance and broadened eligibility for Medicaid.

▶ Cost Containment

By increasing people's access to medical care, national health insurance has the capacity to cause a rapid increase in national health expenditures, as did Medicare and Medicaid (see Chapter 2). By the 1990s, policymakers recognized that an increase in access must be balanced with measures to control costs.

Different national health insurance proposals have vastly disparate methods of containing costs. As noted above, individual- and employment-based proposals tend to use patient cost sharing as their chief cost control mechanism. In contrast, government-financed plans look more to global budgeting and regulation of fees to keep expenditures down. Single-payer plans, which concentrate health care funds in a single public insurer, can more easily establish a global budgeting approach than can plans with multiple private insurers.

Proposals that build on the existing pluralistic financing model of US health care, such as the Clinton health plan and the ACA, face challenges in taming the unrelenting increases in national health care expenditures that seem to be endemic to a fragmented financing system. One of the items that contributed to the demise of President Clinton's health reform proposal before it could even be formally introduced as a bill in Congress was the inclusion of a measure to allow the federal government to cap the annual rates of increases in private health insurance premiums. President Obama eschewed such a regulatory approach in developing the ACA, and the ACA includes much weaker language about private insurance plans needing to "justify" premium increases to be able to continue to participate in state health insurance exchanges. In an effort to control costs, the ACA limits the percentage of health insurance premiums that can be retained by an insurance company in the form of overhead and profits (a concept known as the "medical loss ratio," whereby a greater loss ratio means more premium dollars being "lost" by the company in the form of payments for actual health care services). The ACA also caps the amount that an employer can contribute toward a health insurance premium as a nontaxable benefit to the employee ($10,200 for an individual policy and $27,500 for a family policy), in an attempt to discourage enrollment in the most expensive plans. Many of the savings in the ACA are expected to come from slowing the rate of growth in expenditures for Medicare through measures such as reducing payments to Medicare Advantage HMO plans and appointing an Independent Payment Advisory Board to recommend methods to contain Medicare costs. Yet another strategy of the ACA for addressing costs is to redesign health care delivery to achieve better value, discussed next.

▶ Reform of Health Care Delivery

Throughout the history of national health insurance proposals in the United States, reformers viewed their primary goal as modifying the methods of financing health care to achieve universal coverage. Addressing how providers were paid often emerged as a closely related consideration because of its importance for making universal coverage affordable. However, intervening in the way in which health care was organized and delivered was typically not something that featured prominently in reform proposals. Reformers tended to have their work cut out to overcome the strong opposition of the AMA and hospital associations to health insurance reform without further antagonizing those interests by challenging professional sovereignty over health care organization and delivery. Even many advocates of single payer reform in the United States looked to the lessons of the introduction of government insurance programs in the Canadian provinces, where until recently government took great pains to largely focus on insurance financing and payment rate regulation and not on reforming models for care delivery.

The ACA went considerably farther than most previous major reform proposals in the United States in including measures to shape health care delivery. The ACA created an Innovation Center in the Centers for Medicare and Medicaid Services to spearhead efforts to redesign care models in the United States. One of the charges to the Innovation Center is to promote Accountable Care Organizations. As discussed in Chapter 6, Accountable Care Organizations are intended to be provider-organized systems for delivering care that can emphasize more integrated and coordinated models of care for defined populations of patients, with financial incentives to reward higher value care. The Innovation Center also has responsibility for encouraging development of primary care Patient-Centered Medical Homes, also discussed in Chapter 5. Other measures in the ACA call for pilot programs to expand the roles of nurses, pharmacists, and other health care professionals in redesigned care models.

WHICH FINANCING MODEL FOR NATIONAL HEALTH INSURANCE PLAN IS BEST?

Historically, in the United States the government-financed single payer road to national health insurance is the oldest and most traveled of the three approaches. Advocates of government financing cite its universality: Everyone is insured in the same plan simply by virtue of being a US resident. Its simplicity creates a potential cost saving: The 25% of health expenditures spent on administration could be reduced, thus making available funds to extend health insurance to the uninsured. Employers would be relieved of the burden of providing health insurance to their employees. Employees would regain free choice of physician, choice that is being lost as employers are choosing which health plans (and therefore which physicians) are available to their workforce. Health insurance would be delinked from jobs, so that people changing jobs or losing a job would not be forced to change or lose their health coverage. Single-payer advocates, citing the experience of other nations, argue that cost control works only when all health care moneys are channeled through a single mechanism with the capacity to set budgets (Himmelstein and Woolhandler, 1989). While opponents accuse the government-financed approach as an invitation to bureaucracy, single-payer advocates point out that private insurers have average administrative costs of 14%, far higher than government programs such as Medicare with its 2% administrative overhead. A cost-control advantage intrinsic to tax-financed systems in which a public agency serves as the single payer for health care is the administrative efficiency of collecting and dispensing revenues under this arrangement.

Single-payer detractors charge that one single government payer would have too much power over people's health choices, dictating to physicians and patients which treatments they can receive and which they cannot, resulting in waiting lines and the rationing of care. Opponents also state that the shift in health care financing from private payments (out of pocket, individual insurance, and employment-based insurance) to taxes would be unacceptable in an antitax society. Moreover, the United States has a long history of politicians and government agencies being overly influenced by wealthy private interests, and this has contributed to making the public mistrustful of the government.

The employer mandate approach—requiring all employers to pay for the health insurance of their employees—is seen by its supporters as the most logical way to raise enough funds to insure the uninsured without massive tax increases (though employer mandates have been called hidden taxes). Because most people younger than 65 years now receive their health insurance through the workplace, it may be less disruptive to extend this process rather than change it.

The conservative advocates of individual-based insurance and the liberal supporters of single-payer plans both criticize employer mandate plans, saying that forcing small businesses—many of whom do not insure their employees—to shoulder the fiscal burden of insuring the uninsured is inequitable and economically disastrous; rather than purchasing health insurance for their employees, many small businesses may simply lay off workers, thereby pitting health insurance against jobs. Moreover, because millions of people change their jobs in a given year, job-linked health insurance is administratively cumbersome and insecure for employees, whose health security is tied to their job. Finally, critics point out that under the employer mandate approach, "Your boss, not your family, chooses your physician"; changes in the health plans offered by employers often force employees and their families to change physicians, who may not belong to the health plans being offered.

Advocates of the individual mandate assert that their approach, if adopted as the primary means of financing coverage, would free employers of the obligation to provide health insurance, and would grant individuals a stable source of health insurance whether they are employed, change jobs, or become disabled. There would be no need either to burden small businesses with new expenses and thereby disrupt job growth or to raise taxes substantially. While opponents argue that low-income families would be unable to afford the mandatory purchase of health insurance, supporters claim that income-related tax credits are a fair and effective method to assist such families (Butler, 1991).

The individual mandate approach is criticized as inefficient, with each family having to purchase its own health insurance. To enforce a requirement that every person buy coverage could be even more difficult for health insurance than for automobile insurance. Moreover, to reduce the price of their premiums, many families would purchase "bare-bones insurance" plans with low-cost, high-deductible coverage and a scanty benefit package, thereby leaving lower- and middle-income families with potentially unaffordable out-of-pocket costs.

CONCLUSION

The concept of national health insurance rests on the belief that everyone should contribute to finance health care and everyone should benefit. People who pay more than they benefit are likely to benefit more than they pay years down the road when they face an expensive health problem. In 2009, national health insurance took center stage in the United States with the fierce debate over health reform legislation that resulted in the ACA. This debate revealed a wide gulf between those who believe that all people should have financial access to health care and those who do not. The fate of the ACA will determine which of those two beliefs holds sway in the United States, until now the only developed nation that does not insure virtually all its citizens for health care.

REFERENCES

Bodenheimer T, Grumbach K. Financing universal health insurance: Taxes, premiums, and the lessons of social insurance. *J Health Polit Policy Law.* 1992;17:439.

Butler SM. A tax reform strategy to deal with the uninsured. *JAMA.* 1991;265:2541.

Clark CR et al. Lack of access due to costs remains a problem for some in Massachusetts despite the state's health reforms. *Health Aff.* 2011;30:247.

Emanuel EJ, Fuchs VR. Health care vouchers—a proposal for universal coverage. *N Engl J Med.* 2005;352:1255.

Himmelstein DU, Woolhandler S. Writing Committee of Physicians for a National Health Program: A national health program for the United States: A physicians' proposal. *N Engl J Med.* 1989;320:102.

Kaiser Family Foundation. Summary of New Health Reform Law, 2010. http://www.kff.org/healthreform/upload/8061.pdf. Accessed August 22, 2011.

Kingsdale J, Bertko J. Insurance exchanges under health reform: Six design issues for the states. *Health Aff.* 2010;29:1158.

Long SK, Stockley K. Sustaining health reform in a recession: An update on Massachusetts as of Fall 2009. *Health Aff.* 2010;29:1234.

Morone J. Presidents and health reform: From Franklin D. Roosevelt to Barack Obama. *Health Aff.* 2010;29:1096.

Starr P. *The Social Transformation of American Medicine.* New York: Basic Books; 1982.

Conflict and Change in America's Health Care System

As this book enters its closing chapters, it is worth stepping back from the detailed workings of the US health care system to view the system as a larger whole. Who are the major actors? How have they interacted over the past few decades? What might the future bring?

THE FOUR MAJOR ACTORS

The health care sector of the nation's economy is a 2.5 trillion dollar-plus system that finances, organizes, and provides health care services for the people of the United States. Four major actors can be found on this stage (Table 16–1).

1. The *purchasers* supply the funds. These include individual health care consumers, businesses that pay for the health insurance of their employees, and the government, which pays for care through public programs such as Medicare and Medicaid. All purchasers of health care are ultimately individuals, because individuals finance businesses by purchasing their products and fund the government by paying taxes. Nonetheless, businesses and the government assume special importance as the nation's *organized* purchasers of health care.

2. The *insurers* receive money from the purchasers and reimburse the providers. Traditional insurers take money from purchasers (individuals or businesses), assume risk, and pay providers when policyholders require medical care. Yet some insurers are the same as purchasers; the government can be viewed as an insurer or purchaser in the Medicare and Medicaid programs, and businesses that self-insure their employees can similarly occupy both roles.

(In previous chapters, we have used the term "payer" to refer to both purchasers and insurers.)

3. The *providers*, including hospitals, physicians, nurses, nurse practitioners, physician assistants, pharmacists, social workers, nursing homes, home care agencies, and pharmacies, actually provide the care. While health maintenance organizations (HMOs) are generally insurers, some are also providers, owning hospitals and employing physicians.

4. The *suppliers* are the pharmaceutical, medical supply, and computer industries, which manufacture equipment, supplies, and medications used by providers to treat patients.

Insurers, providers, and suppliers make up the health care industry. Each dollar spent on health care represents an expense to the purchasers and a gain to the health care industry. In the past, purchasers viewed this expense as an investment, money spent to improve the health of the population and thereby the economic and social vitality of the nation. But over the past 35 years, a fundamental conflict has intensified between the purchasers and the health care industry: The purchasers wish to reduce, and the health care industry to increase, the number of dollars spent on health care. We will now explore the changing relationships among purchasers, insurers, providers, and suppliers.

THE YEARS 1945 TO 1970: THE PROVIDER–INSURER PACT

During this period, independent hospitals and small private physician offices populated the US health delivery system (see Chapter 6). Some large institutions

Table 16–1. The four major actors

Purchasers
    Individuals
    Employers
    Government
Insurers
Providers
    Hospitals
    Nursing homes
    Home care agencies
    Pharmacies
    Physicians
    Other caregivers
Suppliers
    Pharmaceutical companies
    Medical supply companies
    Computer equipment

existed that combined hospital and physician care (eg, the Kaiser–Permanente system, the Mayo Clinic, and urban medical school complexes), but these were the exception (Starr, 1982). Competition among health care providers was minimal because most geographic areas did not have an excess of facilities and personnel. The health care financing system included hundreds of private insurance companies, joined by the governmental Medicare and Medicaid programs enacted in 1965. The United States had a relatively dispersed health care industry.

Bert Neighbor was a 63-year-old man who developed abdominal pain in 1962. Because he was well insured under Blue Cross, his physician placed him in Metropolitan Hospital for diagnostic studies. On the sixth hospital day, a colon cancer was surgically removed. On the fifteenth day, Mr. Neighbor went home. The hospital sent its $1200 bill to Blue Cross, which paid the hospital for its total costs in caring for Mr. Neighbor. In calculating Mr. Neighbor's bill, Metropolitan Hospital included a small part of the cost of the 80-bed new building under construction.

At a subsequent meeting of the Blue Cross board of directors, the hospital administrator (also a Blue Cross director) was asked whether it was reasonable to include the cost of capital improvements when preparing a bill. Other Blue Cross directors, also hospital administrators with construction plans, argued that it was proper, and the matter was dropped. In the same meeting, the directors voted a 34% increase in Blue Cross premiums. Sixteen years later, a study revealed that the metropolitan area had 300 excess hospital beds, with hospital occupancy down from 82% to 60% over the past decade.

A defining characteristic of the health care industry was an alliance of insurers and providers. This provider–insurer pact was cemented with the creation of Blue Cross and Blue Shield, the nation's largest health insurance system for half a century (see Chapter 2). Blue Cross was formed by the American Hospital Association, and Blue Shield was run by state medical societies affiliated with the American Medical Association. In the case of the Blues, the provider–insurer relationship was more than a political alliance; it involved legal control of insurers by providers. As in the example of Metropolitan Hospital, the providers set generous rules of reimbursement, and the Blues made the payments without asking too many questions (Law, 1974). Commercial insurers usually played by the reimbursement rules already formulated by the physicians, hospitals, and Blues, paying for medical services without asking providers to justify their prices or the reasons for the services.

By the 1960s, the power of the provider–insurer pact was so great that the hospitals and Blue Cross virtually wrote the reimbursement provisions of Medicare and Medicaid, guaranteeing that physicians and hospitals would be paid with the same bountiful formulas used for private patients (Law, 1974). With open-ended reimbursement policies, the costs of health care inflated at a rapid pace.

The disinterest of the chief organized purchaser (business) stemmed from two sources: the healthy economy and the tax subsidy for health insurance. From 1945 through 1970, US business controlled domestic and foreign markets with little foreign competition. Labor unions in certain industries had gained generous wages and fringe benefits, and business could afford these costs because profits were high and world economic growth was robust (Kuttner, 1980; Kennedy, 1987). The cost of health insurance for employees was a tiny fraction of total business expenses.

Moreover, payments by business for employee health insurance were considered a tax-deductible business expense, thereby cushioning any economic drain on business (Reinhardt, 1993). For these reasons, increasing costs generated by providers and reimbursed by insurers were passed on to business, which with few complaints paid higher and higher premiums for employees' health insurance, and thereby underwrote the expanding health care system. No countervailing forces "put the brakes" on the enthusiasm that united providers and the public in support of a medical industry that strived to translate the proliferation of biomedical breakthroughs into an improvement in people's lives.

THE 1970S: TENSIONS DEVELOP

Jerry Neighbor, Bert Neighbor's son, developed abdominal pain in 1978. Because Blue Cross no longer paid for in-hospital diagnostic testing, his physician ordered outpatient x-ray studies. When colon cancer was discovered, Jerry Neighbor was admitted to Metropolitan Hospital on the morning of his surgery. His total hospital stay was 9 days, 6 days shorter than his father's stay in 1962. Since 1962, medical care costs had risen by approximately 10% per year. Blue Cross paid Metropolitan Hospital $460 for each of the 9 days Jerry Neighbor spent in the hospital, for a total cost of $4140. The Blue Cross board of directors, which in 1977 included for the first time more business than hospital representatives, submitted a formal proposal to the regional health planning agency to reduce the number of hospital beds in the region, in order to keep hospital costs down. The planning agency board had a majority of hospital and physician representatives, and they voted the proposal down.

In the early 1970s, the United States fell from its postwar position of economic dominance, as Western Europe and Japan gobbled up markets (not only abroad but in the United States itself) formerly controlled by US companies. The United States' share of world industrial production was dropping, from 60% in 1950 to 30% in 1980. Except for a few years during the mid-1980s, inflation or unemployment plagued the United States from 1970 until the early 1990s.

The new economic reality was a critical motor of change in the health care system. With less money in their respective pockets, individual health care consumers, business, and government became concerned with the accelerating flow of dollars into health care. Prominent business-oriented journals published major critiques of the health care industry and its rising costs (Bergthold, 1990). A new concern for primary care, which seemed underemphasized in relation to specialty and hospital care, spread within the health professions. These developments produced tensions within the health industry itself.

Faced with Blue Cross premium increases of 25% to 50% in a single year, angry Blue Cross subscribers protested at state hearings in eastern and midwestern states and challenged hospital control over Blue Cross boards (Law, 1974). Some state governments began to regulate hospital construction, and a few states initiated hospital rate regulation. The federal government established a network of health planning agencies, in an attempt to slow hospital growth. Peer review was established to monitor the appropriateness of physician services under Medicare. Thus, the purchasers took on an additional role as health care regulators. But the health care industry resisted these attempts by purchasers to control health care costs. Medical inflation continued at a rate far above that of inflation in the general economy (Starr, 1982).

Nonetheless, these early initiatives from the purchasers made an impact on the provider–insurer pact. As pressure mounted on insurers not to increase premiums, insurers demanded that services be provided at lower cost. Blue Cross, widely criticized as playing the role of an intermediary that passed increased hospital costs on to a helpless public, legally separated from the American Hospital Association in 1972 (Law, 1974). State medical societies were forced to relinquish some of their control over Blue Shield plans. Conflicts erupted between providers and insurers as the latter imposed utilization review procedures to reduce the length of hospital stays. Hospitals, which had hitherto purchased the newest diagnostic and surgical technology desired by physicians or their medical staff, began to deny such requests because insurers would no longer guarantee their reimbursement. Moreover, the glut of hospital beds and specialty physicians, which had been produced by the attractive reimbursements of the 1960s and the influence of the biomedical model on medical education (see Chapter 5), turned on itself as half-empty hospitals and half-busy surgeons began to compete with one another for patients. Strains were showing within the provider–insurer pact.

By the late 1970s, the deepening of the economic crisis created a nationwide tax revolt. As a result, governments attempted to reduce spending on such programs as health care (Kuttner, 1980). But major change was still awaiting the arrival of the other powerful purchaser: business.

THE 1980S: THE REVOLT OF THE PURCHASERS

In 1989, Ryan Neighbor, Jerry Neighbor's brother, became concerned when he noticed blood in his stools; he decided to see a physician. Six months earlier, his company had increased the annual health insurance deductible to $1000, which could be avoided by joining one of the HMOs offered by the company. Ryan Neighbor opted for the Blue Cross HMO, but his family physician was not involved in that HMO, and Mr. Neighbor had to pick another physician from the HMO's list. The physician diagnosed colon cancer; Ryan Neighbor was not allowed to see the surgeon who had operated on his brother but was sent to a Blue Cross HMO surgeon. While Mr. Neighbor respected Metropolitan Hospital, his surgery was scheduled at Crosstown Hospital; Blue Cross had refused to sign a contract with Metropolitan when the hospital failed to negotiate down from its $1800 per diem rate. Ryan Neighbor's entire Crosstown Hospital stay was 5 days, and the HMO paid the hospital $7500, based on its $1500 per diem contract.

The late 1980s produced a severe shock: The cost of employer-sponsored health plans jumped 18.6% in 1988 and 20.4% in 1989 (Cantor et al, 1991). Between 1976 and 1988, the percentage of total payroll spent on health benefits almost doubled from 5% to 9.7% (Bergthold, 1991). In another development, many large corporations began to self-insure. Rather than paying money to insurance companies to cover their employees, employers increasingly took on the health insurance function themselves and used insurance companies only for claims processing and related administrative tasks. In 1991, 40% of employees receiving employer-sponsored health benefits were in self-insured plans. Self-insurance placed employers at risk for health care expenditures and forced them to pay more attention to the health care issue. These three

developments (ie, a troubled economy, rising health care costs, and self-insurance) catapulted big business into the center of the health policy debate, with cost control as its rallying cry. Business, the major private purchaser of health care, became the motor driving unprecedented change in the health care landscape (Bergthold, 1990). Business threw its clout behind managed care, particularly HMOs, as a cost-control device. By shifting from fee-for-service to capitated reimbursement, managed care could transfer a portion of the health expenditure risk from purchasers and insurers to providers (see Chapter 4).

Individual health care consumers, in their role as purchasers, also showed some clout during the late 1980s. Because employers were shifting health care payments to employees, labor unions began to complain bitterly about health care costs, and major strikes took place over the issue of health care benefits. More than 70% of people polled in a 1992 Louis Harris survey favored serious health care cost controls (Smith et al, 1992). The growing tendency of private health insurers to reduce their risks by dramatic premium increases and policy cancellations for policyholders with chronic illnesses created a series of horror stories in the media that turned health insurance companies into highly unpopular institutions.

During the 1980s, the government was facing the tax revolt and budget deficits, and it took measures designed to slow the rising costs of Medicare and Medicaid, with limited success. The 1983 Medicare Prospective Payment System (diagnosis-related groups [DRGs]) reduced the rate of increase of Medicare hospital costs, but outpatient Medicare costs and costs borne by private purchasers escalated in response. In 1989, Medicare physician payments were brought under tighter control, resulting in Medicare physician expenditures growing at only 5.3% per year from 1991 to 1993, compared with 11.3% per year from 1984 to 1991 (Davis and Burner, 1995). Numerous states scaled back their Medicaid programs, but because of the economic recession and the growing crisis of uninsurance (see Chapter 3), the federal government was forced to expand Medicaid eligibility, and Medicaid costs rose faster than ever before. Governments began to experiment with managed care for Medicare and Medicaid as a cost-control device.

The most significant development of the 1980s was the growth of selective contracting. Purchasers and insurers had usually reimbursed any and all physicians and hospitals. Under selective contracting, purchasers and insurers choose which providers they will pay and which they will not (Bergthold, 1990). In 1982, for example, California passed a law bringing selective contracting to the state's Medicaid program and to private health insurance plans. The law was passed because large California corporations formed a political coalition to challenge physician and hospital interests, and because insurers deserted their former provider allies and joined the purchasers (Bergthold, 1990). The message of selective contracting was clear: Purchasers and insurers will do business only with providers who keep costs down. This development, especially when linked with capitation payments that placed providers at risk, changed the entire dynamic within the health care industry. For patients, it meant that like Ryan Neighbor, they had lost free choice of physician because employers could require employees to change health plans and therefore physicians. For the health care industry, selective contracting meant fierce competition for contracts and the crumbling of the provider–insurer pact.

As a result of the purchasers' revolt, managed care became a burgeoning movement in US health care. By 1990, 95% of insured employees were enrolled in some form of managed care plan, including fee-for-service plans with utilization management, preferred provider organizations (PPOs), and HMOs. The growth of managed care plans, especially HMOs, competing against one another for contracts with business and the government, changed the entire political topography of US health care (Table 16–2).

THE 1990S: THE BREAKUP OF THE PROVIDER–INSURER PACT

In 1994, Pamela Neighbor, Ryan's cousin, developed constipation. Earlier that year, her law firm had switched from Blue Cross HMO to Apple a Day HMO because the premiums were lower; all employees of the firm were forced to change their physicians. Apple a Day contracted only with Crosstown Hospital, whose rates were lower than those of Metropolitan, resulting in Metropolitan losing patients and closing its doors. Ms. Neighbor's new physician diagnosed colon cancer and arranged for her admission to Crosstown Hospital for surgery. The physician's office was across the street from the now-closed Metropolitan Hospital.

Four days before the procedure, a newspaper headline proclaimed that Apple a Day and Crosstown had failed to agree on a contract. The colonoscopy was canceled. Pamela Neighbor waited to see what would happen next.

During the 1990s, many metropolitan areas in the United States, and some smaller cities and towns, experienced upheavals of their medical care landscape. Independent hospitals began to merge into hospital systems. In the most mature managed care markets, three or four health care networks were competing for those patients with private insurance, Medicare, or Medicaid. Selective contracting allowed purchasers and insurers to set reimbursement rates to health care providers. HMOs that demanded higher premiums from employers did not get contracts and lost their enrollees. Providers who demanded higher payment from HMOs were cut out of HMO contracts and lost many of their patients.

Selective contracting tended to disorganize rather than organize medical care patterns. Physicians were forced to admit patients from one HMO to one hospital and those from another HMO to a different hospital. Laboratory, x-ray, and specialist services close to a primary care physician's office were sometimes not covered under contracts with that physician's patients' HMO, forcing referrals to be made across town. In one highly publicized case with a tragic outcome, the parents of a 6-month-old infant with bacterial meningitis were told by their HMO to drive the child almost 40 miles to a hospital that had a contract with that HMO, passing several high-quality hospitals along the way (Anders, 1996).

The 1990s was a period of purchaser dominance over health care. The federal government stopped Medicare inflation in its tracks through the tough provisions of the Balanced Budget Act of 1997. The average annual growth in Medicare expenditures declined from 12% in the early 1990s to zero in 1999 and 2000. On the private side, employers bargained hard with HMOs, causing insurance premium annual growth to drop from 13% in 1990 to 3% in 1995 and 1996. In California, employer purchasers consolidated into coalitions to negotiate with HMOs. The Pacific Business Group on Health, negotiating on behalf of large companies for 400,000 employees, and California Public Employee Retirement System (CalPERS), representing a million public employees, forced HMO premiums to go down during the 1990s. Enrollment in HMOs

Table 16–2. Historical overview of US health care

1945–1970: Provider–insurer pact
- Independent hospitals and small private practices
- Many private insurers
- Providers tended to dominate the insurers, especially in Blue Cross and Blue Shield
- Purchasers (individuals, businesses, and, after 1965, government) had relatively little power
- Reimbursements for providers were generous

The 1970s: Tensions develop
- Purchasers (especially government) become concerned about costs of health care
- Under pressure from purchasers, insurers begin to question generous reimbursements of providers

The 1980s: Revolt of the purchasers
- Purchasers (business joining government) become very concerned with rising health care costs
- Attempts are made to reduce health cost inflation through Medicare DRGs, fee schedules, capitated HMOs, and selective contracting

The 1990s: Breakup of the provider–insurer pact
- Spurred by the purchasers, selective contracting spreads widely as a mechanism to reduce costs
- Price competition is introduced
- Large integrated health networks are formed
- Large physician groups emerge
- Insurance companies dominate many managed care markets
- For-profit institutions increase in importance
- Insurers gain increasing power over providers, creating conflict and ending the provider–insurer pact

The new millennium: provider power reemerges
- HMOs fade in importance
- Hospitals consolidate into hospital systems, forcing insurers to pay them more
- Insurers respond by consolidating, with a few large national insurers dominating many markets
- Many specialists form single specialty groups
- Specialists move profitable procedures out of hospitals into specialist-owned centers
- A crisis develops in primary care
- Hospital–physician relations are in flux
- Pharmaceutical companies come under attack
- The paradox of excess and deprivation deepens

DRG, diagnosis-related group; HMO, health maintenance organization.

grew rapidly in the 1990s, expanding from 40 million enrollees in 1990 to 80 million in 1999.

THE NEW MILLENNIUM: PROVIDER POWER RE-EMERGES

In 2005, Pamela Neighbor, who was feeling well, made an appointment for her yearly colon cancer follow-up. The IPA in which her physician practiced had recently gone bankrupt and closed its doors. Ms. Neighbor's employer had switched its employees from Apple a Day Insurance Company's HMO product to Apple a Day PPO, allowing patients to access most of the physicians and all the hospitals in town. Ms. Neighbor had a difficult time finding a new primary care physician, and when she found one, it took several weeks to get an appointment. Eventually, a colonoscopy was scheduled at a diagnostic center owned by a group of *gastroenterologists. She was diagnosed with a second colon cancer and her primary care physician arranged for her admission to Crosstown Hospital. Ms. Neighbor never saw her primary care physician in the hospital; a surgeon plus a salaried inpatient physician called a hospitalist cared for Ms. Neighbor during her 4-day hospital stay. Apple a Day paid Crosstown Hospital $7200, $1800 per diem.*

Several trends characterize the first decade of the twenty-first century: the counter-revolution by providers, consolidation in the health care market, growing power of specialists and specialty services, increasing physician–hospital tensions, an emerging crisis in primary care, growing criticism of pharmaceutical companies, and a steady increase in the uninsured and underinsured population.

The Provider Counter-Revolution

In the mid-1990s, most health care analysts were certain that tightly managed care—with purchasers and insurers dominating health care providers—had become the new paradigm for health care in the United States. By 2001, this certainty had evaporated (Robinson, 2001). From 2000 to 2010, HMO enrollment dropped from 32% to 19% of insured employees, with only 19% of HMOs affiliated with an integrated delivery system. During those years, preferred provider organization (PPO) enrollment grew from about 30% to 60% of insured employees (Claxton et al, 2010). Tightly managed care was faltering.

The first decade of the twenty-first century could be called the era of the provider counter-revolution. Hospitals consolidated into hospital systems and demanded large price increases from insurers. Physicians balked at tight managed care contracts. Negotiations between health care providers and insurers became increasingly hostile, with one side or the other often refusing to sign contracts. As hospitals and providers gained an upper hand in negotiations with health plans, HMOs in turn demanded more money from employers. Insurance premiums for family coverage went from an average of $6,000 per year in 2000 to almost $14,000 in 2010, with virtually no difference between HMO and PPO premiums (Claxton et al, 2010). Purchasers lost faith that HMOs could control costs.

At the same time, individuals have been stuck with a greater proportion of health care costs. Twenty percent of insured employees, up from 10% in 2006, have a deductible of $1000 or more for individual coverage. The percent of insured employees with high-deductible plans has risen from 5% in 2006 to 13% in 2010; in a typical high-deductible plan, employees pay over $3000 for their portion of the premium plus a deductible of $4000 (Claxton et al, 2010). Employees' out-of-pocket health care costs increased 34% from 2004 to 2007 (Gabel et al, 2009).

Consolidation in the Health Care Market

The intense competition of the 1990s stimulated consolidation among insurers and providers, as each vied to improve its bargaining power. Large HMOs bought up smaller ones and merged with one another. In most states, three large insurance companies control more than 60% of the market (Robinson, 2004). These companies generally offer a variety of products including HMO, PPO, high deductible, and Medicare Advantage plans. Three huge insurers, all for-profit, are Wellpoint with 34 million enrollees in 2010, United Healthcare with 32 million, and Aetna with 18 million.

Providers also consolidated. By 2001, 65% of hospitals were members of multihospital systems or networks (Bazzoli, 2004), and consolidation continued, though at a slower pace, through 2008. In many cities, two or three competing hospital systems encompass all hospitals. Hospital prices often rise rapidly after consolidation has taken place since payers are forced to contract with dominant hospital systems (Vogt, 2009). Specialists increasingly joined single-specialty groups, with the majority of cardiologists or orthopedists in some cities belonging to a dominant group (Liebhaber and Grossman, 2007). Private primary care and specialty practices are being acquired by hospital systems hoping to increase their market clout (Iglehart, 2011).

Consolidation went hand in hand with organizations converting from nonprofit to investor-owned "for-profit" status as they sought to raise capital for buy-outs, market expansion, and organizational infrastructure. For decades, for-profit companies have played a prominent role in health care, with the rise in the 1970s of the "medical–industrial complex" (Relman, 2007). For-profits, which owned 35% to 40% of health care services and facilities in 1990, expanded their reach during the 1990s. Nine of the largest 10 HMOs were for-profit by 1994. HMO stocks soared in the early

1990s and executives were rewarded with enormous compensation packages (Anders, 1996). Already in 1990, 77% of nursing homes and 50% of home health agencies were for-profit. Between 1993 and 1996, more than 100 nonprofit hospitals were taken over by for-profit hospital chains, though several financial scandals slowed down this trend. For-profit hospitals provide less charity care, treat fewer Medicaid patients, have higher administrative costs, and lower quality than nonprofit hospitals (Relman, 2007). By 2009, most specialty hospitals, imaging centers, ambulatory surgery centers were investor-owned (Relman, 2009).

▶ The Quest for Profitability and the Growing Power of Specialists and Specialty Services

That hospitals, physicians, and other providers respond to financial incentives is hardly a new phenomenon. As discussed in Chapter 5, more lucrative third-party payment for procedurally oriented specialty care has been one of the key factors shaping a physician workforce weighted toward nonprimary care fields and a hospital sector filled with tertiary care facilities. However, twenty-first-century health care in the United States is becoming characterized by a single-minded quest for profitability that is threatening traditional notions of professionalism and community service. Emblematic of this trend is the emergence of a new type of for-profit hospital, the specialty hospital fully or partially owned by groups of specialist physicians. As of 2010, 265 of these hospitals existed in the United States, typically limiting their services to cardiac and orthopedic procedures—service lines that are well reimbursed (Perry, 2010). Physician owners of these hospitals doubly benefit financially, receiving income from both the payment for the services they directly provide and their share of hospital profits. Moreover, physician owners often channel well-insured patients from nonprofit general hospitals to their own for-profit specialty hospitals. In one example, 16 cardiac surgeons and cardiologists shifted their patients with heart disease from a university medical center to a new hospital only caring for patients with heart disease; the number of cardiac surgeries performed at the university medical center dropped from over 600 to below 200 between 2002 and 2004, resulting in the loss of $12 million in revenues. Uninsured patients continued to have cardiac

procedures at the university hospital (Iglehart, 2005). For the community as a whole, the opening of a cardiac hospital is associated with increased rates of coronary revascularization (coronary artery bypass surgery and angioplasty), raising questions about whether all the additional procedures are medically appropriate (Nallamothu et al, 2007). Because of these problems with specialty hospitals, the Affordable Care Act of 2010 barred new specialty hospitals from receiving Medicare payments (Perry, 2010).

Similar financial incentives have attracted specialist physicians to set up many thousands of ambulatory surgery, diagnostic, and imaging centers that they own. A growing proportion of profitable services—cataract surgery and orthopedic procedures, diagnostic studies such as colonoscopies, and CT or MRI studies—have been shifted from hospital facilities to these physician-owned ambulatory centers. As with specialty hospitals, physicians earn income from both the services they directly provide and the facility's profits. Because general hospitals formerly earned considerable income from these procedures, this phenomenon has created major tensions between hospitals and specialists (Berenson et al, 2006b). The common practice of physicians referring patients for imaging tests at a facility owned by the same physician is associated with higher volumes of imaging services, increasing costs, and exposing patients to unnecessary radiation (Sunshine and Bhargavan, 2010).

Single-specialty groups have grown markedly since the late 1990s. Two major drivers of this growth are (1) the ability of organized specialists with market power in a local area to negotiate for high reimbursement rates from insurers and (2) the bringing together of capital to invest in specialist-owned surgery, diagnostic, and imaging centers. As a result of these trends, the income of specialists who offer procedural or imaging services has far outpaced the growth in earnings for primary care physicians (Bodenheimer et al, 2007). Multispecialty groups, which include primary care physicians and tend to have the best scores on quality report cards, are not growing in part because specialist physicians in multispecialty groups are expected to share their high revenues with lower-reimbursed primary care physicians (Casalino et al, 2004; Mehrotra et al, 2006).

Nonprofit community hospitals are responding to competition from specialist physicians by creating "specialty service lines" to attract specialist physicians and well-insured patients to their institutions. To create capacity for these profitable service lines, hospitals are de-emphasizing traditional medical-surgical wards. Whether the hospital is a nonprofit community hospital, a for-profit hospital, or a physician-owned specialty hospital, filling a hospital bed with a patient receiving an organ transplant or spine surgery is much more financially rewarding than filling the same bed with an elderly patient with pneumonia and heart failure, even if the latter patient has insurance. Strategic planning by hospitals increasingly focuses on how to maximize the most profitable service lines, rather than on how to provide the services most needed in the community (Berenson et al, 2006a).

Compounding this situation is the weakening claim hospitals can make on physicians for community service. Surgeons, diagnostic cardiologists, gastroenterologists, ophthalmologists, and radiologists can successfully run a medical practice without ever setting foot in a hospital by focusing their work on ambulatory centers of which these physicians are owners. Because these specialists no longer need the hospital, they feel little obligation to be on call for hospital emergency departments or for patients in intensive care. Hospitals are forced to pay specialists large sums to provide nighttime emergency department backup or are employing specialists to perform the duties formerly done for free by specialists on the hospital medical staff. The divorce of physicians from the community hospital is not limited to specialists. As a result of the hospitalist movement, many primary care physicians are never seen in a hospital. Hospitalists are physicians who specialize in the care of hospitalized patients. Most are employees of a hospital or hospital system; others are members of single-specialty hospitalist groups, which contract with hospitals to supply hospitalist physicians. Hospitalists are the fastest growing specialty in the history of medicine in the United States; the 500 hospitalists existing in 1997 have multiplied into about 30,000 hospitalists in 2010.

The quest for profitability is further aggravating the primary care-specialist imbalance in the physician workforce in the United States. In 2007, only 7% of US medical school graduates planned careers in adult primary care, with an adult primary care physician shortage projected at about 40,000 by 2020. Nurse practitioners and physician assistants help mitigate this shortage but their numbers are not sufficient to solve the problem. As a result, patients are having increasing difficulty gaining timely access to primary care or finding a new primary care physician. Although the causes of the declining career interest in primary care are multifactorial, the gap between primary care and specialty incomes is one reasons why growing numbers of US medical students and residents—many of whom have more than $150,000 in personal debts from medical school expenses—have turned away from careers in primary care (Bodenheimer and Pham, 2010).

These trends pull health care in the United States farther away from a primary care-based, community-responsive model. Evidence suggests that this trend will fuel continued inflation in health care costs without yielding commensurate benefits for the health of the public. A major reform of payment policies in the United States, along with a rethinking of the role of investor-owned enterprises in health care, will be required in order to realign financial incentives with the values that make for a well-functioning system.

▶ The Pharmaceutical Industry Comes Under Criticism

The rising tensions among purchasers, insurers, and providers spilled over to engulf health care's major supplier: the pharmaceutical industry. In 1988, prescription drugs accounted for 5.5% of national health expenditures. With 71% of drug costs borne out of pocket by individuals and only 18% paid by private insurance plans, these costs had little impact on insurers. In contrast, by 2009, prescription drug costs had risen to 10.1% of total health expenditures, with only 21% paid out of pocket, the rest covered by employers, insurers, and governmental purchasers. The growing cost of pharmaceuticals for the elderly became a major national issue. Because of its unaffordable prices and high profits, the pharmaceutical industry was becoming public enemy number one (Spatz, 2010).

For years, drug companies have been the most profitable industry in the United States, earning net profits after taxes close to 20% of revenues (19.3% in 2008), compared with 5% for all Fortune 500 firms. The pharmaceutical industry argues that high drug prices are justified by its expenditures on research and development of new drugs, yet the National Science Foundation estimates that true R&D spending is half of what the pharmaceutical industry claims (Congressional Budget Office, 2006). R&D for the largest drug companies consumed 14% of revenues in 2002, while marketing and administration accounted for 33% and after-tax net profits 21% (Reinhardt, 2004). Unlike many nations, the US government does not impose regulated prices on drugs; as a result of drug industry lobbying, the Medicare prescription drug coverage law passed in 2003 forbid the government to regulate drug prices (see Chapter 2). From 2006 to 2008, the health industry spent more money on lobbying than any other sector of the economy, and the drug industry was the largest contributor within the health industry (Steinbrook, 2008).

Companies developing a new brand-name drug enjoy a patent for 20 years from the date the patent application is filed, during which time no other company can produce the same drug. Once the patent expires, generic drug manufacturers can compete by selling the same product at lower prices. Some drug companies have waged legal battles to delay patent expirations on their brand name products or have paid generic drug manufacturers not to market generic alternatives (Stolberg and Gerth, 2000; Hall, 2001). In addition, the industry attempts to persuade physicians and patients to use brand-name products, spending $7 billion in 2009 on sales representatives' visits to physicians, journal advertising, and sponsorship of professional meetings, plus $4 billion on direct-to-consumer television ads (Kaiser Family Foundation, 2010). The federal Food and Drug Administration (FDA) has sent hundreds of letters to drug manufacturers, citing advertising violations including minimizing side effects and exaggerating benefits (Donohue et al, 2007). Four out of five physicians have some type of financial relationship with the pharmaceutical industry, ranging from accepting gifts to serving as a paid lecturer on behalf of a company. These physician–industry relationships influence physicians to prescribe new drugs that are the most expensive and whose safety has not been adequately evaluated (Campbell, 2007). Drug firms may pay medical school faculty physicians tens of thousands of dollars to participate on their corporate boards (Lo, 2010).

Most trials to determine the efficacy of prescription drugs are funded by that drug's manufacturer, and trials funded by industry are more likely than those with nonindustry funding to report results favorable to the funding company (Bero, 2007). Yet physicians base treatment decisions on these trials, which inform clinical practice guidelines. Authors of clinical practice guidelines often have ties to the pharmaceutical industry (Abramson and Starfield, 2005). From 2006 to 2010, at least 18 relatively new drugs were removed from the market because of serious side effects; in some cases, the manufacturer knew of the problems but hid them from the FDA and the public; in other cases, the FDA ignored the evidence. Some members of FDA committees recommending approval of a drug have ties to that drug's manufacturer, and these members are often not recused from the process (Angell, 2004).

These revelations have tainted the image of the pharmaceutical industry in the eyes of the medical profession and the public. Private health insurance companies have mounted the most effective response to the drug industry by creating tiered formularies in which generic drugs have lower copayments than brand-name drugs. As a result, 75% of all prescriptions filled in the United States in 2009 were for generic products (Spatz, 2010). This development has slowed the rate of growth of pharmaceutical costs. However, some brand-name drug companies are starting to produce generics, and the generic industry is starting to consolidate into fewer and larger companies; these trends could mean that generic prices may rise to levels not far below brand name prices.

THE CHALLENGE

The health care system has been dominated by a series of unstable power relationships among purchasers, insurers, providers, and suppliers. One of these actors may take center stage for a time, only to be pushed into the corner by another actor. Which entity has the leverage to get its way varies from city to city, depending on who has consolidated into larger institutions. Larger institutions can (in the case of providers and suppliers) demand to receive more money, or (in the case of purchasers and insurers) succeed in paying out less money. Patients continue to be at the mercy of these powerful institutions, as health care costs rise and as individuals bear a greater share of those costs.

Inequities in insurance coverage and in access to care continue, and cost control remains elusive. Whether the Affordable Care Act of 2010 will succeed in improving access and containing costs remains to be seen. The drive to make money—whether for specialist physicians, for-profit and nonprofit hospitals, insurers, or pharmaceutical companies—increasingly determines what happens in health care. For physicians, this economic motivation may clash with the professional commitment to patient welfare. The commitment of all health care professionals to the ethical principles of beneficence, nonmaleficence, patient autonomy, and distributive justice is tested on a daily basis in the profit-oriented environment of twenty-first century health care in America.

Chapter 1 introduced the paradox of excess and deprivation: Some people get too little care while others receive too much, which is costly and may be harmful. The first decade of the twenty-first century saw a sharpening of this paradox, with the number of uninsured climbing from 40 million to 50 million at the same time as the increasing number of specialist physicians owning their facilities was associated with growing volumes of expensive procedures, many of questionable appropriateness (Brownlee, 2007; Welch et al, 2011). Overcoming this paradox remains the fundamental challenge facing the health care system of the United States.

REFERENCES

Abramson J, Starfield B. The effect of conflict of interest on biomedical research and clinical practice guidelines. *J Am Board Fam Pract*. 2005;18:414.

Anders G. *Health Against Wealth: HMOs and the Breakdown of Medical Trust*. Boston, MA: Houghton Mifflin Company; 1996.

Angell M. *The Truth About the Drug Companies*. New York: Random House; 2004.

Bazzoli G. The corporatization of American hospitals. *J Health Polit Policy Law*. 2004;29:885.

Berenson RA et al. Specialty service lines: Salvos in the new medical arms race. *Health Affairs Web Exclusive*. 2006a; 25(5):w337.

Berenson RA et al. Hospital–physician relations: Cooperation, competition, or separation? *Health Aff Web Exclusive*. 2006b;26(1):w31.

Bergthold L. *Purchasing Power in Health*. New Brunswick, NJ: Rutgers University Press; 1990.

Bergthold L. The fat kid on the seesaw: American business and health care cost containment, 1970–1990. *Annu Rev Public Health*. 1991;12:157.

Bero L et al. Factors associated with findings of published trials of drug–drug comparisons. *PLoS Med*. 2007;4:e184.

Bodenheimer T et al. The primary care-specialty income gap: Why it matters. *Ann Intern Med*. 2007;146:301.

Bodenheimer T, Pham HH. Primary care: Current problems and proposed solutions. *Health Aff*. 2010;29:799.

Brownlee S. *Overtreated. Why Too Much Medicine Is Making Us Sicker and Poorer*. New York, NY: Bloomsbury; 2007.

Campbell EG. Doctors and drug companies—scrutinizing influential relationships. *N Engl J Med*. 2007;357:1796.

Cantor JC et al. Business leaders' views on American health care. *Health Aff*. 1991;10(1):98.

Casalino L et al. Growth of single-specialty medical groups. *Health Aff*. 2004;23(2):82.

Claxton G et al. Health benefits in 2010: Premiums rise modestly, workers pay more toward coverage. *Health Aff*. 2010;29:1942.

Congressional Budget Office. *Research and Development in the Pharmaceutical Industry*. 2006. www.cbo.gov/ftpdocs/76xx/doc7615/10-02-DrugR-D.pdf. Accessed November 26, 2011.

Davis MH, Burner ST. Three decades of Medicare: What the numbers tell us. *Health Aff*. 1995;14(4):231.

Donohue JM et al. A decade of direct-to-consumer advertising of prescription drugs. *N Engl J Med*. 2007;357:673.

Gabel JR et al. Trends in underinsurance and the afford-ability of employer coverage, 2004–2007. *Health Aff*. 2009;28:w595.

Hall SS. Prescription for profit. *New York Times Magazine*. March 11, 2001.

Iglehart JK. The emergence of physician-owned specialty hospitals. *N Engl J Med*. 2005;352:78.

Iglehart JK. Doctor-workers of the world, unite! *Health Aff*. 2011;30:556.

Kaiser Family Foundation. Prescription drug trends, 2010. www.kff.org.

Kennedy P. *The Rise and Fall of the Great Powers*. New York: Random House; 1987.

Kuttner R. *Revolt of the Haves*. New York, NY: Simon & Schuster; 1980.

Law SA. *Blue Cross: What Went Wrong?* New Haven, CT: Yale University Press; 1974.

Liebhaber A, Grossman JM. Physicians moving to mid-sized, single-specialty practices. Tracking Report No. 18. Washington, DC: Center for Studying Health System Change; August 2007.

Light DW, Warburton R. Demythologizing the high costs of pharmaceutical research. *Biosocieties*. 2011;6:34.

Lo B. Serving two masters—conflicts of interest in academic medicine. *N Engl J Med*. 2010;362:669.

Mehrotra A et al. Do integrated medical groups provide higher-quality medical care than individual practice associations? *Ann Intern Med*. 2006;145:826.

Nallamothu BK et al. Opening of specialty cardiac hospitals and use of coronary revascularization in Medicare beneficiaries. *JAMA*. 2007;297:962.

Perry JE. A mortal wound for physician-owned specialty hospitals? 2010. www.academia.edu.

Reinhardt UE. Reorganizing the financial flows in US health care. *Health Aff*. 1993;12(suppl):172.

Reinhardt UE. An information infrastructure for the pharmaceutical market. *Health Aff*. 2004;23(1):107.

Relman AS. *A Second Opinion. Rescuing America's Health Care*. New York, NY: Public Affairs; 2007.

Relman AS. The health reform we need & are not getting. *New York Rev Books*. 2009;56(11):38.

Robinson JC. The end of managed care. *JAMA*. 2001;285:2622.

Robinson JC. Consolidation and the transformation of competition in health insurance. *Health Aff*. 2004;23(6):11.

Smith MD et al. Taking the public's pulse on health system reform. *Health Aff*. 1992;11(2):125.

Spatz ID. Health reform accelerates changes in the pharmaceutical industry. *Health Aff*. 2010;29:1331.

Starr P. *The Social Transformation of American Medicine*. New York: Basic Books; 1982.

Steinbrook R. Campaign contributions, lobbying, and the US health sector. *N Engl J Med*. 2008;359:1313.

Stolberg SG, Gerth J. How companies stall generics and keep themselves healthy. *NY Times*. 2000.

Sunshine J, Bhargavan M. The practice of imaging self-referral doesn't produce much one-stop service. *Health Aff*. 2010;29:2237.

Vogt WB. *Hospital Market Consolidation: Trends and Consequences*. National Institute for Health Care Management. November 2009. http://nihcm.org/pdf/EV-Vogt_FINAL.pdf. Accessed November 26, 2011.

Welch HG et al. *Overdiagnosed. Making People Sick in the Pursuit of Health*. Boston, MA: Beacon Press; 2011.

Conclusion: Tensions and Challenges

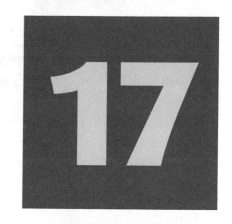

The perfect health care system is like perfect health—a noble aspiration but one that is impossible to attain. In the preceding chapters, we have discussed many fundamental issues and principles involved in formulating health care policy. A recurrent theme has been the notion that "magic bullets" are hard to come by. As stated in Chapter 2, policies tend to evolve in a cyclic process of finding solutions that create new problems that require new solutions. Policy changes may offer a degree of relief for a pressing problem, such as inadequate access to care, but frequently also give rise to various side effects, such as stimulating health care cost inflation.

All health care systems face the same challenges: improving health, controlling costs, prioritizing allocation of resources, enhancing the quality of care, and distributing services fairly. These challenges require the management of various tensions that pull at the health care system (O'Neil and Seifer, 1995). The goal of health policy is to find the points of equilibrium that produce the optimal system of health care (Table 17–1).

Dr. Madeleine Longview is chief resident in critical care medicine and supervises the intensive care unit of a large municipal hospital. It's 5:30 AM, and the intensive care unit team has finally stabilized the condition of a 15-year-old admitted the previous evening with gunshot wounds to the abdomen and chest. Dr. Longview sits by the nursing desk and surveys the other patients in the unit: a 91-year-old woman admitted from a nursing home with sepsis from a urinary tract infection, a 50-year-old man with shock lung caused by drugs

ingested in a suicide attempt, and a 32-year-old woman with lupus erythematosus who is rejecting her second kidney transplant. Dr. Longview feels personally responsible for the care of every one of these patients. She tells herself that she will do her best to help each of them survive.

As Dr. Longview gazes out of the windows of the intensive care unit, the apartment houses surrounding the hospital take shape in the breaking dawn. She wonders: Which block will be the scene of the next drive-by shooting or episode of spouse abuse? Which window shade hides a homebound elder lying on the floor dehydrated and unable to move, waiting for someone to find him and bring him to the emergency department? Which one of the unvaccinated kids in the neighborhood will one day be rushed into the unit limp with meningitis? In which room is someone lighting up the first cigarette of the day? Dr. Longview somehow feels responsible for all those patients-to-be, as well as for the patients lying in the hospital beds around her. After these sleepless nights on duty, the doubts about the value of all the work she does in the intensive care unit creep into her thoughts. She has visions of shutting down the unit and putting all the money to work hiring public health nurses in the community, or maybe just paying for a better grammar school in the neighborhood. But then what would happen to the patients needing her care right now?

One of the most basic tensions affecting physicians and other caregivers is the tension between caring for

Table 17–1. Major tensions in health care

Health of the individual patient	Health of the population
Tertiary care	Primary care
Acute care	Chronic and preventive care
Cost unawareness in medical practice	Cost awareness
Unlimited expectations for care	Affordability of care
Individual physician	Organized health care team
Professional management	Corporate management
Market competition	Government regulation
Inequity in distribution	Fair distribution

Source: Data from O'Neil E, Seifer S. Health care reform and medical education: Forces towards generalism. *Acad Med*. 1995;70:S37.

the individual patient and caring for the larger community or population. Many of the most important decisions to be made in health policy—decisions such as allocating health care resources, addressing the social context of health and illness, and augmenting activities in prevention and public health—depend on broadening the practitioner's view to encompass the population health perspective. The challenge for physicians and other clinicians will be to make room for this broader perspective while preserving the ethical duty to care for the individual patients under their charge.

Like Dr. Longview, the health care system as a whole will continue to struggle over finding the proper balance between the provision of acute care services and preventive and chronic care services, as well as striking the right balance between the levels of tertiary and primary care. Few observers would encourage Dr. Longview to succumb to her despair, close all the intensive care units, and expel all the critical care subspecialists from the health care system. Yet most would agree that health care in the United States has drifted too far away from the primary care end of the tertiary care–primary care axis.

Dr. Tom Ransom has performed what he believes to be a reasonably thorough workup for Zed's abdominal pain and decreased appetite, including a detailed history and physical examination, blood tests, and abdominal ultrasound—all of which

were normal. When Dr. Ransom tells Zed that they will have to work together to manage Zed's symptoms, Zed tells Dr. Ransom that he wants one more test, an abdominal CT scan. Zed says that he had a cousin with similar symptoms who was eventually diagnosed with advanced-stage lymphoma after complaining of pain for over a year.

Dr. Ransom is in a quandary. He believes it extremely unlikely that Zed has serious pathologic changes in his abdomen that will be detected on CT scan. He could order the scan, but then there's the issue of the cost. He can't recall whether Zed is covered by a fee-for-service plan or by one of the health maintenance organizations (HMOs) that pays on a capitated basis and puts Dr. Ransom at financial risk for all radiologic tests ordered. He starts to ask Zed about his coverage but feels a pang of guilt that he should allow these economic considerations to intrude into his clinical judgment.

The desire (and in many instances, expectation) of patients to receive all potentially beneficial care, and the unwillingness of these same individuals in their role as purchasers to spend unlimited amounts to finance health care, creates a strain for all caregivers and systems of care. Physicians increasingly are being called upon to incorporate considerations of costs when making clinical decisions. Debate will continue about the best ways to encourage physicians to be more accountable for the costs of care in a manner that is socially responsible and does not unduly intrude on the physician's ability to serve the individual patient. Is it necessary to use payment methods that place physicians at individual financial risk for their treatment decisions in order to control costs? Are more global methods available to induce physicians and other caregivers to practice in a more cost-conscious manner? If Zed does not get a CT scan, does that constitute painless or painful cost control?

On the eve of his retirement, Dr. Melvin Steadman reminisces with his son, Dr. Kevin Steadman. The elder Dr. Steadman has practiced as a solo pediatrician for more than 40 years in the same town. The only boss he has known in his professional life has been himself. He has served as president of the local medical society, helped spearhead efforts to build a special children's wing of the local hospital, and antagonized several of his colleagues when he pushed for a change in hospital policy that required physicians to attend extra continuing medical education courses in order to maintain their hospital privileges. Mel swore that he'd never retire; but he also swore that he'd never let the insurance companies "tell me how to practice medicine." He has refused to sign any managed care contracts. Facing a dwindling supply of patients, Mel has decided to call it quits.

His son Kevin is also a pediatrician, working as a staff physician for a large for-profit multispecialty group that recently opened up an office in town. Kevin remembers the many nights when his father didn't get home from work until after he had gone to bed. Kevin's work hours are more regular at the group practice, and he is on call for only one weekend every 2 months. He considers his father's approach to medicine old-fashioned in many ways—excessively paternalistic toward patients and irrationally scornful of the pediatric nurse practitioners who work with Kevin. He does, however, envy his father's professional independence. Just this week, the group practice notified Kevin that he would have to divide his time between his current office and a new site that would soon open in a suburban mall. His schedule will be limited to 10-minute drop-in appointments at the new site, rather than the style of practice that promotes a sense of continuity, one that allows him to get to know his patients over time.

A system of health care formerly managed according to a professional model by independent practitioners is being pulled toward a corporate model of care featuring large organizations managed by administrators. As the role of corporate entities expands, traditional responsibilities toward patients and local communities are vying with new obligations to shareholders. Power relationships are changing, with insurance companies and organized purchasers challenging the dominance of the medical profession. A shift toward multidisciplinary group practice may provide more opportunity for health care professionals to work collegially and implement new approaches to quality improvement to elevate the competence of all health care providers. At the same time, a competitive, for-profit health care environment may induce physicians to compromise their humanity and turn toward the "homo economicus" model, basing clinical decisions in part on monetary considerations.

> *Aurora can't wait any longer in the crowded county hospital emergency department. She's already been there for 6 hours, and the physician hasn't seen her yet. Her lower abdomen still hurts, but she figures she'll just have to put up with it for a few more days. She really doesn't have much choice. Poor and uninsured, where else could she go? Aurora has two young children at home who need to be put to bed. In half an hour, their father has to get to his night job as a security officer. As she enters her apartment, she collapses, the pregnancy in her fallopian tube having ruptured, producing internal hemorrhage. Her husband frantically dials 911, praying that his wife won't die.*

Perhaps no tension within the US health care system is as far from reaching a point of satisfactory equilibrium as the achievement of a basic level of fairness in the distribution of health care services and the burden of paying for those services. Many more people in the country were uninsured in 2011 than in 1991. Because of persistent financial barriers, patients do not benefit from early detection of potentially curable cancers, patients with chronic diseases are hospitalized because of lack of timely primary care, hypertensive patients forego the medications that might avert the occurrence of strokes and kidney failure, and babies are born prematurely and spend their first weeks of life in a neonatal intensive care unit. The poor pay a greater proportion of their income for health care than do more affluent families. The Affordable Care Act of 2010 would greatly reduce the number of uninsured. However, implementation of the Act faces political, judicial, and financial challenges, and coverage would fall short of truly universal even if fully implemented.

People providing and receiving care in the United States must work together to achieve a brighter future for the nation's health care system. Changing the future will require that people look beyond their immediate self-interest to view the common good of a health care system that is accessible, affordable, and of high quality for all. A heightened level of public discourse will be needed, with a populace that is better informed and more actively engaged in shaping the future of their health care system. Concepts in health policy based on established facts rather than ideologically driven myths will need to be discussed and debated in a manner that connects with the daily realities experienced by patients and caregivers. The attitudes and actions of physicians and other health care professionals will play a major role in determining the future of health care in the United States. With leadership and foresight among the community of health care professionals, our nation may yet achieve a system that allows the most honorable features of the healing professions to flourish.

REFERENCE

O'Neil E, Seifer S. Health care reform and medical education: Forces towards generalism. *Acad Med*. 1995;70:S37.

Questions and Discussion Topics

CHAPTER 2: PAYING FOR HEALTH CARE

1. What are the four modes of financing health care? Describe each.

2. Describe regressive, proportional, and progressive financing. Explain how each of the following is regressive, proportional, or progressive: out-of-pocket payments, experience-rated individual private insurance, community-rated individual private insurance, health insurance purchased 100% by the employer (assuming that employees actually pay for health insurance as explained in the text), and the federal income tax.

3. Harvey, who has worked all his life for General Electric, reaches 65 years of age. He does not retire. Is he eligible for Medicare Part A? Part B? Six months later, his wife, who has never worked, reaches 65 years of age. Is she eligible for Medicare Part A? Part B? How are Parts A and B paid for?

4. Hubert has received social security disability for 24 months because he has AIDS. Is he eligible for Medicare?

5. Rena developed chronic renal failure and started renal dialysis 2 weeks ago. She feels fine and is working. Is she eligible for Medicare?

6. Heidi, aged 72 years, on Medicare Part A and B without Medicaid or a Medigap policy, is hospitalized for a stroke complicated by a deep vein thrombosis of the leg and a pulmonary embolus. She is in the acute hospital for 70 days and cared for by a family practitioner and a neurologist. She improves somewhat and is then transferred to the skilled nursing facility (SNF) for rehabilitation. She remains in the SNF for 30 days and is still severely disabled and unable to go home. She is sent to a nursing home for custodial care, where she stays for 3 months. Surprisingly, she improves and goes home, where she receives skilled physical therapy services from a home care agency and also has a homemaker come in for 4 hours a day to buy food, cook, and clean the house. She is on three prescription medications at home. What does Heidi pay and what does Medicare pay? Acute hospital? SNF? Nursing home? Home care? Physicians? Prescriptions while in hospital? Prescriptions while at home?

▶ Discussion Topics

1. Discuss your experiences with health insurance that was provided through a job. How did you obtain the insurance? Did you pay part of the premium? Were there deductibles or copayments? How many choices of plans did you have? What happened if you left your job?

2. Divide into two groups: one insurance company selling community-rated health insurance policies and the other selling experience-rated policies. Each side should try to convince the instructor to buy its policy, first with the instructor as a young, healthy person, and then with the instructor as an older person with diabetes. Which policy is the young person more likely to choose, and which the older person?

CHAPTER 3: ACCESS TO HEALTH CARE

1. Describe the two main categories of people without health insurance.

2. Why did uninsurance increase during the period 1980 to 2010?

3. Compare access to health care for people with private insurance, for Medicaid recipients, and for people without insurance. Give examples.

4. Compare health outcomes for people with private insurance, for Medicaid recipients, and for people without insurance. Give examples.

▶ Discussion Topics

1. What are some explanations as to why Ace Banks was healthy at age 48 while Bill Downes died at that age?

2. Women on average have more visits than men to physicians. Does that mean that women receive better health care than men?

3. Discuss possible reasons why minority patients receive poorer quality of care than white patients for many diseases.

4. What is the relationship between socioeconomic status (including factors such as income, education, and occupation) and health? Why does such a relationship exist?

5. What would be the best strategies to improve the health status of African Americans in the United States?

CHAPTER 4: REIMBURSING HEALTH CARE PROVIDERS

1. Explain each mode of physician reimbursement: fee-for-service, episode of illness, capitation, and salary. Explain each mode of hospital reimbursement: fee-for-service, per diem, episode of illness (diagnosis-related group [DRG]), and global budget.

2. How does capitation payment free insurers of risk? How does capitation payment shift risk to providers of care?

3. What are the arguments for risk-adjusting capitation payments?

▶ Discussion Topics

1. You are a primary care physician (PCP) caring for a young woman with new onset of severe headaches and amenorrhea and a normal physical examination. What are the financial incentives and disincentives that would lead you to order or not to order a

magnetic resonance imaging (MRI) scan in a case in which the need for the MRI was equivocal?

(a) under traditional fee-for-service practice;

(b) under fee-for-service practice with utilization review;

(c) under an independent practice association (IPA)-model health maintenance organization (HMO) in which you receive a capitation payment that places you at risk for laboratory and x-ray studies and specialty referrals;

(d) under a staff model HMO that has a two-month waiting list for elective MRI scans?

In the case of the staff model HMO, what would you do if you felt you needed to obtain the MRI within 48 hours?

2. You are a hospital administrator and your hospital is in financial difficulty. You are about to address the medical staff, imploring them to help the hospital financially. In the old days, all you had to say was, in effect: "Admit as many patients as possible and keep them in the hospital as long as you can," but times have changed. For some methods of reimbursement, you want physicians to admit more patients; for others, you don't. For some methods, you want patients to stay long, for others, you don't. What do you tell the medical staff regarding the following:

(a) Medicare (DRG) patients

(b) Medicaid (per diem) patients

(c) HMO (per diem) patients

(d) HMO (capitated) patients

For each of these categories of patients, does it help or hurt the hospital for physicians to

(a) admit more patients;

(b) keep them in the hospital more days;

(c) order more diagnostic studies?

CHAPTER 5: HOW HEALTH CARE IS ORGANIZED—I: PRIMARY, SECONDARY, AND TERTIARY CARE

▶ Discussion Topics

1. You are 63 years old and you begin to experience chest pain when walking. You do not have a physician. A friend suggests that you need a coronary

artery bypass and recommends a cardiac surgeon at the medical school. What do you do

(a) under a dispersed model of health care delivery?

(b) under a regionalized model?

2. Give some examples of the statement, "Common disorders commonly occur and rare ones rarely happen." What are the implications of this statement for the ratio of generalist to specialist physicians in the United States?

3. In Great Britain, 65% of physicians are general practitioners. In Canada, 50% of physicians are generalists. In the United States, approximately one-third of physicians are generalists (general and family practitioners, general internists, and general pediatricians). Assume you are Chair of the Health Subcommittee of the US House of Representatives Ways and Means Committee. What legislation might you propose to increase the proportion of generalist physicians?

4. Discuss the pros and cons of requiring everyone to enter the health care system through a "gatekeeper" health care provider (generalist physician, nurse practitioner, or physician assistant).

5. What are some advantages of a primary-care-based health system?

CHAPTER 6: HOW HEALTH CARE IS ORGANIZED—II: HEALTH DELIVERY SYSTEMS

1. What are the two generations of HMOs? Give examples of each (if possible, in your community).

2. What is vertical integration? What is virtual integration?

3. What is an ACO? What is a medical home and a medical neighborhood? Is a medical neighborhood the same as an ACO?

CHAPTER 7: THE HEALTH CARE WORKFORCE AND THE EDUCATION OF HEALTH PROFESSIONALS

Describe past and future trends in the physician, "mid-level," nursing, and pharmacist workforce.

CHAPTER 8: PAINFUL VERSUS PAINLESS COST CONTROL

1. Give examples of medical interventions that lie on the steeper portions of the cost–benefit curve, and

interventions that lie on the flatter portions. Is the elimination of the latter painful or painless cost control?

2. Give examples of painless cost control. Are these painless for everyone?

▶ Discussion Topics

1. CABGville has four cardiac surgery units; one unit performs 300 coronary artery bypass graft (CABG) surgeries each year, and the other units perform an average of 40 per year. Cardiac surgeons can schedule a CABG anytime they wish. The small units have an operative mortality of 7% compared with 4% for the large unit. To control costs, the health planning council of CABGville closes the three less productive cardiac surgery units. Elective CABG surgeries now have a 1-month waiting list, and because of tight scheduling, surgeons are less likely to operate; the number of CABGs goes down from 420 to 340 per year; both the overall costs of CABG surgery and the unit cost per CABG operation drop, as does the mortality rate. Did CABGville achieve painful or painless cost control?

2. Pretend that total US health care expenditures have been capped and are controlled by a health services commission. Because of tight budgetary constraints, the commission must decide whether to fund an all-out program of mammography or to limit mammography and finance in its place high-cost chemotherapy regimens for patients with metastatic breast cancer, treatments whose effectiveness has not been proven, but which might help certain subgroups of women. Under the first option, several thousand cases of early-stage breast cancer could be treated with curative surgery each year, but women currently suffering from advanced-stage breast cancer would receive no benefit. Which is the more painful cost control option from the point of view of women without breast cancer? From the perspective of women with metastatic breast cancer? From the perspective of society as a whole? Which of these two groups of women should have priority in this decision?

CHAPTER 9: MECHANISMS FOR CONTROLLING COSTS

▶ Discussion Topics

1. You are chair of the health planning council of CABGville, a town that continues to have a health

care cost crisis. The town has 30 physicians, each seeing 30 patients a day at a cost of $30 per visit. Total daily cost is $30 \times 30 \times 30 = \$27,000$. What methods are available to reduce the total cost of physician services? Would it work to reduce the fee per visit from $30 to $20? If an expenditure cap strategy (tying fees to volume) were used, how would it work?

2. The CABGville health planning council changes the mode of physician reimbursement from fee-for-service to capitation: $20 per patient per month to PCPs, with 20 PCPs each having 2000 patients. (PCPs pay specialists from the $20 capitation.) Total cost per month = $800,000 (approximately $27,000 per day). How could the health planning council reduce the monthly cost? Could physician costs still increase despite this method of cost control? Why or why not?

3. You have finished your residency in internal medicine and have the choice to work at Kaiser or at a private practice that is part of an IPA. You are particularly concerned about your ability to order laboratory tests and x-rays and to obtain specialty consultations. At Kaiser, you learn that you have freedom in ordering tests and obtaining consultations, but that patients may have to wait (except in urgent situations) because of the limited supply of such equipment as MRI scanners and of specialty appointments. At the IPA, you must request prior authorization for expensive diagnostic studies and for specialty consultations, but once prior authorization has been obtained, waiting periods are fairly short. Which work situation would you prefer, and which do you think has the better chance of controlling costs?

4. What are the arguments pro and con patient cost sharing as a cost control strategy?

5. You are the President of the United States, and your first term ends in a year. The cost-control mechanism you instituted 2 years ago, based on patient cost sharing and managed competition, has not worked, and the American people are upset about persistent health care inflation. You are preparing for a major television address on health care costs. What will you propose? Can you convince the public that yours is a painless cost-control strategy?

CHAPTER 10: QUALITY OF HEALTH CARE

▶ Discussion Topics

1. Have you ever experienced or witnessed a medical care encounter of poor quality? What did you do about it? What should you have done?

2. In the vignette about Shelley Rush, who do you think was responsible for the error in giving insulin to the wrong patient?

3. In the vignette about Nina Brown, had the physician been working in a fee-for-service environment rather than a cost-conscious HMO, do you think he or she would have admitted Ms. Brown to the hospital?

4. Reread the example of the 23-year-old graduate student whose x-ray report was lost. If you were the administrator of the hospital, what would you do to prevent such an error from taking place again? If you were the office manager of the internist's office that never received the x-ray report, what would you do to avoid a recurrence of this problem?

5. What is wrong with the malpractice system? What would you do to fix it?

CHAPTER 11: PREVENTION OF ILLNESS

1. Why did tuberculosis (TB) decline prior to the identification of the TB bacillus? Why did polio morbidity and mortality decline? Why did Hodgkin disease mortality fall in the late twentieth century?

2. What are the first and the second epidemiologic revolutions?

▶ Discussion Topics

1. Two people are campaigning for the consumer board of their group practice. The incumbent is running on a platform of charging tobacco users higher premiums than nonusers, because their use of tobacco costs the group practice more money. The opponent believes that society rather than the individual is responsible for tobacco addiction and that the group practice should become involved in social action against cigarette smoking. Conduct a debate between these two views.

2. How do you explain the fact that a large number of heart attacks occur at early ages in people with

cholesterol levels below the median level for the United States? That heart attacks seldom occur at these ages in Japan? What is the implication for primary prevention of coronary heart disease?

3. You are named as head of the breast cancer prevention section of the US Centers for Disease Control and Prevention. What primary and secondary prevention programs would you favor to reduce the incidence of and mortality from breast cancer?

CHAPTER 12: LONG-TERM CARE

1. What are activities of daily living and instrumental activities of daily living?

2. What percentage of long-term care services are funded by which funding sources?

3. Which long-term care services are covered by Medicare and which are not? Which are covered by Medicaid?

▶ Discussion Topics

1. You are president of LTC Insurance Company and are testifying before a Senate committee on long-term care. You are asked two questions: Why do only a few million people carry private long-term care insurance? How do you answer the complaints that senior citizen advocacy groups make about the terms of private long-term care insurance policies? What do you say to the committee?

2. Your mother's Alzheimer's disease is getting worse; she wanders around the neighborhood, sometimes unable to find her way home; she sleeps during the day and stays up most of the night; and she has become incontinent. Your father died 2 years ago. You and your spouse both work, you have three school-aged children, and you have an extra room in your home. The hospital social worker calls and says that your mother needs 24-hour-a-day help. Your choices are:

   (a) hiring a homemaker to live with your mother at $16,000 per year;

   (b) placing your mother in a nursing home whose bill will be paid by Medicaid;

   (c) taking your mother home with you. What do you decide?

What reforms in the US long-term care system would have benefited you in this situation? How should such reforms be financed?

CHAPTER 13: MEDICAL ETHICS AND RATIONING OF HEALTH CARE

▶ Discussion Topics

1. Pretend that the Lakeberg family discussed in this chapter belongs to an HMO, and that you are the HMO's medical director. The Lakeberg parents want surgery to separate the Siamese twins at the cost of $1 million. The list of benefits covered in the Lakebergs' HMO policy neither affirms nor denies their right to the surgery, so the responsibility to approve or deny the surgery falls on you. What do you decide? If you approve the surgery, who will end up paying for it? Is an ethical dilemma involved or not?

2. You are Dr. Marco Intensivo, as described in the vignette in the section "What is Rationing?" What do you do?

3. In the case of Mr. Olds and Mr. Younger described in the organ transplant section, which patient should receive the donor heart?

4. You are the PCP for Rodolfo, a 58-year-old man who suffered a cerebral hemorrhage and has been in a persistent vegetative state for 18 months. He lives in a nursing home, requires tube feedings and round-the-clock nursing attention, and his care is paid for by Medicaid. Rodolfo's daughter is a nurse in the intensive care unit of your hospital. Rodolfo's wife is deeply religious and has faith that Rodolfo will get better.

   Approximately every 6 weeks, Rodolfo develops a urinary tract infection with septicemia and must be admitted to the hospital—often to the ICU—for treatment. Over the course of 2 years, Rodolfo's care has cost $260,000. The hospital ethics committee discussed the case and recommended that tube feedings be withdrawn, or that the next episode of septicemia not be treated, thereby allowing Rodolfo to die. When you discussed the ethics committee recommendations with the family, the daughter agreed but the wife demanded that everything possible be done to continue Rodolfo's life. As Rodolfo's physician, what do you do? Which ethical dilemmas are involved? Autonomy versus beneficence?

Autonomy versus nonmaleficence? Autonomy versus distributive justice? Beneficence versus distributive justice? If Rodolfo's care were withdrawn, what would happen to the money saved?

5. Evidence from public opinion polls suggests that people in the United States want the right to health care but don't want to pay for it.

   At midnight, a new mother awakens to hear her 2-week-old infant scream. The mother and baby are Medicaid recipients. If she were experienced, the mother would know that the scream is normal, but she is frightened. She phones the emergency department and asks to bring the baby in to be seen. No amount of telephone advice seems to reassure her. Does the right to health care include society paying for her visit to the emergency department? Who is actually paying? Should the mother be advised to come into the emergency department if she is uninsured and wealthy? Uninsured and poor?

6. In Oregon, the Medicaid program was extended to thousands of Oregonians who had previously been uninsured. To help pay for this extension, the breadth of services available to Medicaid recipients was reduced such that recipients lost access to some care that might have been beneficial. You are the Governor of Oregon and you have to testify in a lawsuit alleging that the program is unfair because it deprives Medicaid recipients of certain services enjoyed by privately insured people. What is your response?

7. Should physicians be responsible to serve one master—their patient—or two masters—their patient and the broader needs of society? In your discussion, draw from the examples of the Lakebergs, Dr. Intensivo, and Rodolfo. How has the distribution system for organ transplantation tried to balance these two masters?

CHAPTER 14: HEALTH CARE IN FOUR NATIONS

1. You are a secretary in a large company in Germany (Canada, United Kingdom, or Japan). How is your health care paid for? You become sick and are forced to retire from your job. How is your health care paid for in Germany (Canada, United Kingdom, or Japan)?

2. If you developed a urinary tract infection, what would you do in Germany (Canada, United Kingdom, or Japan)? What if you needed cataract surgery? What if you had a sudden abdominal pain in the middle of the night? What if you developed leukemia and needed a bone marrow transplant? In each of these cases, which physician would care for you and where would you be cared for?

3. You are a general practitioner in Germany (Canada, United Kingdom, or Japan). How are you paid? You are a specialist in Germany (Canada, United Kingdom, or Japan). How are you paid? You are a hospital administrator in Germany (Canada, UK, or Japan). How is your hospital paid?

4. How are costs controlled in the four countries?

CHAPTER 15: HEALTH CARE REFORM AND NATIONAL HEALTH INSURANCE

1. Describe how a government-financed national health insurance plan, an employer mandate plan, and an individual mandate plan would work.

2. What is the difference between a social insurance and a public assistance approach to government-financed national health insurance? Use Medicare and Medicaid as examples.

3. What are the main features of the 2010 Patient Protection and Affordable Care Act (ACA)?

▶ Discussion Topics

1. You are the speech writer for two candidates for the Democratic presidential nomination. One candidate favors a mixed employer and individual mandate and the other a single-payer approach. What points would you have each candidate make about the strengths of his or her position and the weaknesses of the other candidate's position?

2. Why do you think that there has been such a polarized debate over the ACA?

CHAPTER 16: CONFLICT AND CHANGE IN AMERICA'S HEALTH CARE SYSTEM

1. Describe how the payers of health care services increased their power between 1945 and 1995.

2. Describe changes in the relationships between physicians and insurance companies between 1945 and 1995.

3. Describe the 1995–2000 backlash against managed care.

4. Describe the recently growing power of specialty-oriented providers of care.

▶ Discussion Topics

1. Discuss potential conflicts between the profit motive and the principles of beneficence and nonmaleficence in the following situations:

   (a) a private surgeon receiving fee-for-service reimbursement;

   (b) a primary physician in a small group practice that receives capitation payments covering primary care, laboratory, x-ray, and specialty referrals;

   (c) a physician who is the utilization manager of a large for-profit HMO receiving requests from her employed physicians to authorize expensive MRI scans for their patients;

   (d) the administrator of a nonprofit hospital who has calculated that a new cardiac surgery unit will be profitable even if only one surgery is performed each week;

   (e) the CEO of an HMO deciding whether to accept Medicaid patients, for whom the state government is paying premiums 30% lower than premiums paid for private patients.

   What changes in the organization of health care could be made that would minimize such conflicts?

2. Discuss how health care is organized in your community—who are the payers, insurers, and providers? To what degree has your local health care system moved from a dispersed set of institutions to a small number of vertically or virtually integrated health care conglomerates?

3. Where in the health care system of the twenty-first century would you like to be—as a provider and as a patient? What are yours fears and hopes for the future?

Index

Page numbers followed by f refer to figures; page numbers followed by t refer to tables.